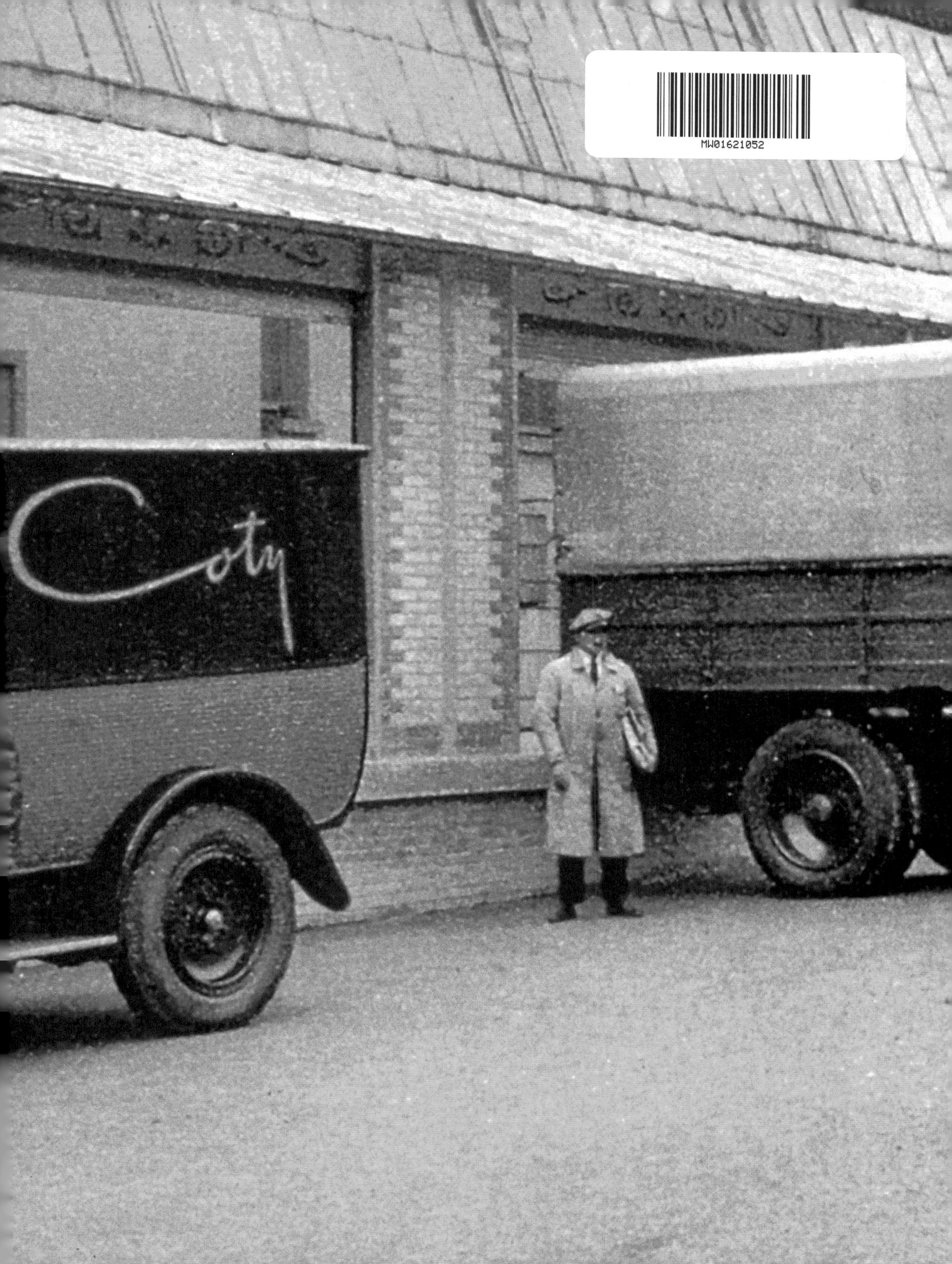

MW01621052

COTY

© Assouline Publishing
601 West 26th Street, 18th Floor
New York, NY 10001, USA
www.assouline.com

ISBN: 2 84323 622 3

Color Separation: Gravor (Switzerland).
Printed by Grafiche Milani (Italy).

All rights reserved.
No part of this publication may be reproduced, stored
in a retrieval system, or transmitted in any form
or by any means, electronic, mechanical, photocopying,
recording, or otherwise, without prior consent from the publisher.

ORLA HEALY

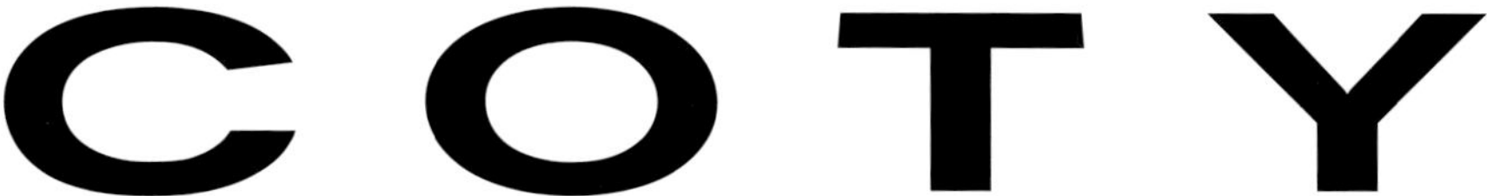

THE BRAND OF VISIONARY

ASSOULINE

“One thing eluded me.
I never managed
to capture the smell
of honeysuckle.”

Introduction

Shortly before he died in 1934, François Coty corrected a friend who said: "You had everything that a man could want, you owned all that you desired." "One thing eluded me," Coty confessed. "I never managed to capture the smell of honeysuckle." He probably wasn't being disingenuous.

Those who believe the craft of perfume-making to be the ultimate in abstract art, regard François Coty as perfumery's first genius, not least because he created enduring, iconoclastic classics such as "Chypre," "Emeraude," "L'Origan," "Paris," and "L'Aimant." In fact, "L'Aimant" so delighted Mme. Jacques Guerlain, that she boldly declared she preferred it to her husband's concoctions. She wasn't alone. The intoxicating allure of Coty perfumes would quickly waft across Europe, the Americas and as far as South Africa and Australia.

From the moment that the young François decided to make perfume his life's work, he did so with his nose attuned to feminine fancies, his eye fixated on an unerringly elegant signature style, and his mind shrewdly intent on revolutionizing an industry. A hundred years after its birth in a small Parisian apartment, Coty Inc. reached its centennial in 2004.

Today it is a global company with operations in over 25 countries, which continues to draw on the creative, entrepreneurial and visionary legacy of its founder, a man whose business card unabashedly listed his occupations as "Artist, Industrialist, Craftsman, Economist, Financier and Social Scientist."

As the fearlessly self-confident grandfather of inspirational marketing, his goal was to build a brand that would produce prestige products at accessible prices or, as he phrased it, to create a dream that was within every woman's reach.

Even in the early 1900s, when François was going around selling samples of his first perfume "La Rose Jacqueminot" to Parisian department stores, he was already aware of the need to cultivate an interest among the trend-setting socialites and actresses of the day. He thought it was indispensable to create the necessary excitement to make "Coty" a desirable purchase for this lucrative, relatively untapped, middle-class market of women who cared about their appearance, yet were not consumed by it. François' strategy was to seduce these women with the kind of enticements usually reserved for the very rich; an elegant presentation and an air of refinement, concentrating on the design of the perfume bottles, and later on the packaging, as much as to their contents.

Endowed with a rabid curiosity that stretched far beyond the world of potions, lotions and test tubes, François was determined to work with the brightest talents the new century had to offer. Long before the international corporate world came to rely heavily on cutting-edge design as the lynchpin for successful marketing campaigns, François Coty had intuitively understood that the packaging for his Coty collection was as important as the perfume itself. Flaunting his disdain for the rules, ignoring the business formulas of the past and gleefully upsetting the status quo within the industry with an absolute refusal to acknowledge the word compromise, François' first, most legendary and groundbreaking collaboration was with René Lalique. Initially commissioning the master glass maker and jeweler to create elaborate bottle stoppers, their partnership quickly progressed to the point where Lalique was crafting labels, publicity signs, and by 1914, magnificent wooden presentation cases which were big enough to hold a dozen demonstration flasks. Even the lowly shopkeepers who stocked Coty products were treated like part of the team and tutored by Coty on the specific etiquette of display and merchandizing. "You are," he would grandly salute them, "our ambassadors

[1] Advertising for *Muse* perfume by Coty in the 1940's.

Une Date ...

Muse

LA NAISSANCE D'UN GRAND PARFUM
EST UN ÉVÈNEMENT

Des sons ne font pas une symphonie...

Des traits de pinceau ne font pas un tableau...

Les meilleures essences ne suffisent pas davantage à créer un Parfum.

" Muse " est le fruit de huit ans de recherches : mélanges savants, dosages subtils, expériences délicates. Huit ans d'espoirs et de découragements, couronnés par une éclatante réussite !

" Muse " est une œuvre maîtresse dans l'art du Parfum.

" Muse " est né au cœur de Paris. Une fois encore, c'est la Parisienne qui l'a inspiré ; c'est elle qui, la première, reconnaîtra qu'il s'agit d'une création exceptionnelle ; c'est elle encore qui saura l'imposer au monde entier !

to women." The result was extraordinary brand loyalty and unparalleled customer support, as well as vendors who became skilled in the art of creating dazzling window displays for Coty.

François was inspired by anything beautiful enough to hold his eye—a withered gossamer leaf became the template for cellophane wrapping, an eleventh century manuscript inspired the design for a perfume box. His philosophy of seeking out unexpected talents with whom to collaborate and be able to continue to deliver "the shock of the new," still fuels the entrepreneurial ethos that thrives at Coty today.

Just as François saw the potential of his partnership with Lalique, Coty Inc. currently collaborates with a constellation of superstars from the glamorous worlds of fashion, music, sport and Hollywood to ensure that the echo of François's vision remains clear. François wrote in 1924, that his ultimate dream was for "each woman to have her own subtle fragrance. One which will suit her style and be a true expression of her personality, and which will denote the kind of a woman she is, her emotions and aspirations, as much as enhance her outward appearance." Today's Coty woman, (and man, and teenager) has a veritable worldwide Coty counter replete with choices. Ironically, the scent of honeysuckle, which so poignantly eluded François' grasp, is one of the key notes in "Glow by JLO," one of the industry's greatest success stories and beloved by the singer's millions of young fans across the globe. Edgier, funkier tastes turn to Rimmel, the sassy London-makeup and perfume label that radiates street-smartness, while more sophisticated women gravitate to Jil Sander. Colorful German designer Wolfgang Joop! is also a member of Coty's diverse brand portfolio, as are eccentric British couturier Vivienne Westwood and New York's downtown tastemaker, Marc Jacobs. Kenneth Cole, outfitter to America's upwardly mobile young professionals, also produces perfume with Coty, as does the sports-label turned fashion-staple, adidas. Actress Isabella Rossellini and performer Céline Dion are two other, distinctly different personalities in Coty's vast portfolio.

Beginnings

François Coty was a competitive, stylish man who, at the precocious age of 25 decided that he needed to be at the heart of the action in Paris. Bristling with ambition, he had fled his native Corsica to work as a haberdashery salesman in the pulsating port of Marseilles where, after a stint in the military, he developed a reputation as a pugnacious salesman with a taste for adventure.

In later years, François, a man who spoke in the present and rarely in the past tense, nimbly glossed over the details of his upbringing, which, naturally, intensified the mystique that would shroud his legend.

When he did talk about his childhood, he relied on a nostalgic rendition of his story: François Marie Joseph Spoturno was born on May 3, 1874 in Ajaccio, Corsica. His mother, Marie Coti, died when he was four and his father, Jean-Baptiste Spoturno, passed away three years later. Raised by his grandmother, Anna Maria Spoturno Bellone, François, who was academically bright, was forced to drop out of school due to the family's lack of finances.

Despite the handicap of poverty, François was smugly proud of his family's illustrious links with the Bonaparte family. He was a descendent of Isabelle Bonaparte, who was an aunt of the Emperor. Another of his ancestors had been an officer of Napoleon's, a Captain in the Fusilier Brigade, who, after the Russian campaign, had been awarded the title of Count (he died in 1812 in the Vilnius front). Although François never attempted to use the title, at the peak of his good fortune he had the Spoturno coat of arms printed on his stationery.

Once in Marseilles, François became a journalist with a daily paper and developed an impressive portfolio of contacts. This portfolio became particularly useful following his decision to move to Paris in 1898, when a close friend of the family, Senator Emmanuel Arene, hired him as a parliamentary attaché.

Like Pablo Picasso, who left Barcelona for Paris the same year, François was lured to the French capital by a need to find out what the new century had to offer. It was a glamorous era when anything and everything, seemed possible. The first cars were traveling along the boulevards where a new form of entertainment, the cinema, was generating great excitement.

Other marvels, including the airplane, the phonograph and the first wireless transmission would soon follow. The newspapers were bursting with stories detailing the courageous adventures of Amundsen's expedition to the North Pole, Count von Zeppelin's airship flight around Lake Constance, and the Charcot expeditions to the North and South Pole. Electricity, the greatest marvel, was the star attraction at the 1900 World Fair, where François spent time searching for ideas and opportunities that could lead to a business of his own.

The first scent of success

The perfume industry was extensive but unremarkable at the beginning of the 20th century and François spotted the potential for its development. Weighed down by outmoded ideas, the best-selling perfumers, such as Guerlain, Lubin and Houbigant, all offered overpoweringly florid confections that were distinguishable only by their outlandish names. In addition, François found perfume packaging at the time to be unappealing. The prevailing square, rectangular or cylindrical "rouleaux' bottles spruced up with a profusion of flowery labels and, occasionally, with a festive stopper, miserably failed to evoke the seductive magic of their contents.

Like many who attended the World Fair that year, François was impressed by the creative ferocity of jeweler René Lalique. Already a favorite among style-savvy high society Europeans, (Sarah Bernhardt was among his devoted clientele), Lalique's brooches, tiaras and ankle bracelets were intricately embellished with a menagerie of animal motifs. By 1900, Lalique's work was considered to be such a spectacle of craftsmanship that his collection was singled out for its own pavilion at the Fair. Even more impressively, in François' entrepreneurial mind, the self-sufficient Lalique was one of the few artists who controlled his designs completely – from the sketchpad through to the production process.

Another useful acquaintance was Leon Chirris, Senator of the Alpes Maritimes and Mayor of Grasse, the birthplace of the perfume industry, who introduced François to a pharmacist from Grasse called Dr. Jacques Minot. Minot, who appreciated Coty's qualities and his good taste, invited him to come to Grasse. It was there that Coty discovered the magic of natural and aldehyde essential oils, and where he met a young pharmacist named Raymond Goery who had grown up in the Dubois family. (Alphée Dubois, recipient of the great medal-engraving award in Rome in 1859, was grandfather to Yvonne Le Baron, who François was married in Paris in 1900.) By a twist of fate, several years later, in 1920, Raymond Goery went to work for François, becoming the first pharmacist to work in a perfume factory.

Even though François was uneducated in the craft of matching essential oils or base notes, he instinctively succeeded in concocting a scent that Goery ruefully admitted was a more appealing, harmonious blend than any that he had created.

A curious student, François absorbed as much as he could about the business in just under a year. A regular sight in the jasmine fields at dawn, he spent most of his time in the laboratory, tenaciously educating his nose while learning the intricate steps necessary to express the fragrances conjured up in his mind. Through a process of analysis and synthesis, he learned to recognize the signature of each scent and concentrated on discovering new ways to stylishly blend the seemingly endless options.

Tirelessly studying the offerings of the competition, François aimed to come up with a perfume that was in-keeping with the spirit of the day: a unique concoction that would have at its core, the hallmark of the genuine artist; a subtle simplicity. Using a delicate balance of base notes, he enhanced textures with full-bodied ingredients, and showing remarkable discipline he kept his formulae brief.

Convinced that he had an original and feasible concept, and knowing that his education in Grasse had given him the tools to develop it, François returned to Paris. With a ten thousand franc loan from his grandmother, he set up his first laboratory in a back room of the small apartment he shared with his wife.

With a sense of smell unconstrained by any desire to mimic fragrances that already existed, François considered the possibilities. Other perfumers had rejected the new generation of concentrates, but François was enthralled by the potential of synthetic flower oil extracts. Soon, the couple's tiny apartment started to look like a factory. Yvonne commandeered the living room and under her husband's keen eye, used her millinery skills to embroider silk pouches with velvet ribbon and satin trims for the sample bottles. Each morning, François would swap his white lab coat for a sober salesman's suit and set off on sales appointments.

In one of his earliest marketing decisions, François realized that his surname, Spoturno, didn't exactly roll off the tongue. In searching for a catchy nom de guerre, François took his mother's two-syllable maiden name "Coti" and changed it to the more elegant "Coty." Short and easy to pronounce in any language, it was a recognizable name for the brand he envisioned building. Aware that he had to attract socialites and actresses in order to cultivate the necessary glamour to make "Coty" products desirable, François focused at first on targeting middle class women who could afford perfume, yet for whom it was still a self-conscious, special purchase. Even though he wanted to make the market for his products as wide as possible, he still wanted "Coty" to spell prestige.

Unfortunately, storekeepers who were enjoying a brisk business with trendy perfumes such as Rigaud's "Air Embaume" didn't see why they should risk introducing a new fragrance, especially one without the crucial recognition factor that pleased the olfactory trends of the time.

[2] *L'Eau* by Coty, launched in 1920,
in honor of Napoleon the 1st who tolerated only Eau de Cologne. By Keiichi Tahara.

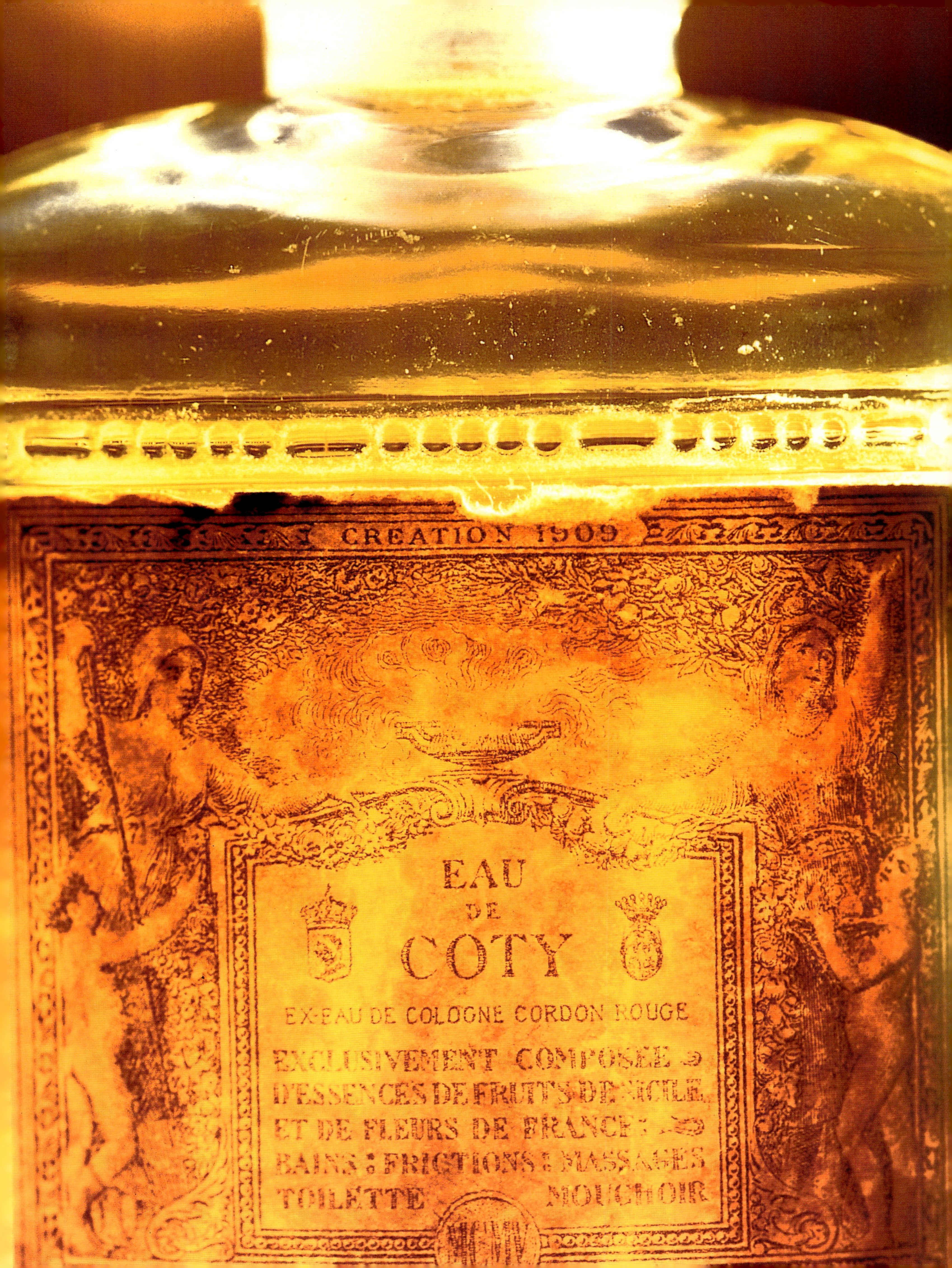

CREATION 1909

EAU
DE
COTY

EX-EAU DE COLOGNE CORDON ROUGE

EXCLUSIVEMENT COMPOSÉE
D'ESSENCES DE FRUITS DE SICILE
ET DE FLEURS DE FRANCE:
BAINS: FRICTIONS: MASSAGES
TOILETTE MOUCHOIR

Coty's first big break, literally, occurred when on a disappointing day, he smashed a bottle of "La Rose Jacqueminot," on a countertop at the Grand Magasins du Louvre, after a snooty store manager tried to eject him without deigning to sniff the proffered perfume. Whether or not François, as is official lore, lost his composure, or whether it was, as is gossip, an inspired marketing ploy, breaking that bottle was a brilliant move. Intoxicated by the creamy rose perfume that filled the store's ground floor, customers rushed to get their hands on a bottle of "La Rose Jacqueminot". His supply disappeared within a matter of minutes. He was, finally, in business. In a matter of two months, "La Rose Jacqueminot" was the must-have scent of both socialites and housewives, and François began making his fortune.

Creative and commercial partnership

This great success financed the new headquarters at 61 Rue de la Boétie, a laboratory in Neuilly, on the outskirts of Paris, and seven sales representatives. Though buoyed, François was still frustrated that he hadn't managed to come up with a remarkable bottle for his perfumes that would stand out from the rest. His arrangement with Baccarat, who produced the slim, classic bottle for "La Rose Jacqueminot," and its follow-up, "L'Origan," wasn't hitting the right note. François was enthralled by the beauty of 18th century flasks, but he knew that they were impossible to mass-produce. Yet, the grace and diversity of their style kept niggling at him.

Meanwhile, almost in creative over-drive, he produced "Vertige," "Idylle," and "Effluve," within months of each other. In 1905 he created three masterpieces "L'Ambre Antique," "L'Origan" and "Le Jasmin de Corse". "L'Origan" was marketed as "warm, rich and luminous; it suits all women and yet is different on each one." It was a heady blend of orange blossom, jasmine, rose and carnation, married with a note of sweet grass, which gave it an exceptionally subtle signature. Overnight, "L'Origan" became the fragrance of choice of fashionable society ladies and an instant best seller.

In 1908, when François opened the first Coty shop at 33 Place Vendôme in the heart of Paris, he had an influential neighbor at number 24: René Lalique. Audaciously, Coty approached Lalique to design a glass vignette to be the signature label for his perfume bottles. Initially, Lalique snubbed the idea of taking on such a menial commission. He was, after all, a legend as both a sculptor and a jeweler. But François persisted and, appealing to the man's ego, convinced Lalique that he was the only person capable of creating a flask that could be perceived as an authentic work of art. "A perfume," Coty argued knowingly, "needs to attract the eye as much the nose."

Sufficiently intrigued and challenged, Lalique eventually agreed to design "an artistic" bottle for Coty. A glass vignette for "L'Effleurt" initiated their partnership in 1908. Astonishingly fluid, it was made from molded and pressed glass with a brownish glow and depicted a woman emerging from the voluptuously curving petals of a blossoming flower, reminiscent of Venus rising from her shell. Coty was captivated and urged Lalique to create a mold to incorporate the design into a flacon.

Coty and Lalique did not have the means for mass-production at that point but were energized by the potential for development and they moved swiftly. In the fall of 1908, Lalique rented a glassworks at Combs-la-Ville on the river Seine, and the next year he produced the bottle for "Cyclamen", decorated with insects whose intricately sculpted wings outlined the delicate curves of the bottle. The impact of the bottle was revolutionary and formed the cornerstone for an entirely new marketing approach that would be copied by the greatest names in perfumes.

The following year, "L'Ambre Antique" was launched. The faint reddish-brown patina of the bottle lit up the figures of the Fates, with their wild hair and long robes, all holding bouquets. Some fifteen extraordinary bottles were conceived during this collaboration. Each was considered a work of art, due in part to the imaginative originality and beauty of each design. The model for "Styx" was a fluted cylinder with a slightly rounded body, crowned with a gold-leaf stopper and adorned with four bees whose unfurled wings joined together in the center, while "Au Coeur de Calices," created in 1913, used an unusual shade of blue. Lalique went on to create elaborate stoppers that assumed the majesty of a tiara and came in a variety of shapes and sizes: capsules, tricornes or globes sculpted with a carnation in bloom or a large bee were as intricately worked as his fabled glass necklaces.

The contrast between smooth and uneven surfaces, subtle finishes, frosted or soft polishes and sharp lines that brought fantasy flora and fauna to life that, reflected the naturalism which governed the "Modern Style," and the art of the master glass maker. The greatest coup, however, was the marriage of form and function: Each glass creation elegantly complemented its potion without impinging on Coty's determination to avoid compromising either the quality of his products or the rapid rate of their production.

Coty and Lalique's collaboration extended to the flacon labels, which were designed in art nouveau graphic style and printed on a golden background. In addition, publicity signs and presentation cases were incorporated into a marketing strategy that was as much a part of Coty's arsenal against the competition as his uniquely packaged, trail-blazing scents.

Marketing, elegance and success

Coty concentrated his efforts on making sure that his retailers understood and applied the message he wanted the brand to communicate. He would deal with his retailers in an esprit de corps that encouraged the notion that they were his business partners, and ensured a loyalty that went beyond stocking the product. In "The Path to Beauty," a comprehensive catalogue of Coty products, retailers were able to show the customers products that were not in stock, but could be specially ordered.

By 1912, the Coty catalogue comprised a list of 22 "handkerchief perfumes," and François Coty was only starting to hit his stride. Later that year, he launched "L'Or," a floral perfume created especially for "pale-eyed blondes, who will love the way this fragrance blends with the smell of blond tobacco." It was Coty, the seductive salesman, at his best. From then on, each perfume would have its own profile, poetically sketching a portrait to reflect the moods and aspirations of the woman for whom it was intended.

In an era when fashion designers such as Balmain, Poiret, Paquin and the Callot sisters dictated the strictures of the day, Coty had a radically opposite and personal stance. His desire to create a different perfume for each individual woman may have been unrealistic, but it was a refreshingly inspiring ideal. In later years, Coty would amplify such musings, imparting pointers that would resound strongly among his faithful. In a 1924 guidebook, Coty expounded on the necessity that "each woman should have her own subtle fragrance; one which will suit her style and which will be a true expression of her personality."

Now, Coty went on to create a range of creams, soaps and bath salts available in fifteen fragrances, so that, as he wrote "...each woman can drape her beauty in one evocative, lingering fragrance leaving behind her an indelible memory."

Increasing production and crossing borders

In 1908 Coty had relocated his burgeoning empire to Suresnes and within a year he purchased the aristocratic Château de la Source, which would become the first building block of what Coty christened "Perfume City," a grandiose gesture, but one that spoke to Coty's vision as much as his ambition. Others including Volnay, Lejeune and Worth would later follow Coty to the area between Saint Cloud and Puteaux, which would become the most modern industrial complex in Europe.

"Perfume City" became its own little world. Fifty thousand square meters of workshops and laboratories nestled alongside a glassworks division capable of making up to one hundred thousand bottles a day. Powder box, metal box, and lipstick manufacturing required 26 000 square meters and 9 000 employees – 80% of whom were women. This factory, designed for the packaging of beauty products hit on a rich, untapped market. Cosmetics were in the first stages of infancy when Coty decided to enter this side of the business, creating yet another arm for an already booming empire and reinforcing his position as a far-sighted market leader.

Among Coty's most groundbreaking cosmetics was an "air spun" face powder. Remarkably high in quality for a mass-produced product, its finesse and success were unrivalled. Packaged in Lalique's sumptuous triangular glass jar, the lid was designed in the form of a veil whose folds envelop the figure of a woman. The Lalique-designed round box, with an iconic white and gold powder-puff motif, became a collector's item.

A follow-up compact version enjoyed a similar success and, by 1914, was selling, an astonishing, thirty thousand a day in America alone. "My powder compact is my own best advertisement," Coty boasted at the time. It wasn't an overstatement. The powder, available in more than twenty shades, would make Coty a legitimate multi-millionaire, inspiring him to aim for his dream: to become an immortal visionary.

Coty commissioned Lalique to create a bas-relief in honor of "Perfume City" (now housed at the François Coty museum in Suresnes), which was grandly embedded at the entrance between two factories. An exalted work of art, it depicted two women kneeling before a perfume-burner – an ancient motif that was also incorporated as the watermark on Coty's vellum writing paper. Lalique's crowning achievement with Coty however was yet to come. In 1913, when Coty became established in a magnificent building at 714 Fifth Avenue, New York which currently houses Henri Bendel, he commissioned Lalique to help liven up the interior and the façade, which had been designed in 1871 by American architect Charles Duggan. Lalique created a series of pressed glass panels, embellished with flowering poppies to decorate the entrance hall and meeting rooms, as well as the large shop windows. It was Lalique's first architectural glasswork in the US and his most celebrated achievement.

By the end of WW1, Lalique was burning on all cylinders. Coty, at that point, had the capability to manufacture up to one hundred thousand bottles per day, and the demanding standards were escalating, as each of the ground glass stoppers used for the majority of flacons was individually fitted, and the bottom of each bottle was numbered to ensure an perfect match.

Soon, Coty established thriving subsidiaries in London and New York. Displaying the canny street-smartness that made him as revered for his business acumen as for his nose, when the United States began imposing heavy duties on all imported products, (with an emphasis on luxury goods) Coty outfoxed the government by transporting his perfumes in detached components. As of 1915, all boxes, empty flasks, stoppers and raw materials were shipped to the U.S. from Suresnes separately.

Birth of a new fragrance and the end of an era

In 1917, Coty hit his highest creative note with the debut of "Chypre." A composition in the literal sense, "Chypre" was heralded as a masterpiece, combining style, energy, subtlety, clarity and volume. Above all, it evoked an ethereal seduction thanks to its capacity to take on new depths when worn. Top light notes were modified by a middle note of jasmine, while a vague powdery edge was balanced by a lingering blend of patchouli, vetiver, sandalwood, bergamot and a unique note of oak moss, which Coty referred to as the "bouillon of moss." Unobtrusive but lingering, both light and luxurious, "Chypre" spoke to the spirit of the times, which was simultaneously expressed by Gabrielle Chanel who, in the spirit of stylish simplicity, designed her first shirtwaist dress that year.

[3] *Following pages:*
I Love Me: name of the Chupa Chups perfumes, launched in 2003.

I LOV

FRAG

EME

RANCE

"Chypre" would become one of Coty's five bestsellers along with "Emeraude," "L'Origan," "Paris," and "L'Aimant," a sensational success, that was endlessly emulated by the competition. Derivatives would include Millot's "Crêpe de Chine," Chanel's "No.5," Rochas' "Femme," Grès' "Cabochard," and most recently "Eau Sauvage."

Despite a new factory in Alsace, René Lalique couldn't keep up with Coty's demands and relations between the men became strained. The problems included delays in production and delivery. Coty grew impatient and irritable. Lalique, who resented being treated like a mere supplier, was equally unhappy. The conflict that would erupt between the two egotistical talents was inevitable. On January 12, 1920 Coty distributed a circular to each of his clients informing them that "my bottle suppliers have finally admitted their inability to deliver," and that he would in the future undertake the glass design and production himself. Lalique was furious when he witnessed the first bottles come off the Coty production line: they were unadulterated copies of his designs. The subsequent courtroom battle, which Lalique ultimately won, soured the relationship between the men. Eventually, the men patched over their troubles and Lalique returned to the Coty fold until 1934, this time to design, but not to manufacture the glassware.

By the early 1920s, François Coty was one of the richest men in the world – an enviable status in which he reveled. Considered something of a parvenu by some, malicious gossip had it that the mysterious mogul always carried handfuls of precious stones in his pocket, carelessly wrapped in paper, so that he could gaze at his riches whenever the desire to contemplate his wealth took him.

From perfume to newsprint

Now at the peak of his success, Coty was known as the Napoleon of perfumery and like many dictators, he believed he could master anything he set out to achieve. Consequently, in 1921, Coty, who understood the power of the press, purchased Le

Figaro newspaper and became as intoxicated by the smell of ink as he was with the power the newspaper gave him. Hooked, he then bought the rival broadsheet Le Gaulois and liquidated it to create an independently spirited publication, L'Ami du Peuple ("The People's Friend"). Intended to be the most widely read newspaper in the world, it sold seven hundred thousand copies a day at ten centimes. Its competitors in the industry, all of who charged 25 centimes for their publications, were so upset that one of them (the Hachette Distribution Company) levied a tax on any kiosks that stocked any Coty newspaper. Undeterred, Coty launched an evening edition of L'Ami du Peuple, followed by a daily sports paper, and established an independent network of newsagents. The move allowed him to thwart his foes and expand his publishing chain nationwide with an explosion of regional newspapers.

Lover and aesthete

Coty's passions included women and property, and he collected mistresses and houses with enviable nonchalance. Coty's generosity with his lovers was legendary. For those who knew how to manipulate the situation, a blank check awaited and, if a child appeared, maintenance was discreetly paid. There was more than one illegitimate Coty running around Paris, a fact which Roland and Christiane, his children by Yvonne, discovered after their father's death when they unearthed a colorful list of allowances on his personal books.

More consuming than his love of women, however, was his obsession with chateaux, which he would remodel to his own grandiose taste. His first significant purchase was the Château de Longchamp, a classical residence with a lake, located on the edge of the Bois de Boulogne on the outskirts of Paris. Coty's piece-de-resistance, however, was his refurbishment of the d'Artigny estate near Tours, in the Loire valley. After demolishing the existing chateau, a clumsy, pseudo-renaissance manor with vulgar Violet-Leduc turrets, Coty employed an army of workers for twelve years to bring to life his fantasy home. It boasted rare extras such as electric gates, air conditioning and ice-making machinery.

A worldwide ambition realized

Coty's personal pleasures and ambitions didn't, however, distract him from his business. In the 1920s he produced over fifteen new perfumes, while also maintaining an iron grip of control over all stages of production, from the activity in the rose fields to minutiae on the assembly line. In 1925, an estimated 36 million women across the world were using Coty powders to dust their faces, and the company returned an enormous 60% profit.

This was also decade when Coty became the pioneer for incorporation of a company throughout Europe. Although the hubs of his operation still lay in France and his native Corsica, Coty established a well-oiled network of subsidiaries to infiltrate the Italian, Swiss, German and Spanish markets. In 1927 he opened a base in Bucharest with the intention of penetrating the Russian market. Turning his eye towards South America, he employed independent distribution networks, using small local factories to circumvent the trade barriers in Brazil, Argentina and Mexico. These markets alone generated a turnover of one hundred million francs a year.

The 1930s saw a dramatic shift in the status of perfume. No longer a secret feminine whim, perfume became a fashionable gift and a blissfully guilt free form of self-indulgence. Magazine editors encouraged their readers to use perfume not only to scent their bodies, but also their clothes, their underwear, their writing paper, books, and cushions – even their bedroom curtains.

Ironically, the year Lalique finally severed his ties with the company, 1934, was the same year that Coty died. François had lived to see the unveiling of his final masterpiece.

[4] Scarab stopper designed by René Lalique
for the *L'Effleurt* perfume by Coty, launched in 1910. By Keiichi Tahara.

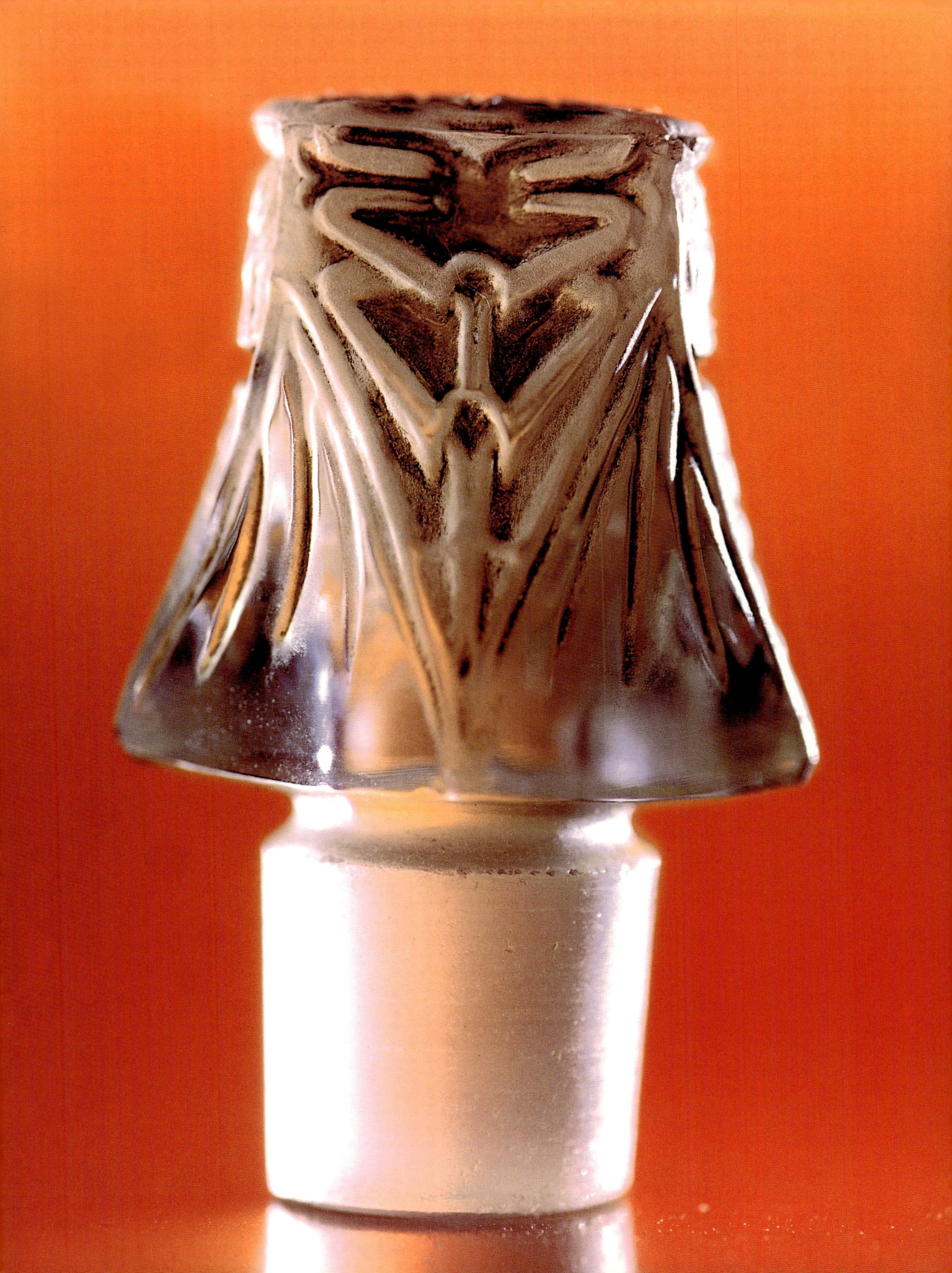

Having replaced Lalique with Pierre Camin, François oversaw the new team's efforts to develop an exciting design change that would result in an extraordinary packaging innovation for the launch of "Vertige."

Instead of presenting the perfume in the customary colored leather box, the faceted crystal bottle was regally placed in a Dresden-motif porcelain case, decorated with a picture of a gentleman and his beloved, painted with the precision of a miniature. The attention-grabbing departure from tradition shook up the industry and marked yet another creative coup for Coty perfumes.

A continuing legacy

Seventy years after the death of François Coty, his philosophy of always keeping an eye on the future, is alive and thriving. Even a man as ambitious as François Coty would find it difficult not to be impressed by the audacious breadth and scope of Coty today. Powered by 6,500 employees, the company has grown dramatically by way of a series of acquisitions and extensions that began in 1963, when positioned as the third largest fragrance company in the US, Coty was acquired by Pfizer Panama Just over three decades later, in 1992, Joh. A. Benckiser GmbH took the company over and boosted Coty's holdings by bringing luxury and fashionable high-profile names such as Lancaster, Davidoff, Jil Sander, adidas and Joop! to the union. Two years later, the company's growth intensified when Coty's US subsidiary acquired Quintessence Inc., a Chicago-based manufacturer of fragrances and personal care, including Jovan and Aspen. In 1996, Benckiser announced that Coty Inc. would encompass all its prestige and mass beauty brands. That same year, Coty acquired Unilever's European make-up brands, including the trend-setting Rimmel collection.

François' raison d'être, to create a collection of prestige products that remain within reach, has probably never been more relevant than it is at present in the fast-paced contemporary marketplace. His belief in the attention-grabbing tactics of eye-catching marketing strategies, and that the beauty of a product is not enough; that every nuance must be glorified in order to transcend the ordinary and thus seduce, continues to be germane. But above all, François' penchant for cultivating the excitement of surprise by collaborating with artistic talents from other fields fuels the entrepreneurial spirit that drives the company today.

Coty's 2002 launch of "Glow by JLO" is a vivid example of how Coty's past meshes with the present, and provides a signpost to the future. Reflecting François' disdain for adhering to business formulae (and the devilish pleasure he took in upsetting the status quo), Coty Inc. ignored the industry belief that celebrity-inspired scents were commercially non-viable.

Convinced that a fragrance reflecting the fresh, sexy aspect of Jennifer Lopez's personality was a perfect fit in a global culture where celebrity influences everything from fashion to home design, Coty began a collaboration with the celebrated superstar. The result "Glow by JLO," is a perfume that tempers the tang of orange flower, grapefruit, and rose with the subtle simplicity of vanilla, musk, and sandalwood (and, poignantly, the honeysuckle that so eluded François). It skillfully captures the dewy, effervescent spirit of young, fun-loving women. "Glow by JLO" has baffled the skeptics by turning out to be one of the greatest success stories in the history of the fragrance industry, generating record-breaking sales of over $80 million within ten months of its debut. The launch also cemented Coty Inc.'s reputation for boldness. The company's short decision-making chains, much like François Coty's brief formulae, have enabled the swift transition from idea to application, taking less than a year to travel from concept to shelf. By contrast, the rest of the industry normally lags behind, anywhere between 18 months to two years.

A second perfume, "Still Jennifer Lopez," was inspired by the idea of "an independent, confident, and modern woman juggling family, relationships, work, clients, and friends all at once—just too many things," explains the multi-faceted actress, singer and dancer. "Yet somehow," she adds, "we make it work." The resulting perfume, a confident yet unpredictable medley of notes infusing mandarin, Earl Grey, sake, pink freesia, rose spiced with white pepper and wild jasmine, appeals to women with a slightly more grown-up sensibility. Recently launched in the US and parts of Europe and Japan, with plans to expand to the rest of the world, "Still Jennifer Lopez" looks set to repeat the stellar performance of "Glow by JLO," which was honored with the fragrance industry's highest distinction: a FiFi Award for the Celebrity Fragrance Star of the Year. (2003)

Dividing to conquer

By the turn of the 21st century, Coty Inc. had grown so quickly that the company had been divided to operate in two separate divisions: Lancaster Group, which develops fragrance, color cosmetics and skincare for the prestige sector, and Coty Beauty, which sells in the mass and masstige distribution sectors.

Both divisions encompass a strong portfolio of vastly distinctive brands, some of which are international best sellers, while others are leaders in key regional markets in Europe, North America and Asia.

The prestige division, Lancaster Group, bears the name of its flagship fragrance, skincare and make-up brand. Established in Monaco in the aftermath of World War II, Lancaster began as a partnership between French entrepreneur Georges Wurtz and chemist Eugène Frezzati. It was named in tribute to the Royal Air Force bombers who played a vital role in the liberation of occupied France. Lancaster Group, headquartered in Paris, is among the world's top ten prestige beauty businesses. It represents some of the global culture's most influential names, from the multi-talented Jennifer Lopez to the red-carpet jewelers, Chopard.

The Coty Beauty division, on the other hand, is widely recognized as the world's number one manufacturer of mass-market fragrances. A trailblazer in the mass and masstige broad distribution sectors, it offers high-quality and value-added products. Ranked among the leaders in color cosmetics, Coty Beauty includes global power brands such as adidas, Rimmel and Céline Dion, another superstar in the Coty lineup.

The world-renowned singer's fragrance, "Celine Dion Parfums" inspired by the restrained elegance of a bouquet of white flowers, is evocative of Dion's warm personality and endearing joie de vivre, and is among the largest selling perfumes in worldwide distribution. Signature fragrance scent strips were inserted into Celine Dion's new CD at the time of the launch of "Celine Dion Parfums," a clever promotional move that was rewarded with instant success. The fragrance sky-rocketed to the number one spot in US mid-level department stores, achieving over double the sales that the previous market leader, Elizabeth Taylor White Diamonds, had attained a decade earlier. Building on the success of Dion's first fragrance, Coty Beauty then launched a second fragrance called "Celine Dion Parfums Notes."

"Glow by JLO" and "Celine Dion Parfums" amplify the impact these celebrities yield. Both of these stars are undeniably glamorous yet, they are viewed as approachable and accessible to their fans. By wearing these fragrances, women feel they are being allowed to share in the passions that fill their idols' lives; which, given that both women were integral in the creation of the scents produced under their names, is true.

"Celine Dion Parfums" and "Glow by JLO" are contemporary examples of how François Coty's obsession with bottle design and packaging continues to thrive. Although "Celine Dion Parfums" is sold in the broader "masstige" market, the style of its chic packaging speaks to what women expect from a prestige fragrance: a decorative box and an elegant, faceted flacon with a two-tone cap. The presentation of "Glow by JLO" perceptibly reflects Jennifer Lopez's personality, with the sensual curves of the bottle evoking a feminine silhouette.

Technology that delivers beauty

Despite the complex infrastructure and geographical vastness of Coty Inc., both divisions operate on a single, fundamental tenet defined by three indelibly linked values: Beauty, Lifestyle and Quality. Developing technologically advanced, aesthetically pleasing products that reflect the consumer's sensibilities, desires and aspirations, Coty Inc. maintains a strategy that it calls "surprising beauty," which is aimed at developing new products. An ambition that is buffered by Coty's concentration on research & development, which has been a sustained priority ever since 1955, when Coty pioneered a revolution in lipstick with the introduction of it's the long-lasting formula, Coty 24.

Renowned for its pioneering sun-care line, which introduced the use of Retinol in skincare, the Lancaster Group has garnered an enviable reputation for scientific innovation, while producing a complete range of care for all skin types. Redolent of the sun-drenched Riviera, Lancaster's Mediterranean-inspired sun-care collection, which debuted in orange bottles in 1971, offers a long-lasting subtle and golden color, while effectively protecting the skin thanks to the exclusive RPF (Radical Protection Factor)—a powerful anti-free radical complex that protects against cell damage and photo-aging. Employing the latest technology has kept the division one cosmeto-scientific step ahead of the competition. The Lancaster laboratories have also developed innovative products including "Re-Oxygen" (a unique transport system that delivers Oxygen directly to the skin cells) and 365 Cellular Elixir Serum (a DNA complex that stimulates the skin's natural repair process).

Leading the charge in anti-aging skincare products, Lancaster pioneered the use of micro-crystals (containing a Retinol complex) in "Excellence," which stimulates the revitalization of the skin. Lancaster's technological precision is also evident, and attractive to a younger generation of women, in "The Body Glow Collection," spawned after the enormous success of the "Glow by JLO" perfume. Using vitamin-powered formulas to aid the skin's firmness, "The Body Glow Collection" also brightens the complexion with a burst of botanical extracts, which infuse the skin with a balanced blend of replenishing moisture and anti-oxidant protection.

Constantly on the lookout for new compounds, the Coty research and development units in the United States and Monaco file more than 500 worldwide patent applications for about 60 new cosmetic technologies each year. They continue to flourish with novel ideas. In 1997, they developed "the healing garden," the first major mass-market line of home-spa aromachology products based on botanical ingredients. In 2003, Coty signed an agreement with Dupont to use LYCRA® technology in cosmetic products, offering a uniquely absorbent nail enamel, for Rimmel and Astor, that delivers great shine in 36 shades. The company has also developed Rimmel's Extreme Definition Comb Mascara, which boasts exceptional application control and has quickly gained market leadership in several countries.

Among Coty's other radical developments was the patented Smart™ Technology, which releases a key ingredient to kill odor-causing bacteria on demand, and is utilized by the personal care collection from adidas (anti-perspirants, body sprays and shower gels), Coty Beauty's largest and fastest-growing brand. As the original adidas clothing brand has evolved from a sports necessity to a street-through-nightclub staple, Coty initiatives have helped shift the brand's lifestyle image up-market. Fragrance by adidas is number one in the male mass market in Europe, while the adidas advanced-performance skin fitness line "adidas Active Skincare for Men," (launched in 2003,) now matches competitors, including Unilever, Procter & Gamble and L'Oreal.

Fragrances from the stars

Just as François Coty aspired to create a different perfume to cater to the vast array of tastes and desires of different women, today Coty concentrates on providing a far-reaching range of products that will speak to women of different ages, lifestyles, personality types and aspirations. Fragrances by teen-style queens Mary Kate and Ashley Olsen attract the young fashion and price-conscious girls, who also gravitate to the cultish trend appeal of high-voltage brands such as "Chupa Chups." Rimmel, which has evolved from being perceived as a cut-price brand into a sassy best-selling fashion-leader, attracts women who are keen to emulate the hip image personified by its super-cool spokeswoman, Kate Moss. Alternatively, fragrances by German designer Wolfgang Joop, an extrovert whose colorful runway presentations routinely generate a great deal of attention appeal to the playful self-assured man (Joop! Homme) and woman (Joop! Muse) while "Celine Dion Parfums" by Celine Dion and "Glow by JLO," perpetuate the charisma of their creators amongst fans of all ages from all corners of the globe.

Meanwhile, "My Manifesto," by Isabella Rossellini, a refreshingly jaunty fragrance that opens with an unusual notion of basil, is typically favored by older women who enjoy channeling the enigmatic, sparkle of its creator. Meanwhile, the haute fashionista will be drawn to the elegant minimalism of Jil Sander's fragrance and make-up lines. More flamboyant tastes are satisfied by "Boudoir" and "Libertine" from Vivienne Westwood, the eccentric British couturier renowned for her punk creations, baroque touches and stridently nonconformist attitude. Park Avenue Princesses, and their legion of imitators, will love must-have Marc Jacobs Perfume and Blush fragrances. The darling of the international fashion flock, Jacobs is the fashion designer favored by Hollywood's hip royalty: Sofia Coppola, Lisa Marie Presley, Winona Ryder and Chloe Sevigny—whom Vogue editor Anna Wintour, has elevated to iconic status by nicknaming them "Marc-olettes." Jacobs signed with Coty in 2002; the same year as the company acquired the license for Kenneth Cole, another luminary on the American style scene.

Coty also shows innovation in the production and marketing of its male fragrance lines. For instance, Davidoff Cool Water, a zesty mix of bergamot, fresh peppermint, lavender and rosemary/, dramatically shifted the perception of men's fragrances when it was launched in 1988. An urbane masculine fragrance, it remains a worldwide best seller today.

The dawning of a new century

"Give a woman the best product you can make," François Coty succinctly proclaimed, "market it in the perfect bottle, beautiful in its simplicity yet impeccable in taste, ask a reasonable price, and you will witness the birth of a business the size of which the world has never seen."

Accordingly, one hundred years after its birth in a small Parisian apartment, Coty Inc. is poised on a high note to begin its second century in the business of setting pulses racing. It continues to draw on its rich heritage while also cultivating the values, mix of talents, and innovative ideas that have propelled it to be a power player at the contemporary global beauty counter. A century after François Coty was first bedazzled by the unlimited potential that greeted him at the beginning of the 1900s in Paris, Coty Inc. heads into its second century, fuelled by the intoxicating excitement of the endless creative, technological and entrepreneurial possibilities that once infused the maverick François Coty's dream: To stylishly seduce the world with enticements that would lead every man and every woman, as he once mused, to "a love affair with oneself."

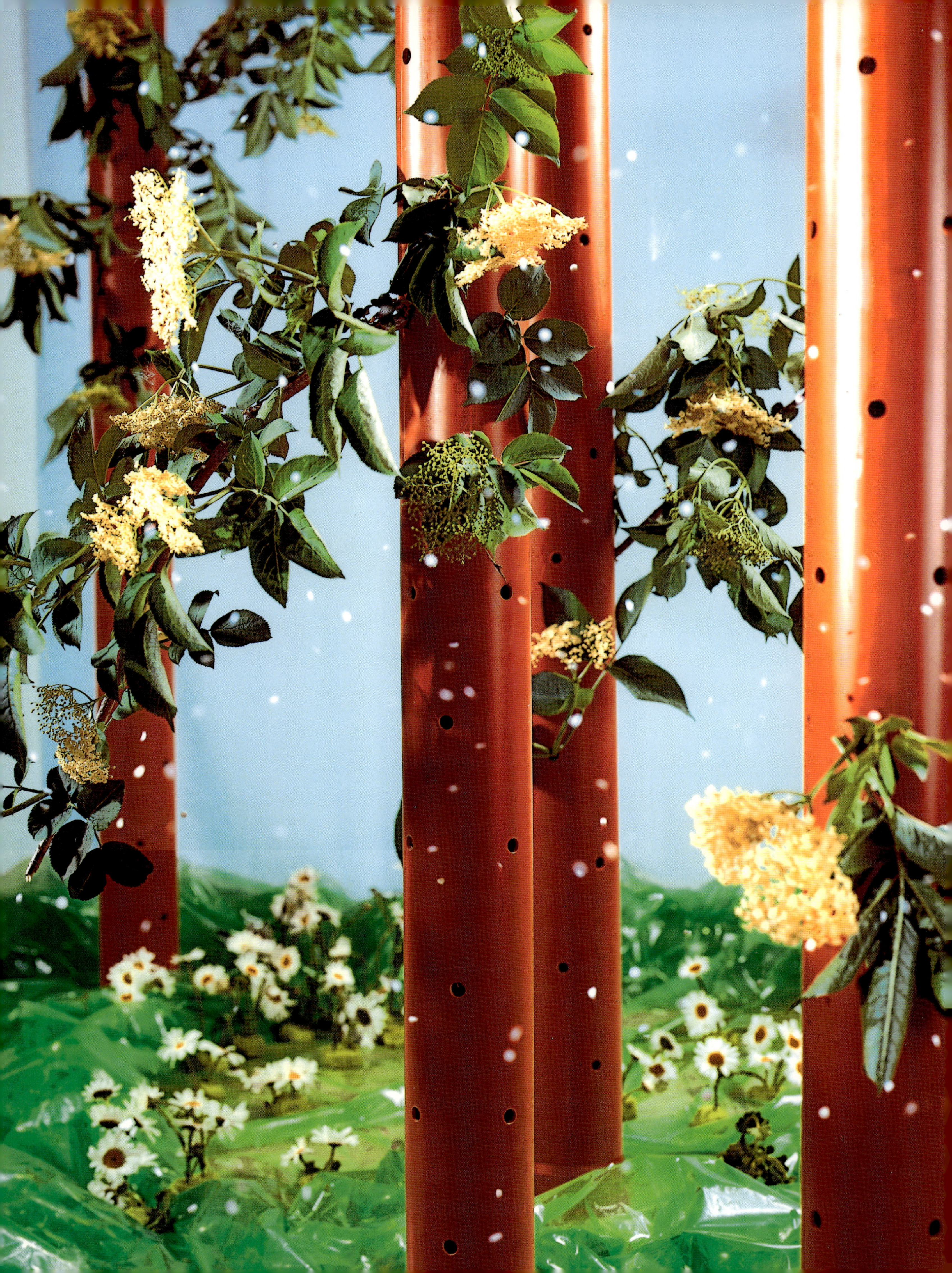

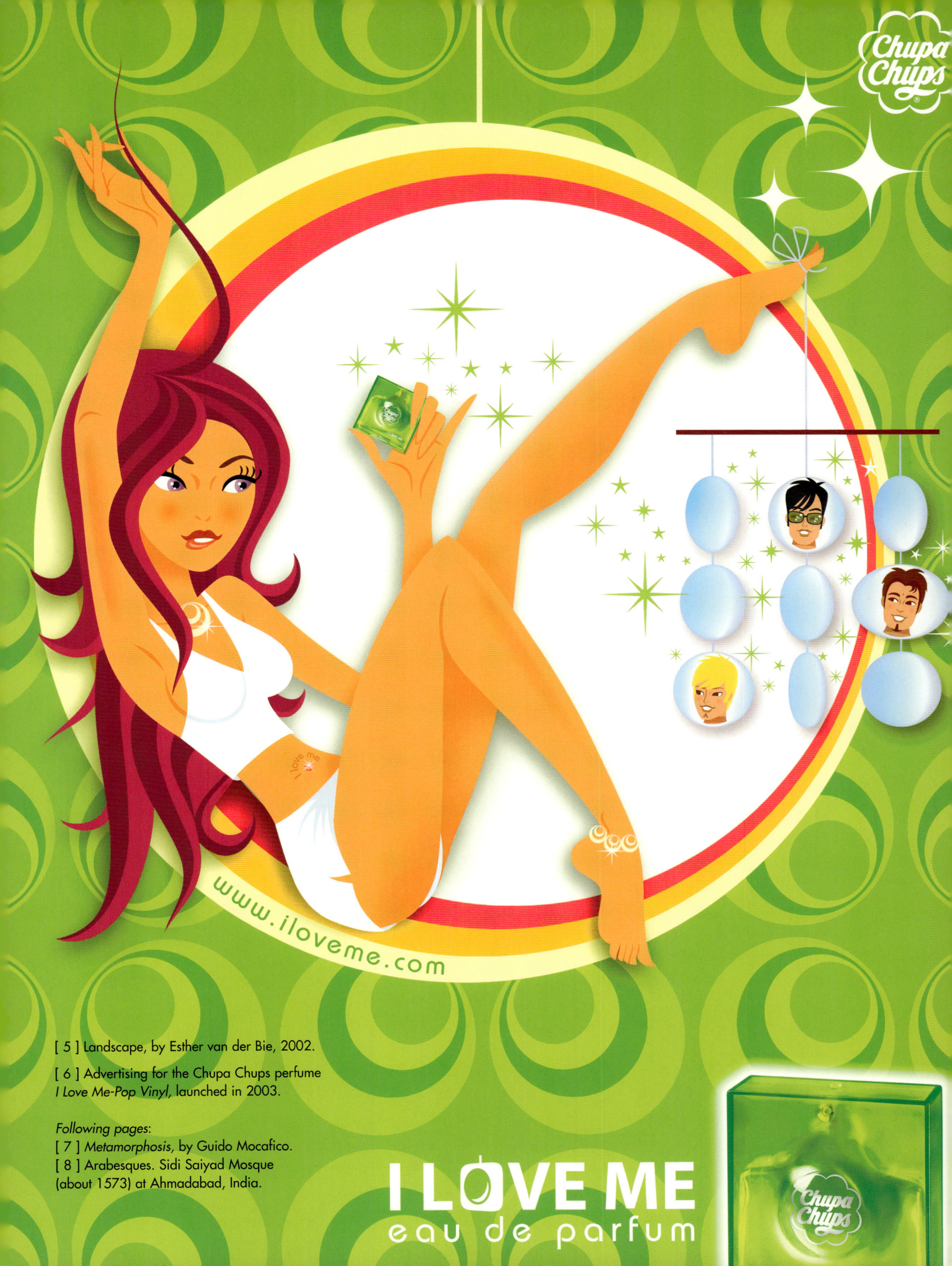

[5] Landscape, by Esther van der Bie, 2002.

[6] Advertising for the Chupa Chups perfume *I Love Me-Pop Vinyl*, launched in 2003.

Following pages:
[7] *Metamorphosis*, by Guido Mocafico.
[8] Arabesques. Sidi Saiyad Mosque (about 1573) at Ahmadabad, India.

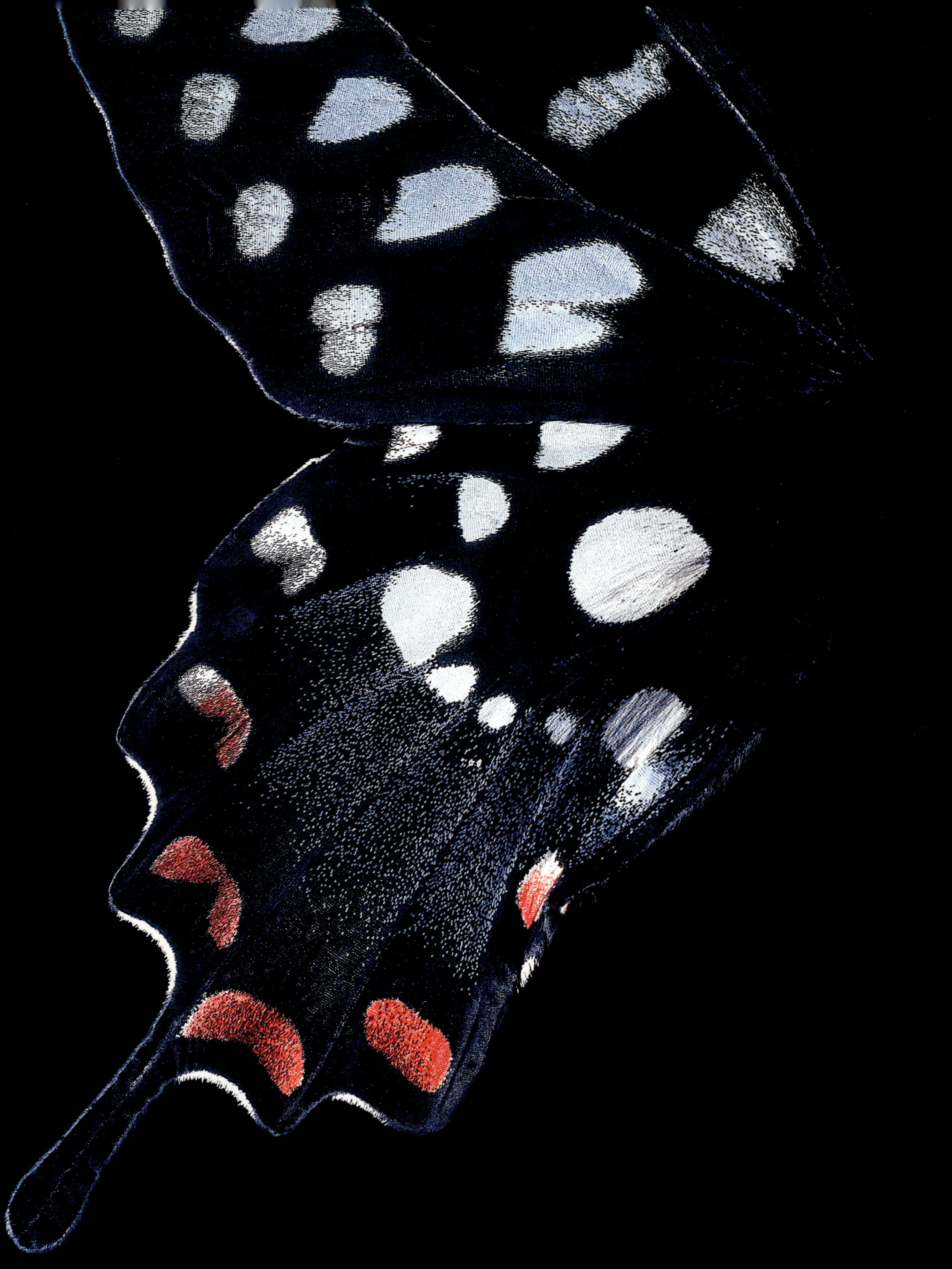

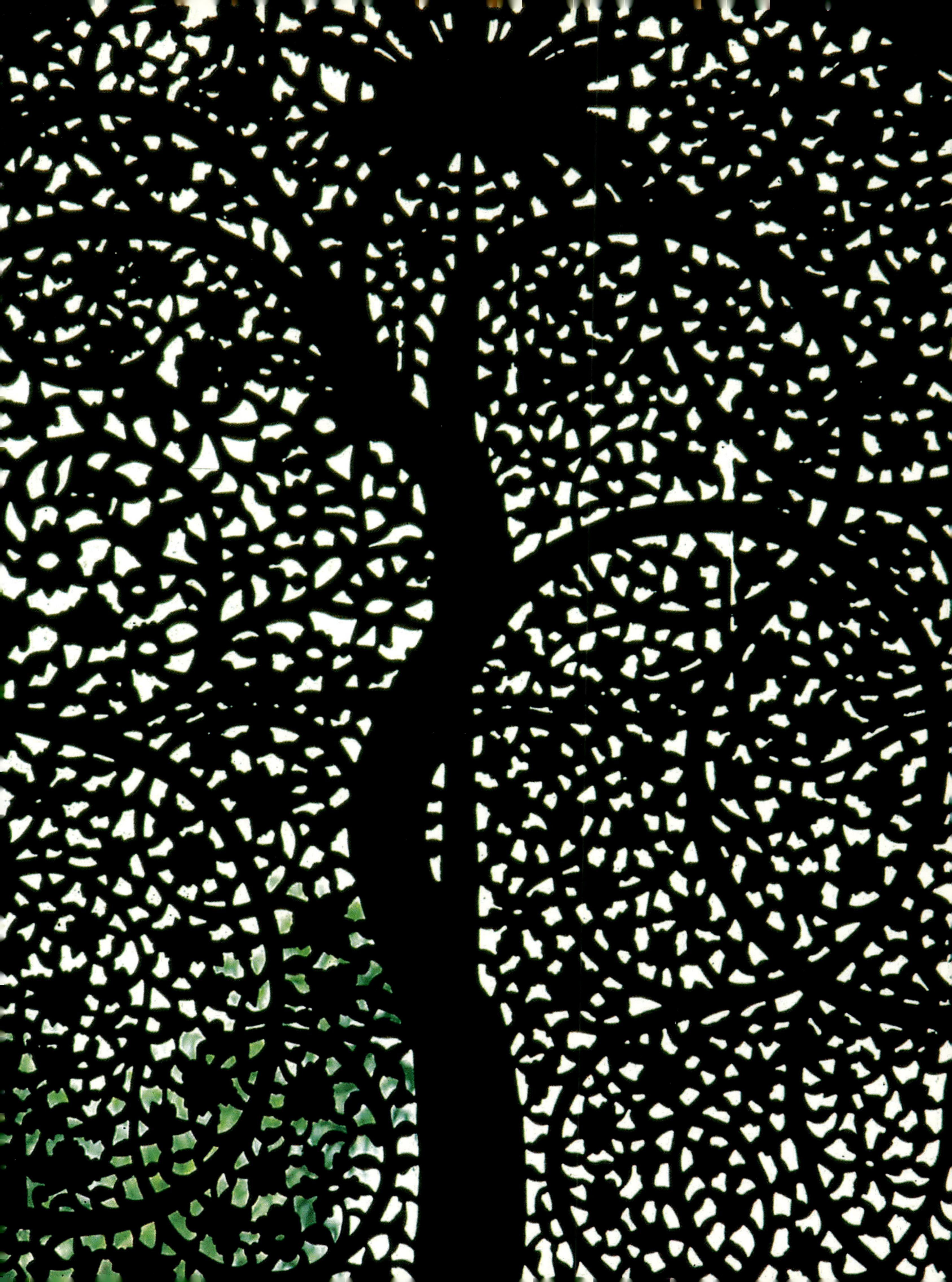

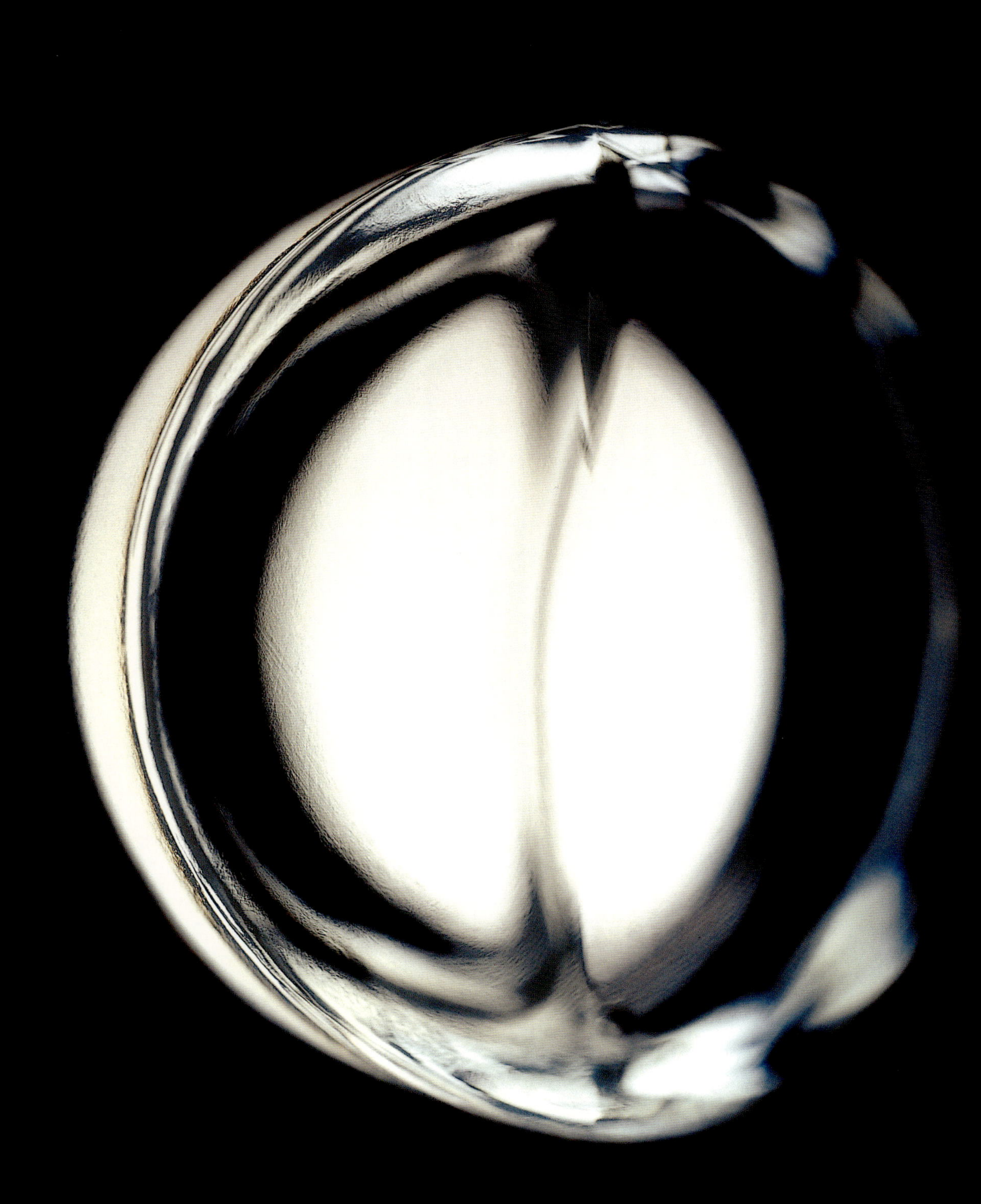

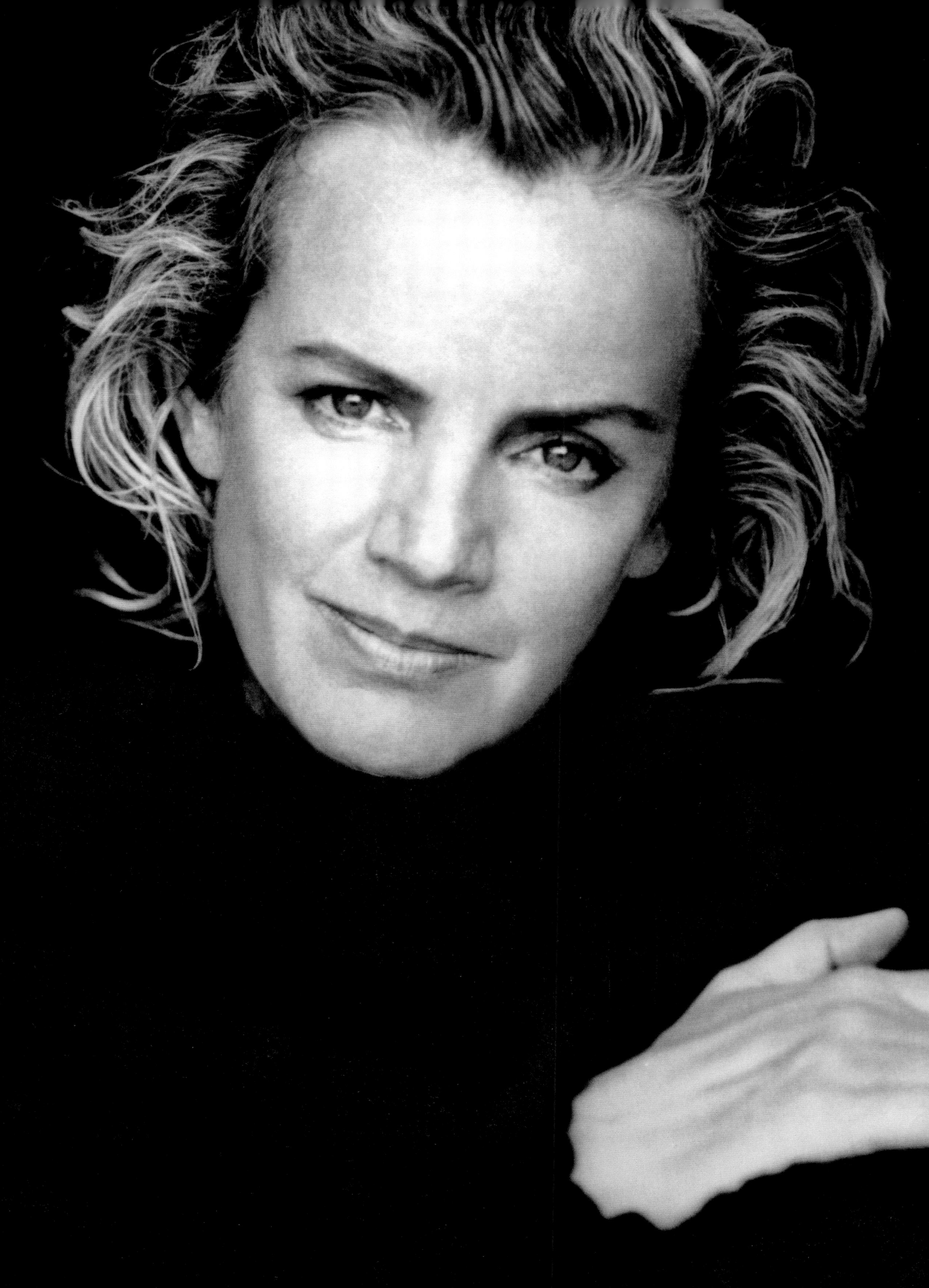

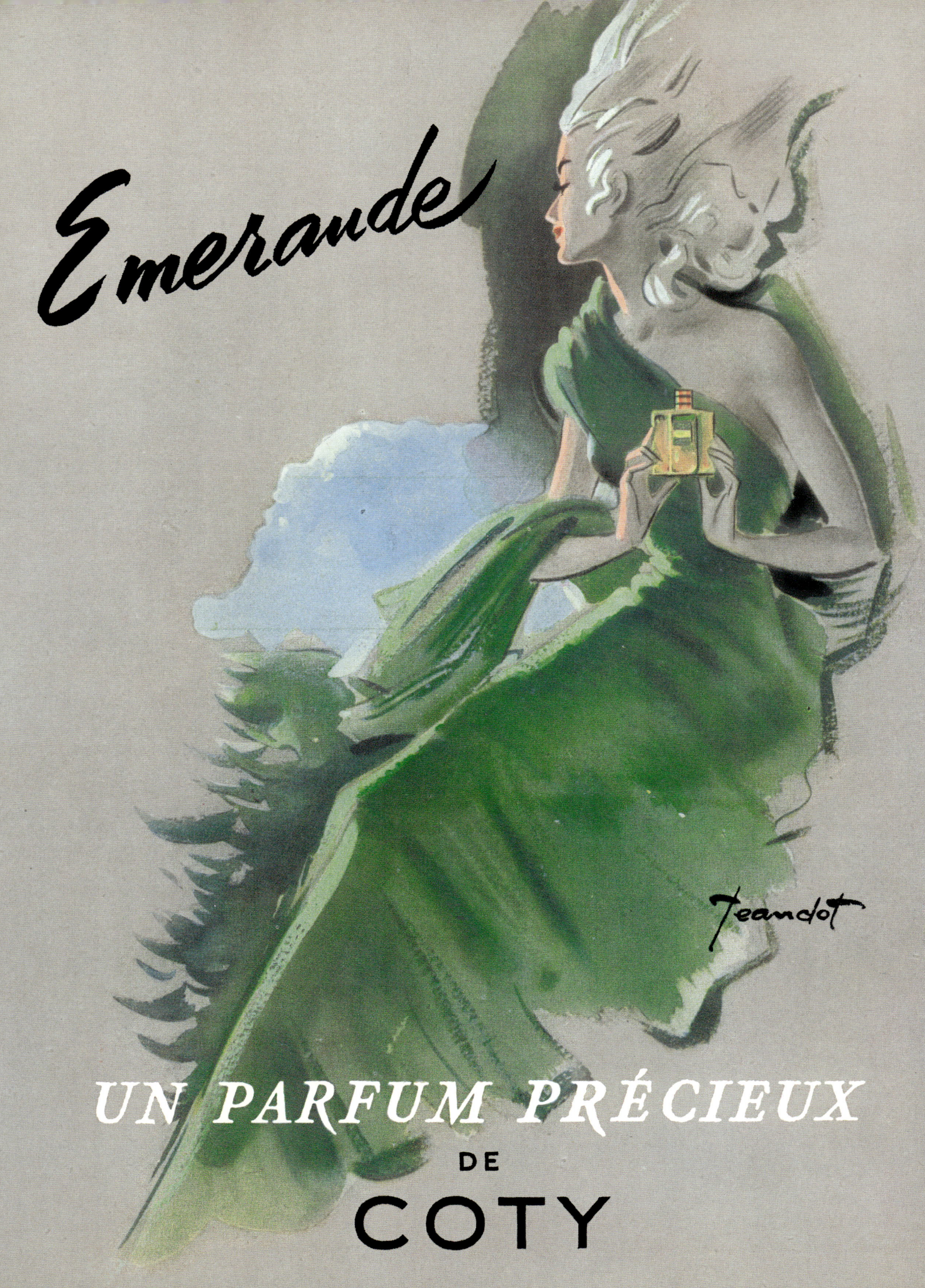
Emeraude
Jeandot
UN PARFUM PRÉCIEUX
DE
COTY

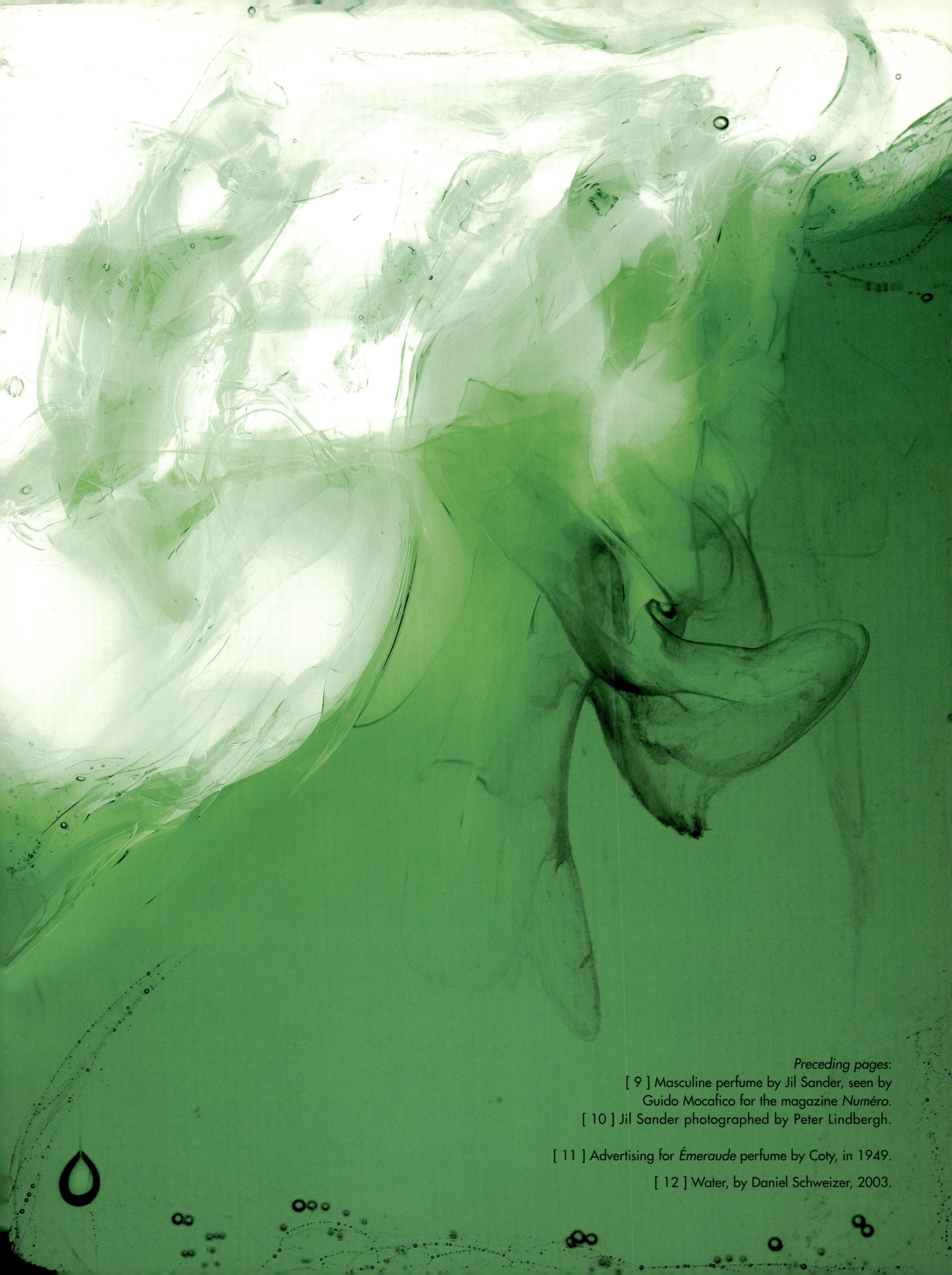

Preceding pages:
[9] Masculine perfume by Jil Sander, seen by Guido Mocafico for the magazine *Numéro*.
[10] Jil Sander photographed by Peter Lindbergh.

[11] Advertising for *Émeraude* perfume by Coty, in 1949.

[12] Water, by Daniel Schweizer, 2003.

RIMME

RIMMEL

Lasting Finish

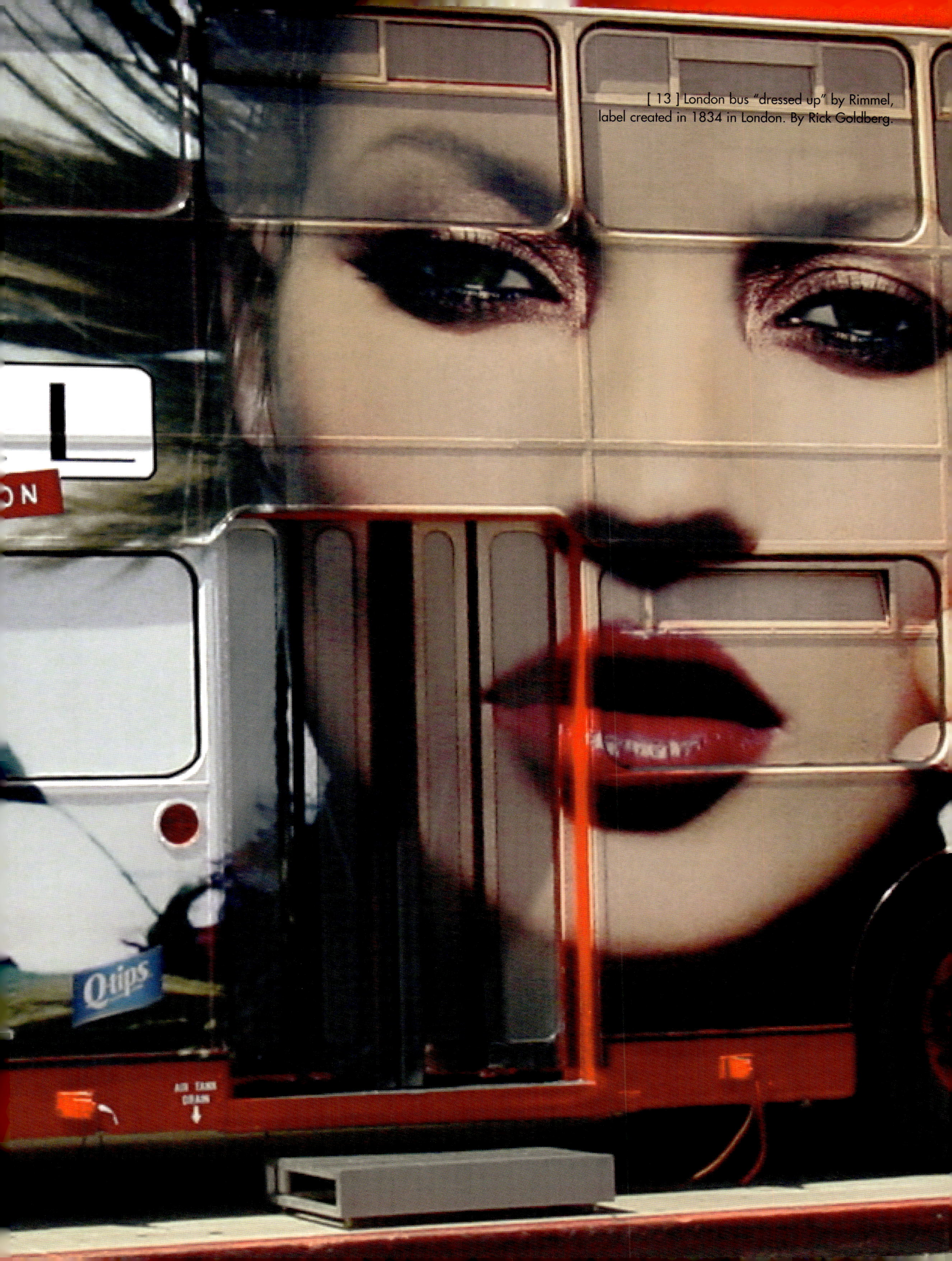

[13] London bus "dressed up" by Rimmel, label created in 1834 in London. By Rick Goldberg.

“From the moment the young François Coty decided to make perfume his life’s work, he did so with his nose attuned to feminine fancies.”

[14] Portrait of Sofia Coppola by Elizabeth Peyton for the advertising of the Marc Jacobs *Essence* perfume.

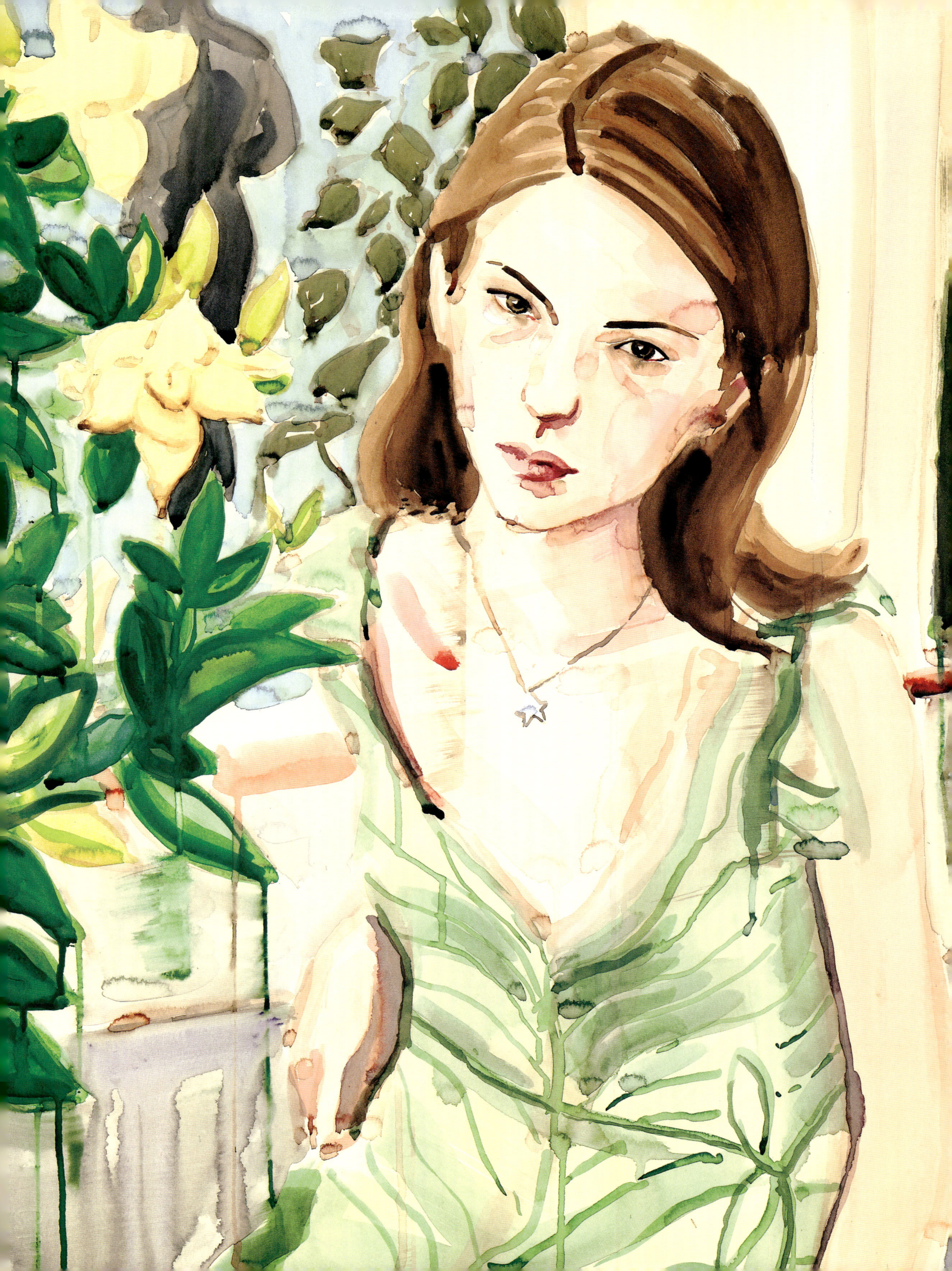

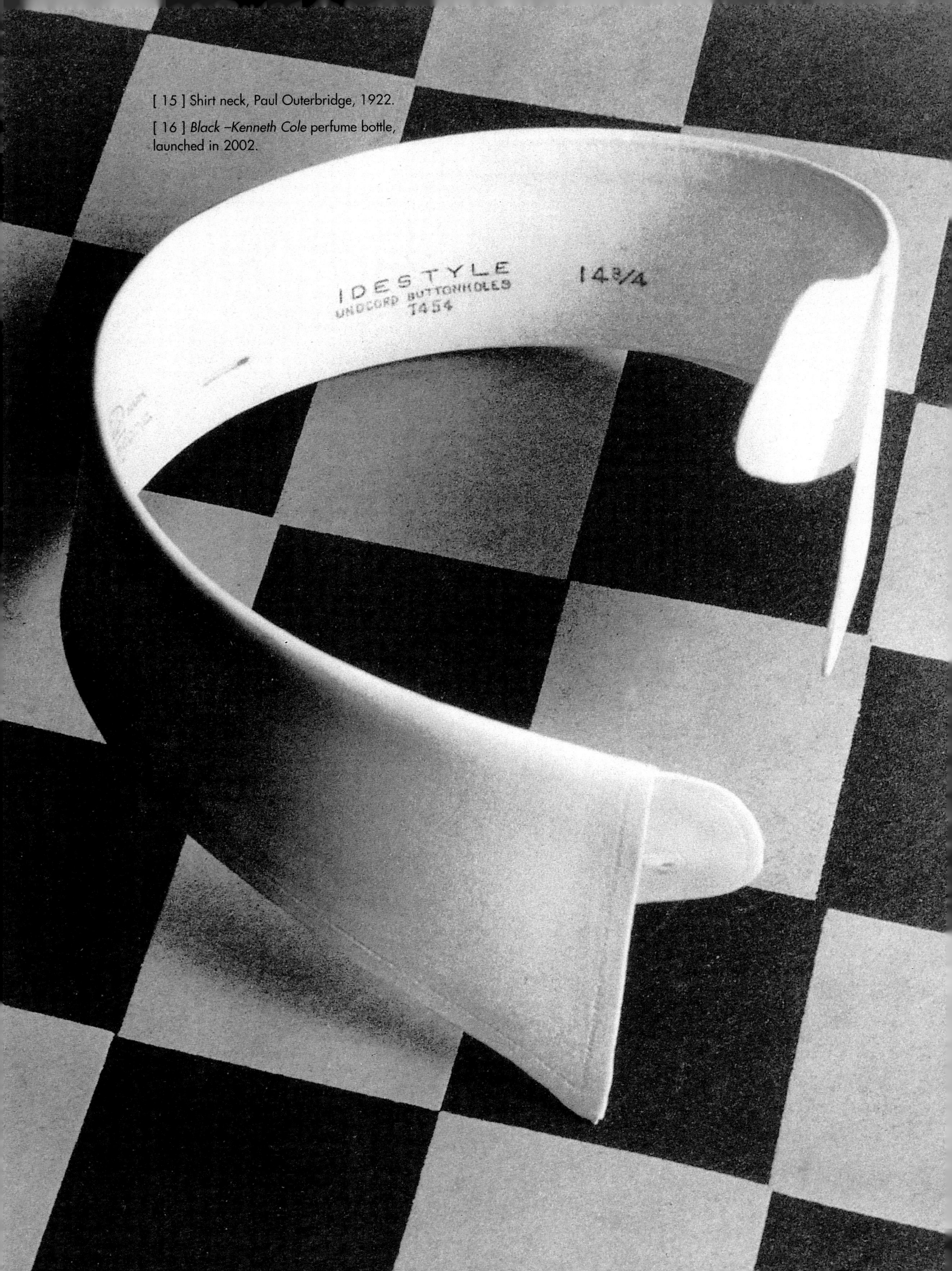

[15] Shirt neck, Paul Outerbridge, 1922.

[16] *Black –Kenneth Cole* perfume bottle, launched in 2002.

BLACK
—KENNETH COLE

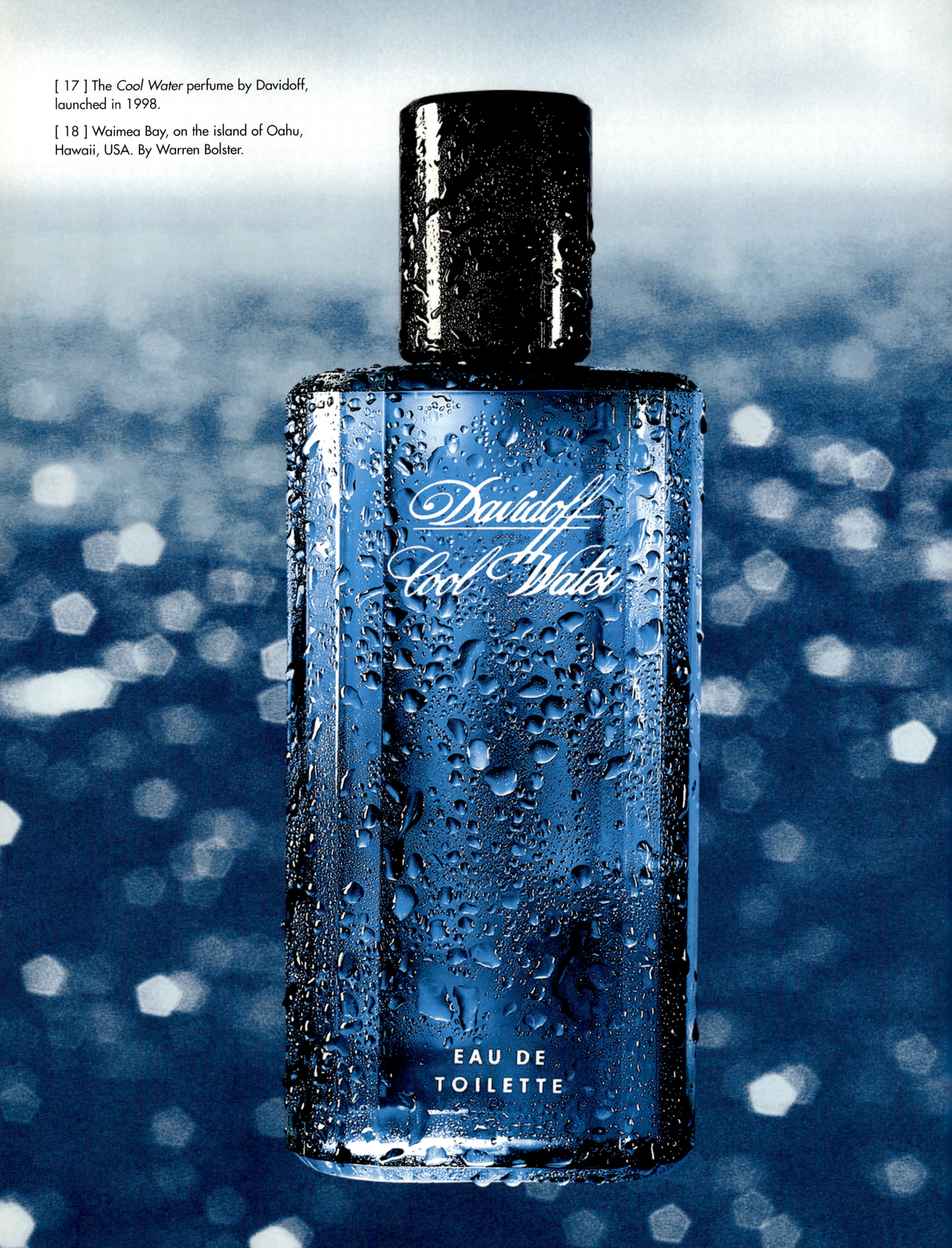

[17] The *Cool Water* perfume by Davidoff, launched in 1998.

[18] Waimea Bay, on the island of Oahu, Hawaii, USA. By Warren Bolster.

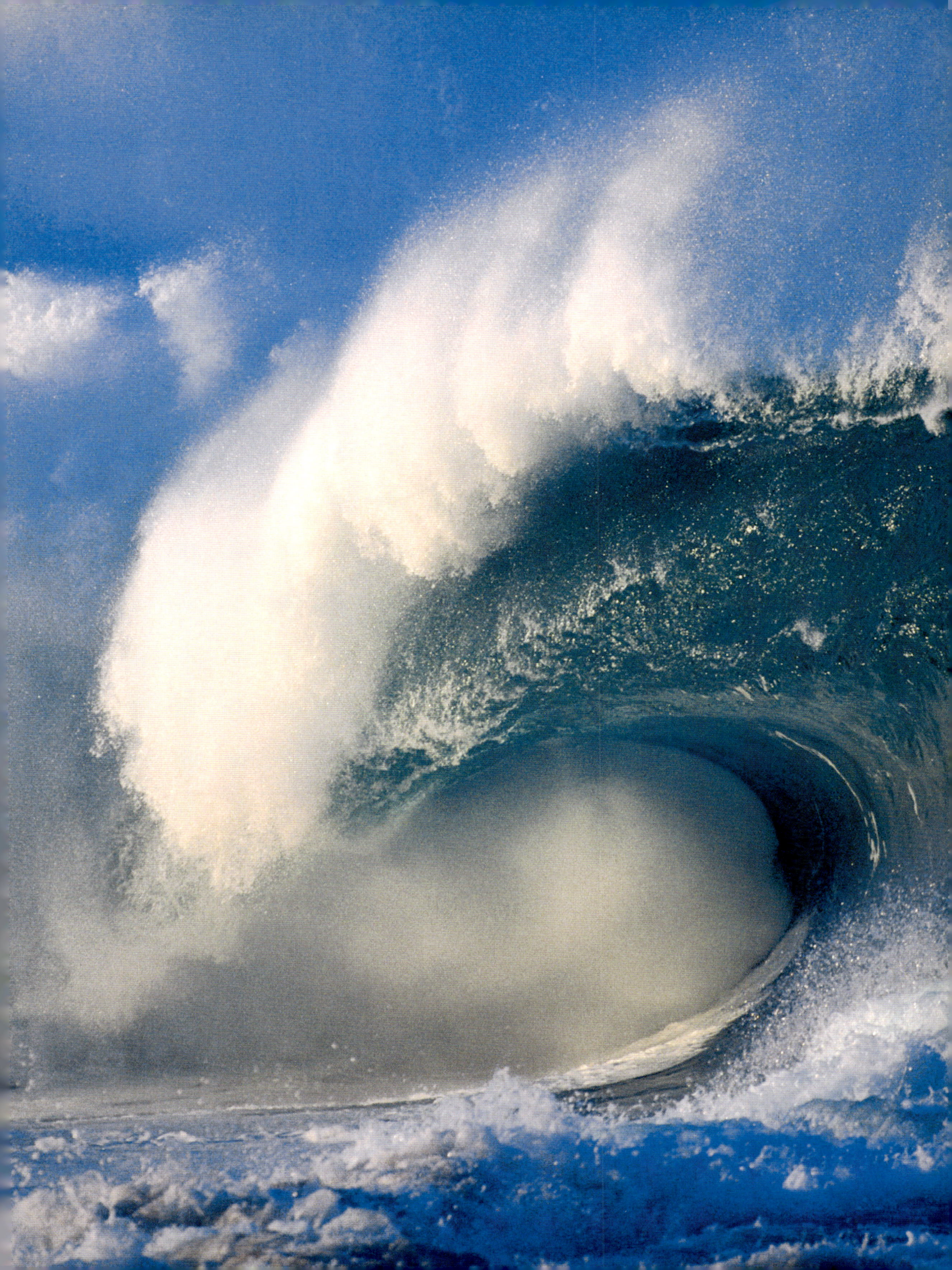

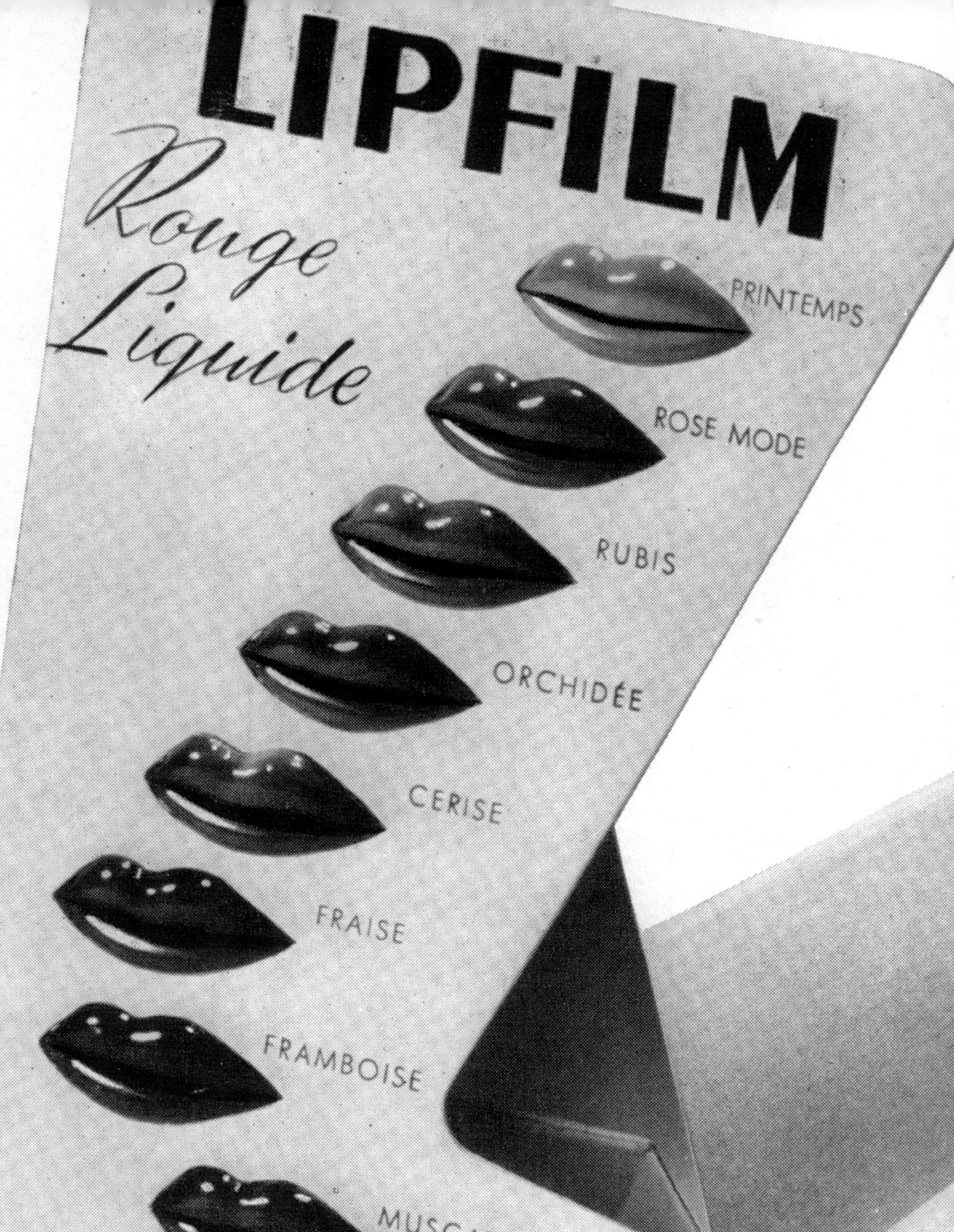

[19] Lancaster advertising from 1954 for lipsticks.

[20] Painting "Under High Voltage", Martial Raysse, 1965.

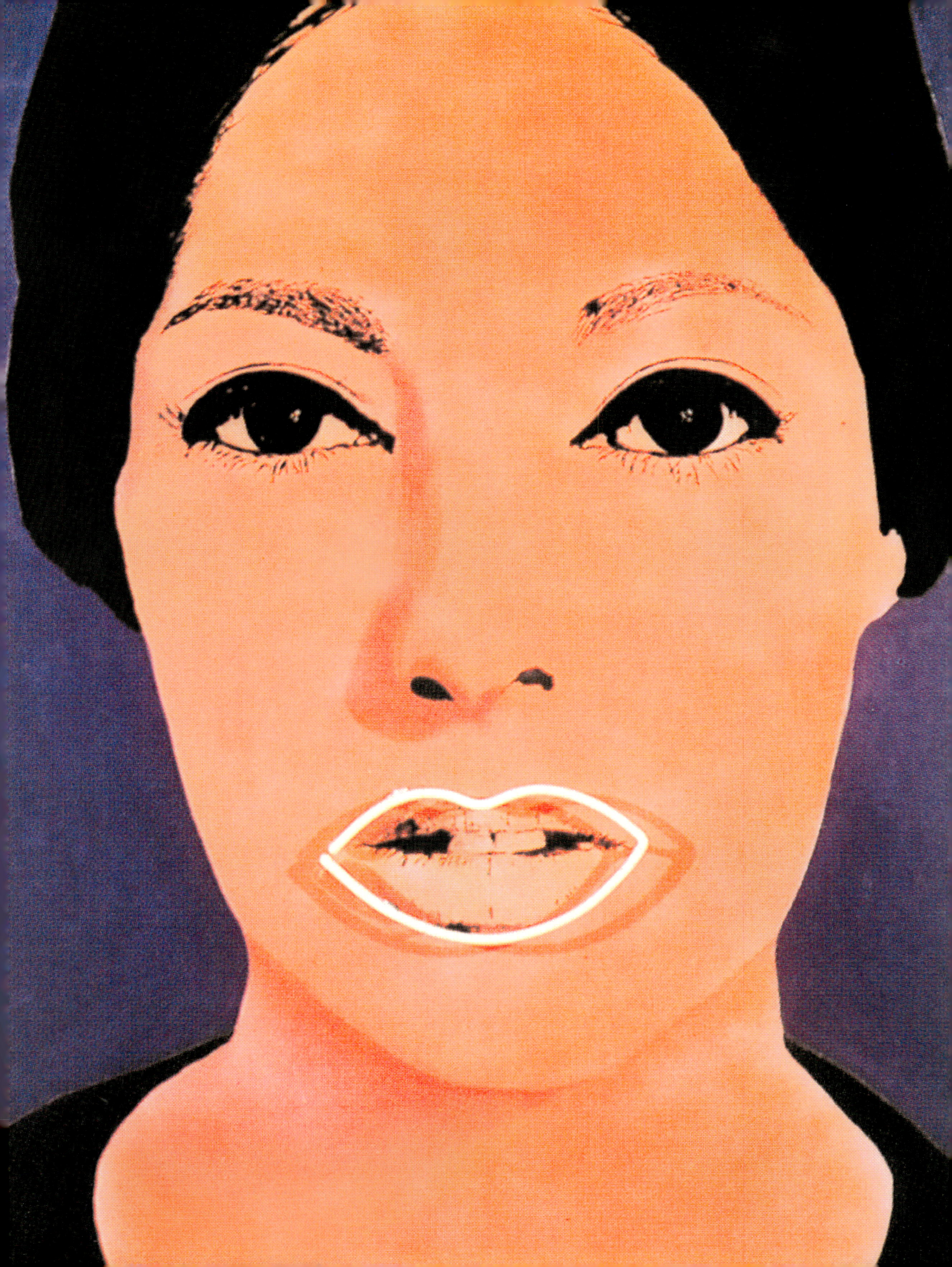

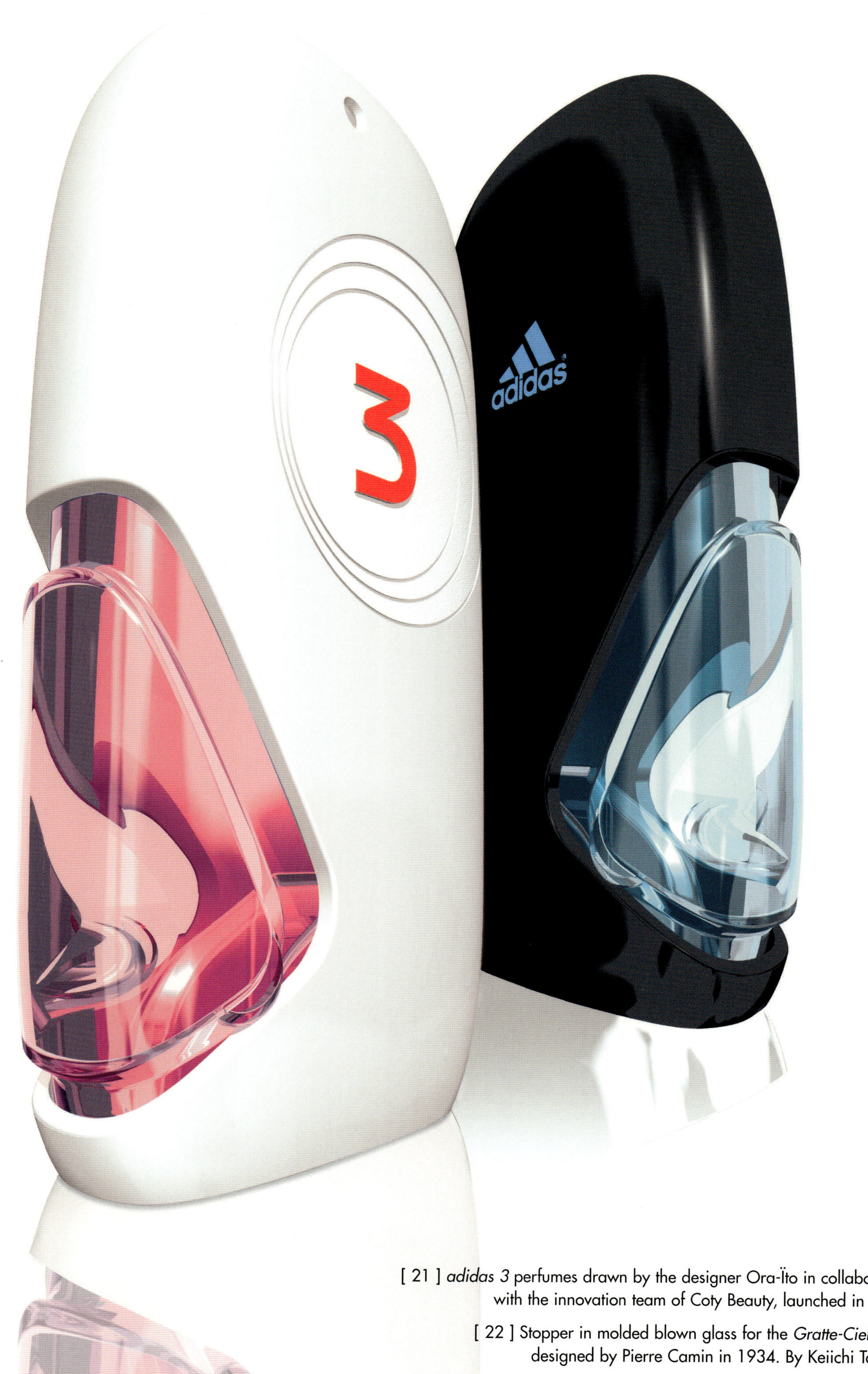

[21] *adidas 3* perfumes drawn by the designer Ora-Ïto in collaboration with the innovation team of Coty Beauty, launched in 2003.

[22] Stopper in molded blown glass for the *Gratte-Ciel* bottle designed by Pierre Camin in 1934. By Keiichi Tahara.

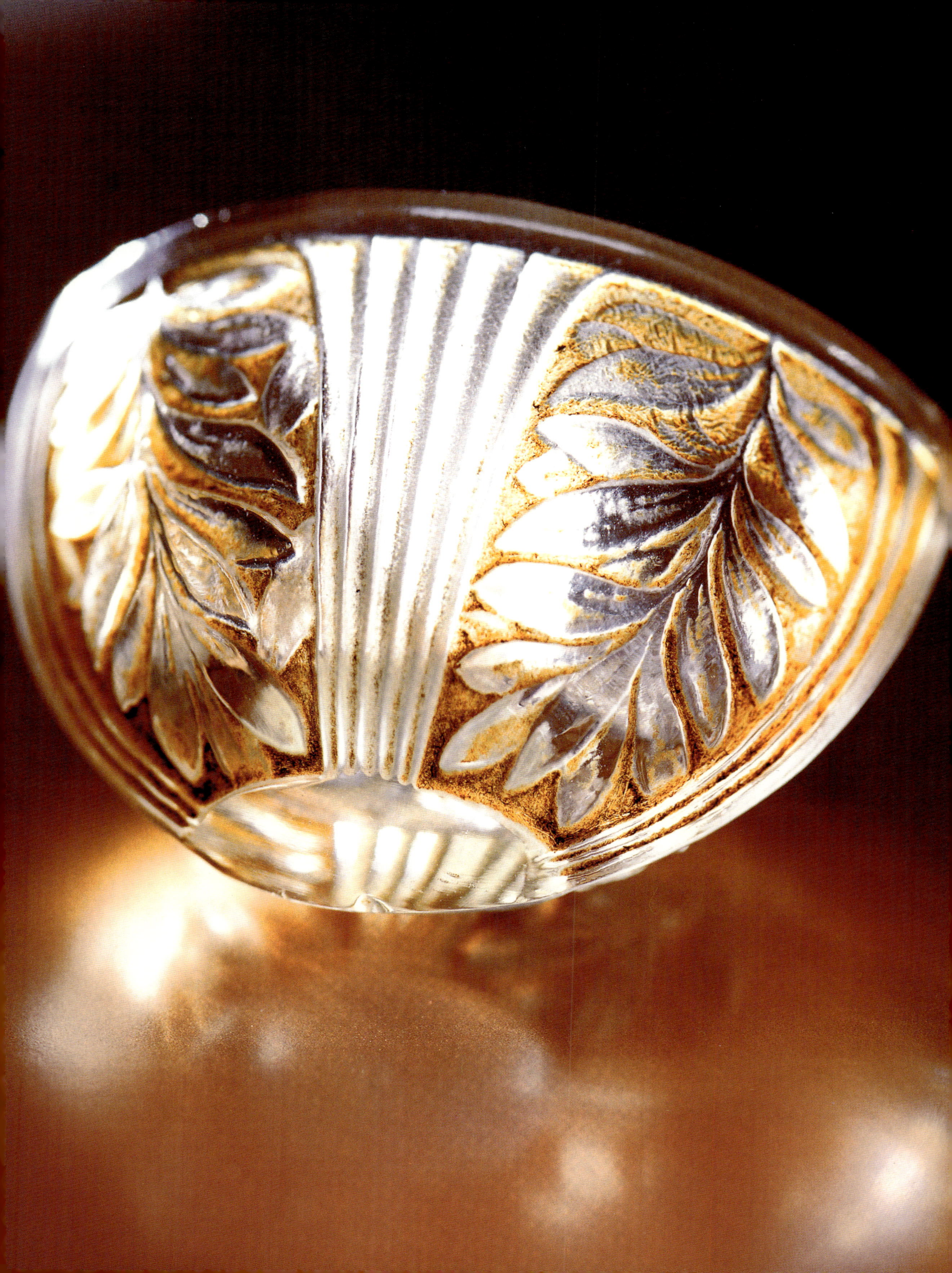

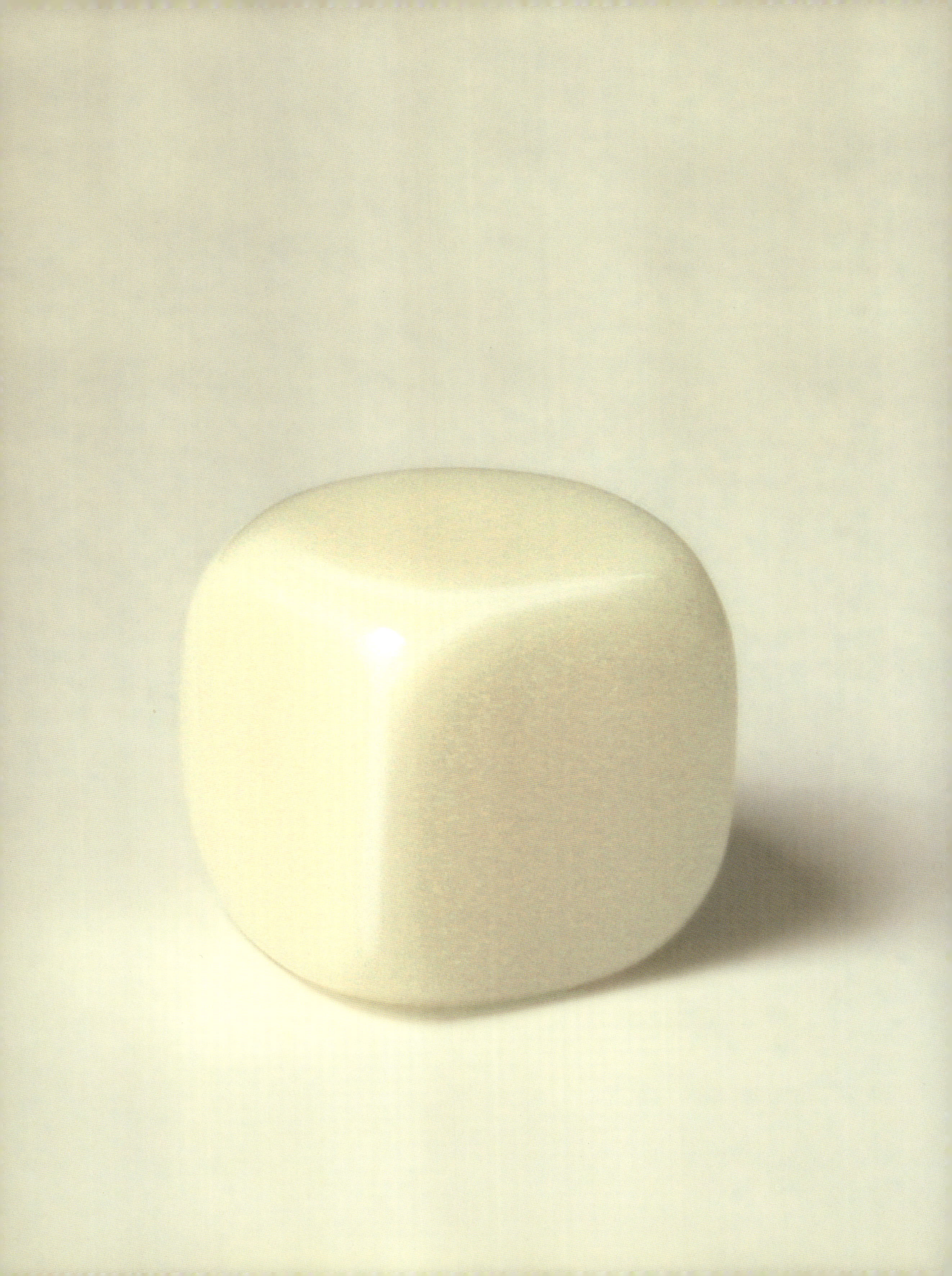

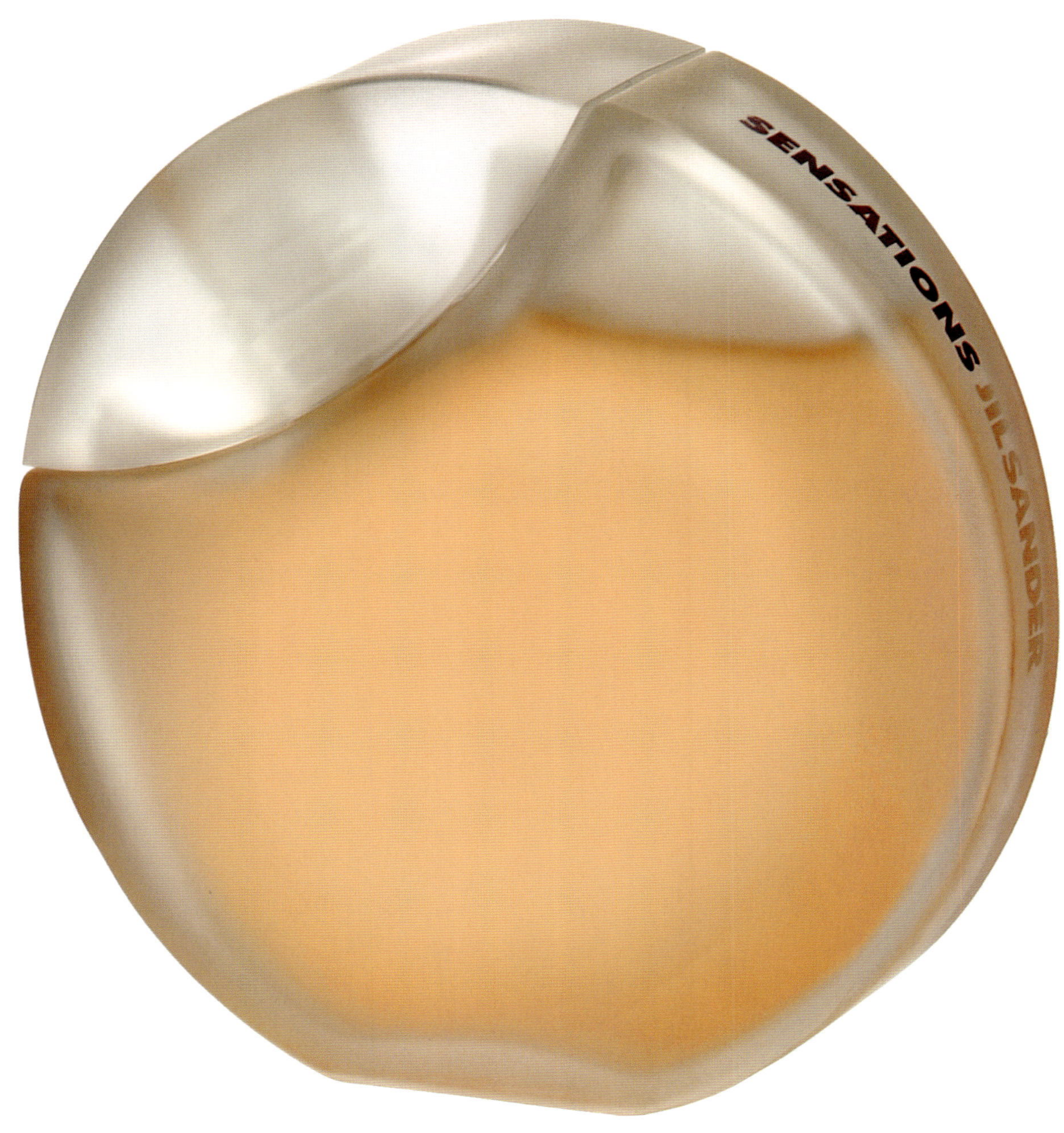

[23] *Blank dice,* Dove Allouche and Evariste Richer, unlimited edition, 2000.

[24] Bottle of *Sensations* perfume by Jil Sander, launched in 2000.

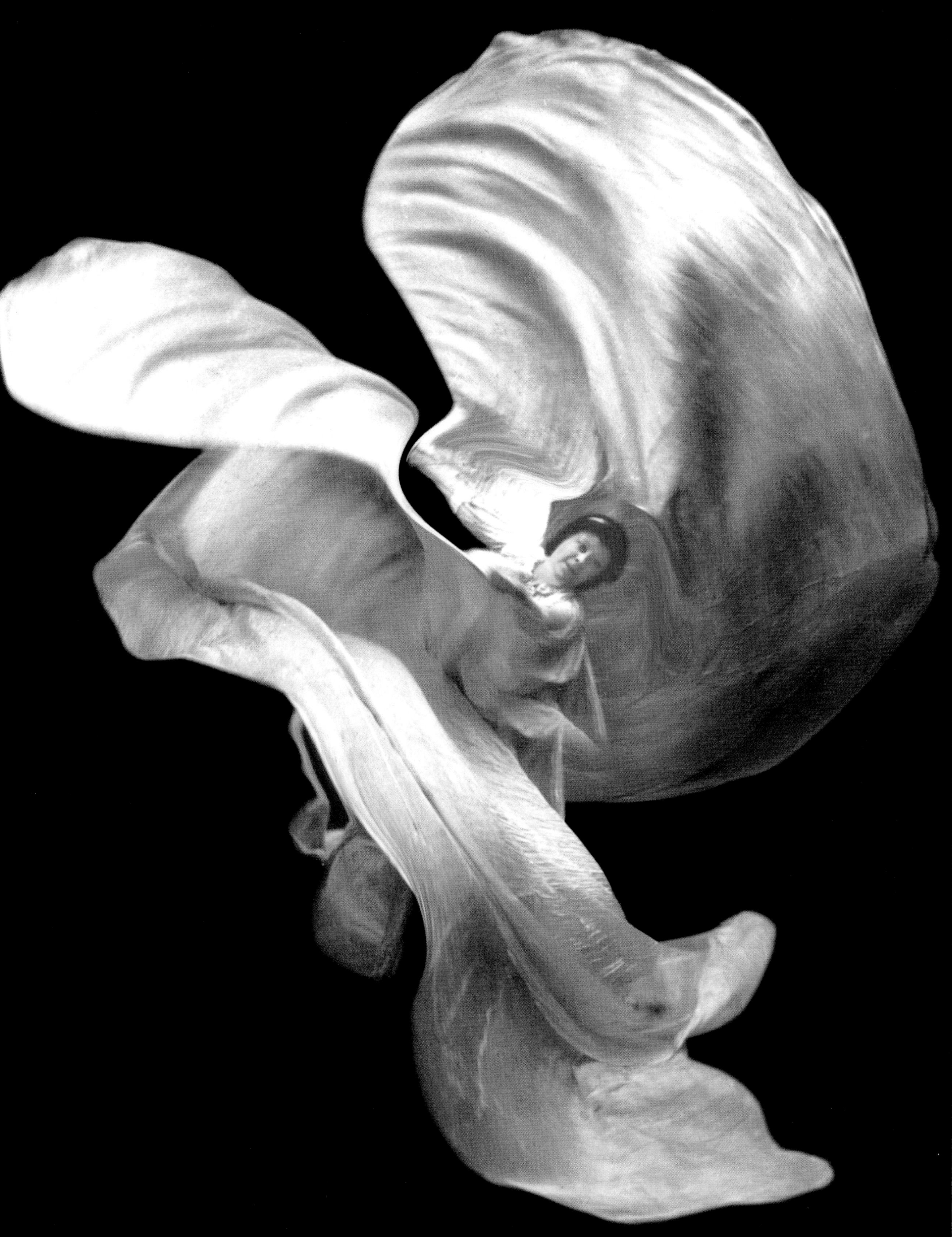

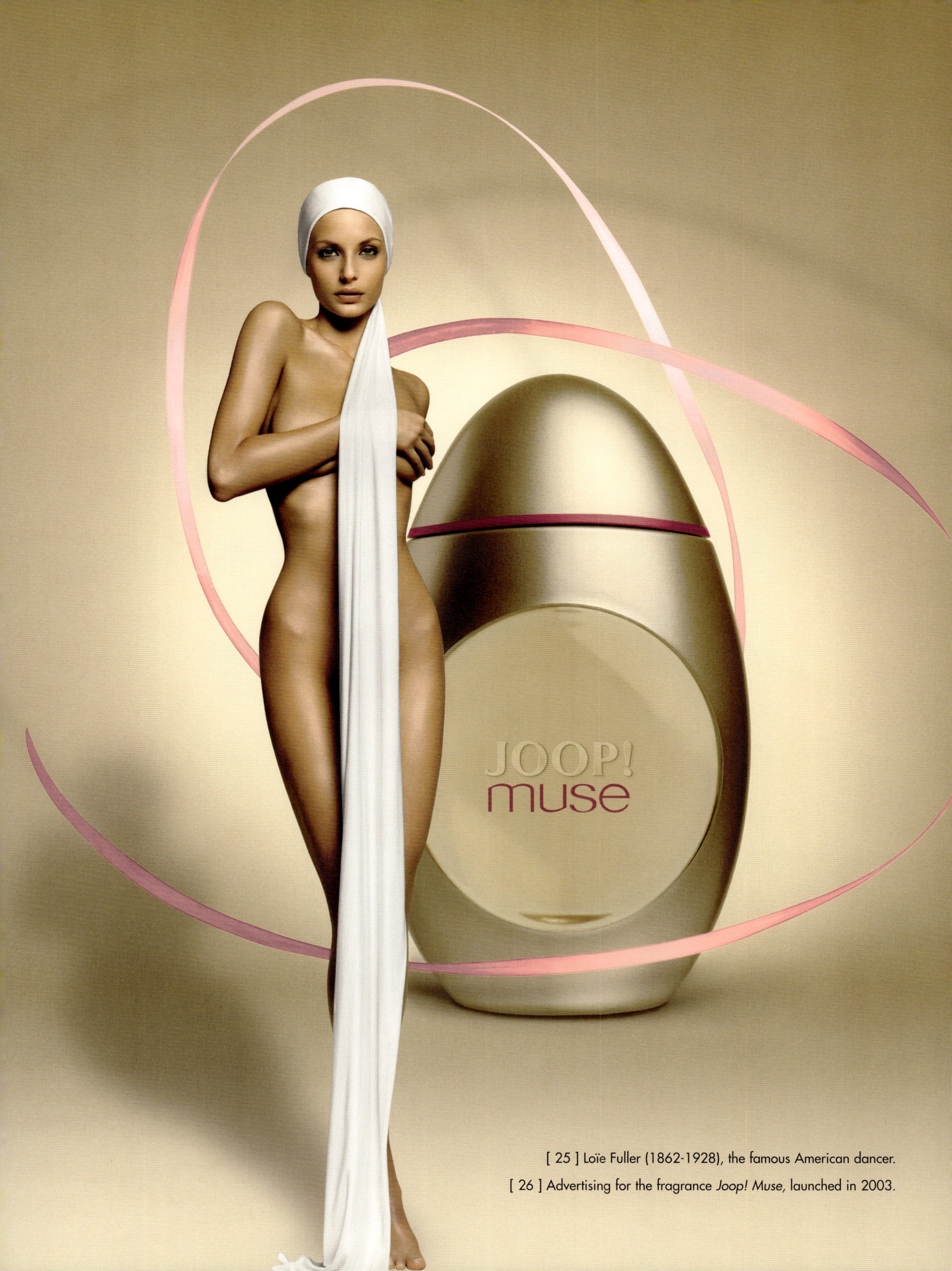

[25] Loïe Fuller (1862-1928), the famous American dancer.

[26] Advertising for the fragrance *Joop! Muse,* launched in 2003.

[27] Rimmel *Lasting Finish* lipsticks,
launched in 2003.

[28] The painter Brice Marden in his studio
by David Seidner, 1993.

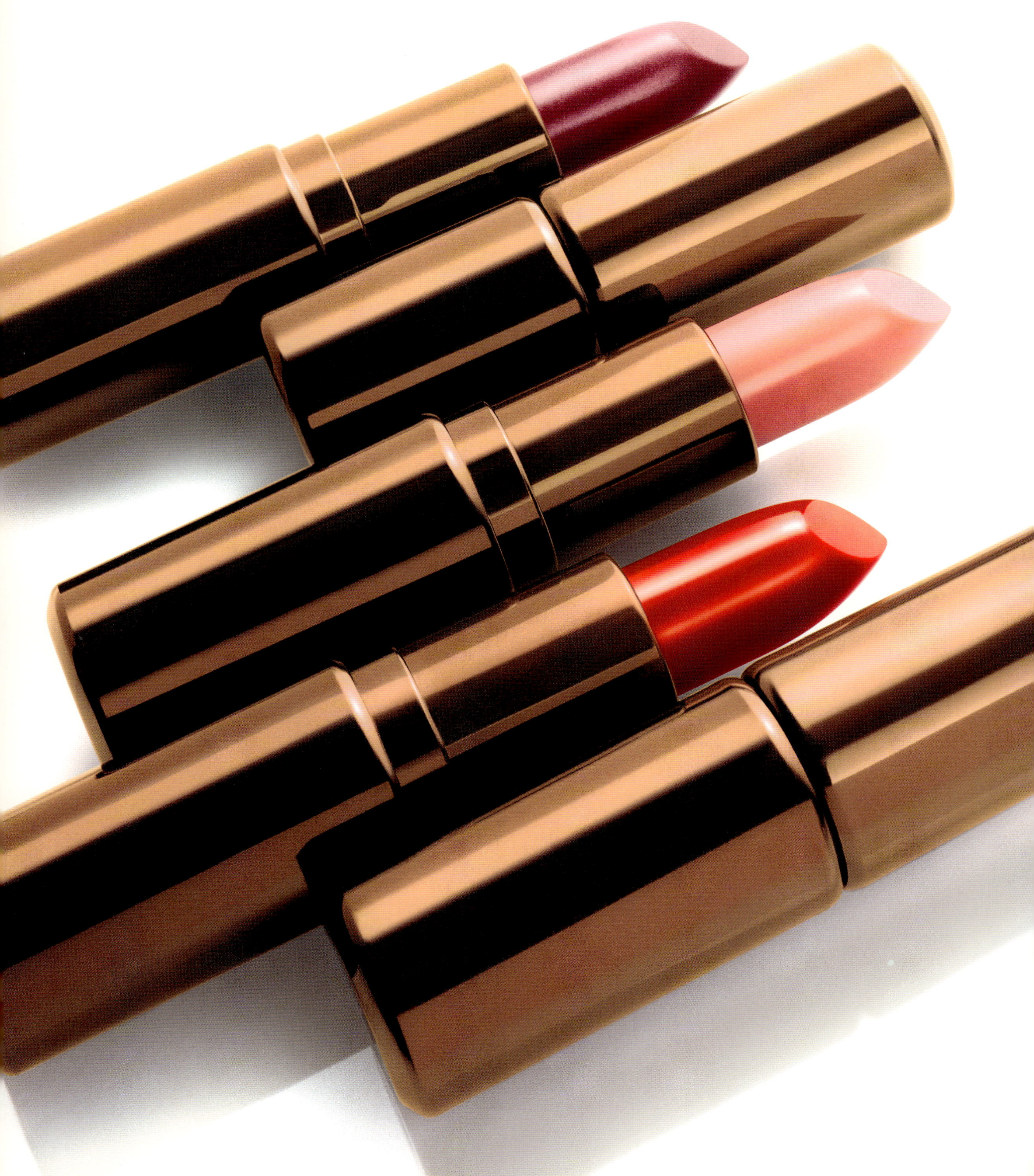

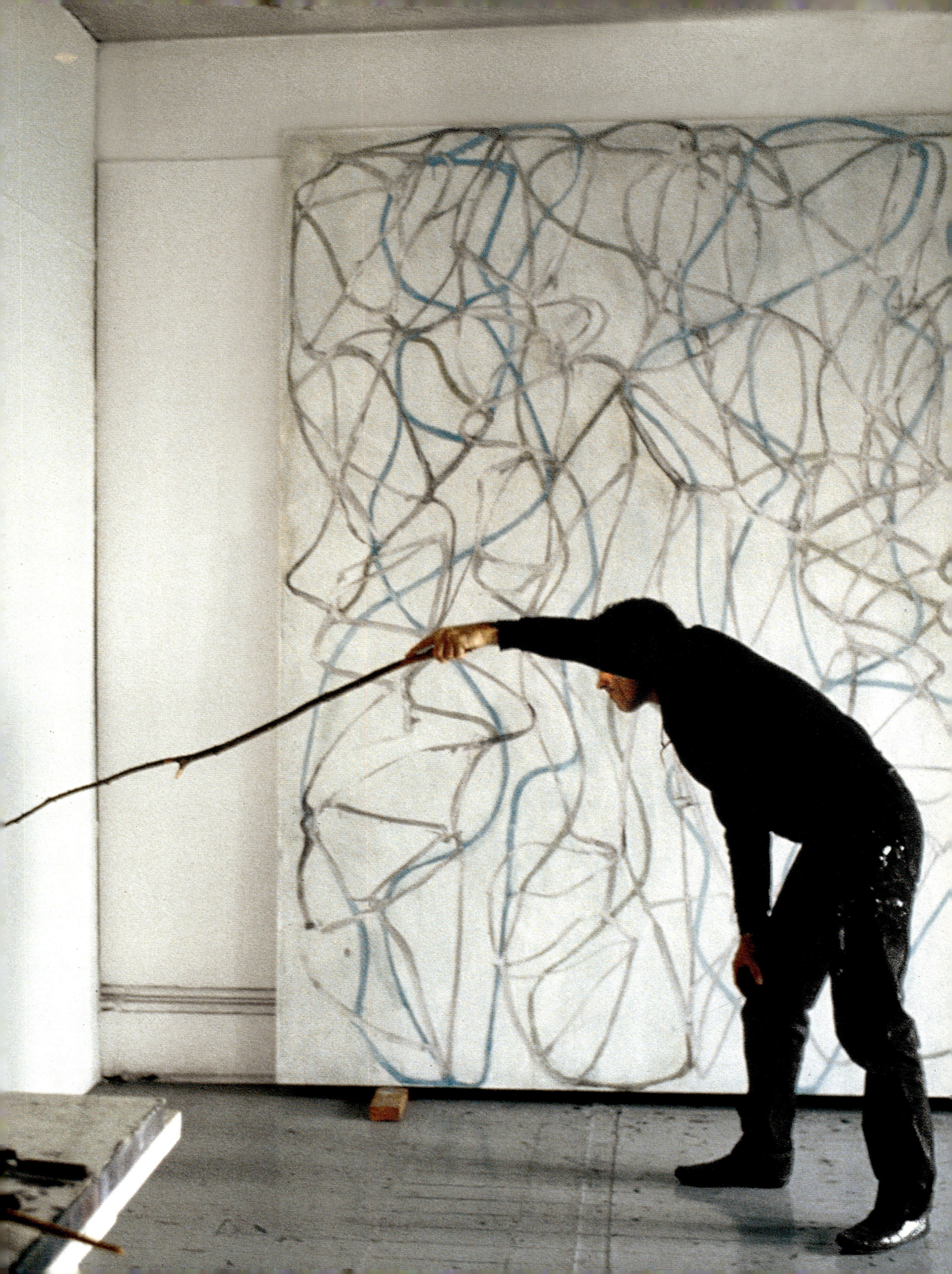

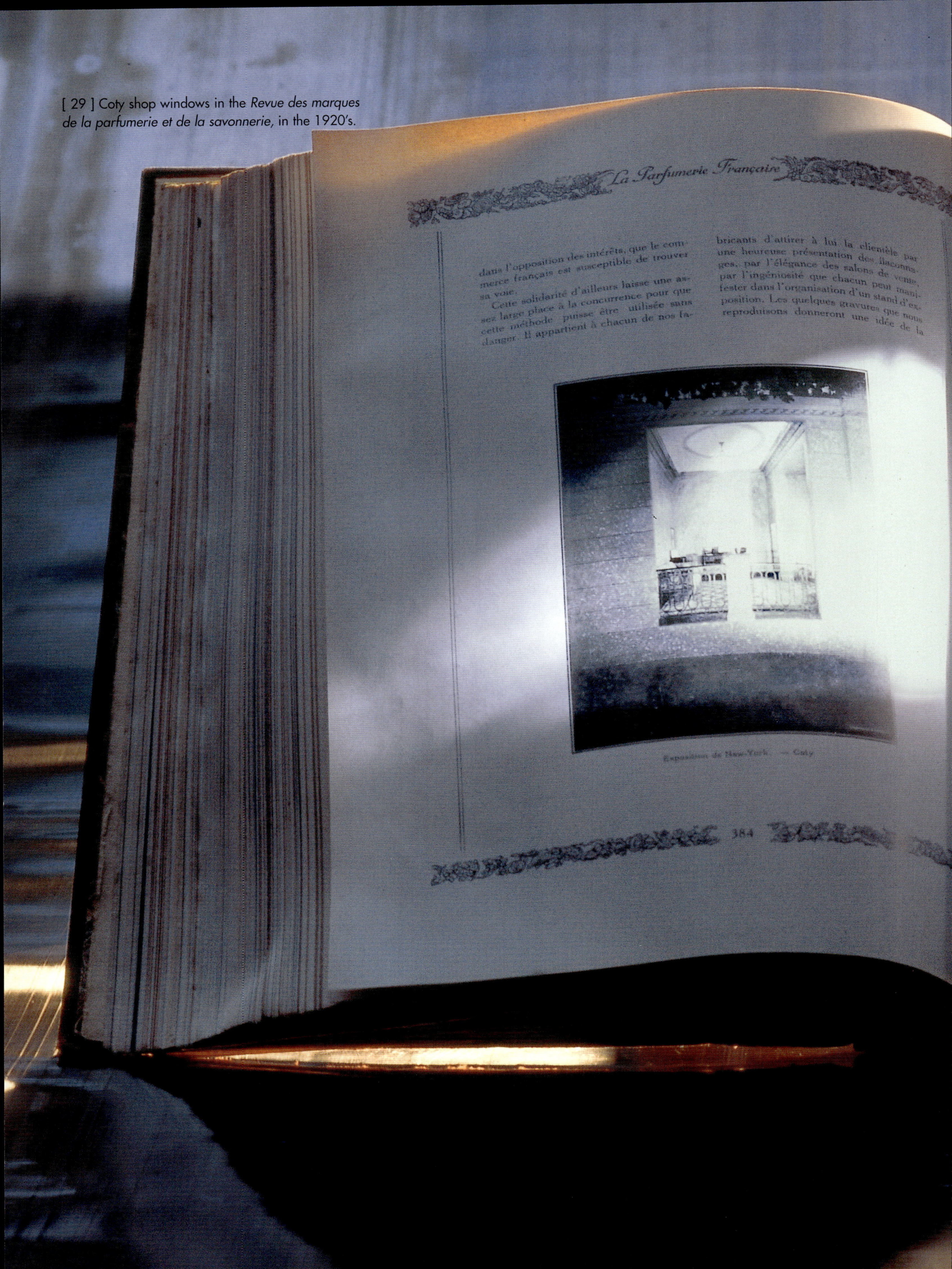

La Parfumerie Française

dans l'opposition des intérêts, que le commerce français est susceptible de trouver sa voie.

Cette solidarité d'ailleurs laisse une assez large place à la concurrence pour que cette méthode puisse être utilisée sans danger. Il appartient à chacun de nos fabricants d'attirer à lui la clientèle par une heureuse présentation des flaconnages, par l'élégance des salons de vente, par l'ingéniosité que chacun peut manifester dans l'organisation d'un stand d'exposition. Les quelques gravures que nous reproduisons donneront une idée de la

Exposition de New-York — Coty

384

[29] Coty shop windows in the *Revue des marques de la parfumerie et de la savonnerie*, in the 1920's.

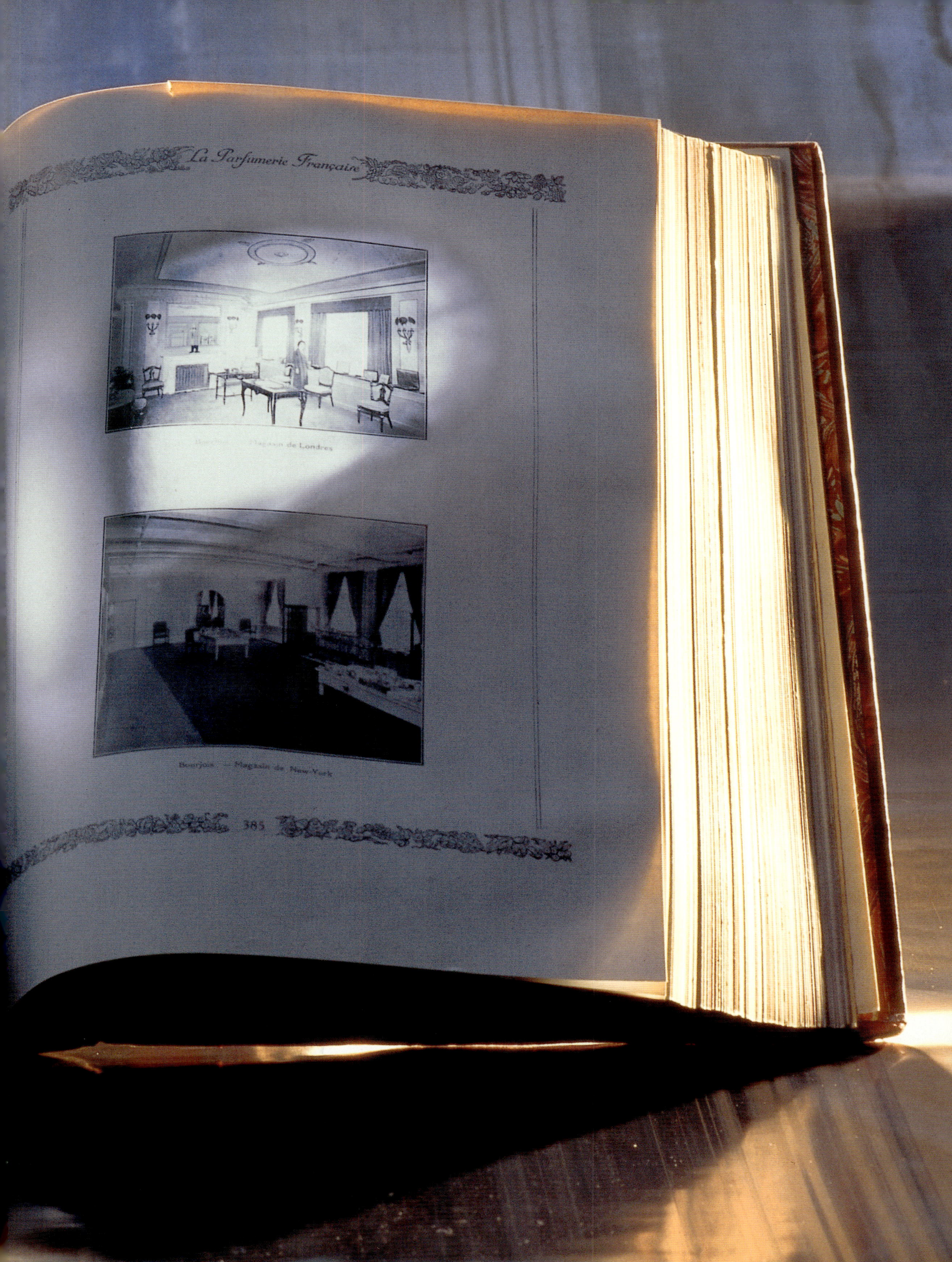
La Parfumerie Française
de Londres
Bourjois — Magasin de New-York
385

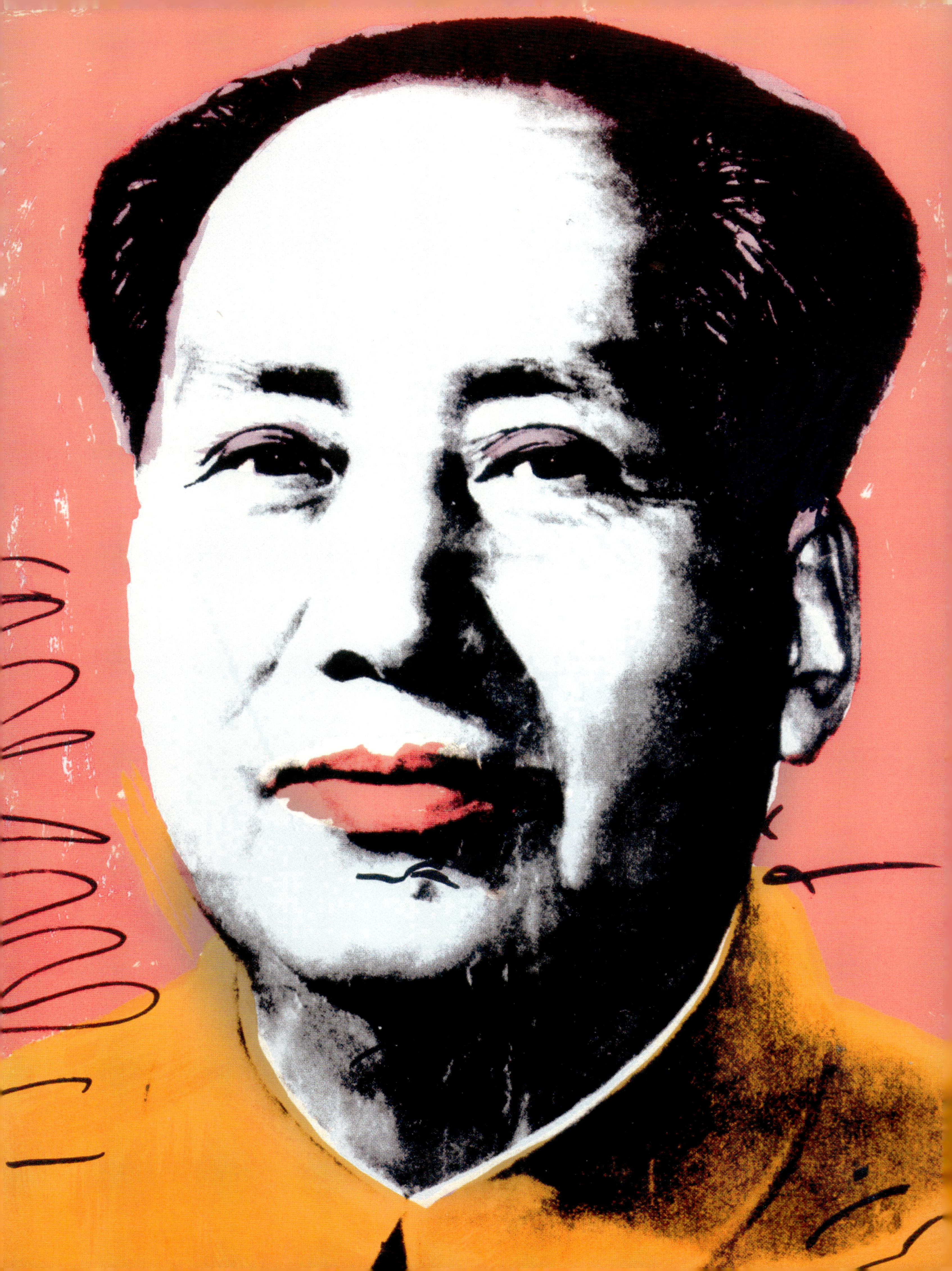

[30] Portrait of Mao-Tse-Tung by Andy Warhol, 1972.

[31] *Rouge Grace* lipstick by Lancaster, launched in 2003.

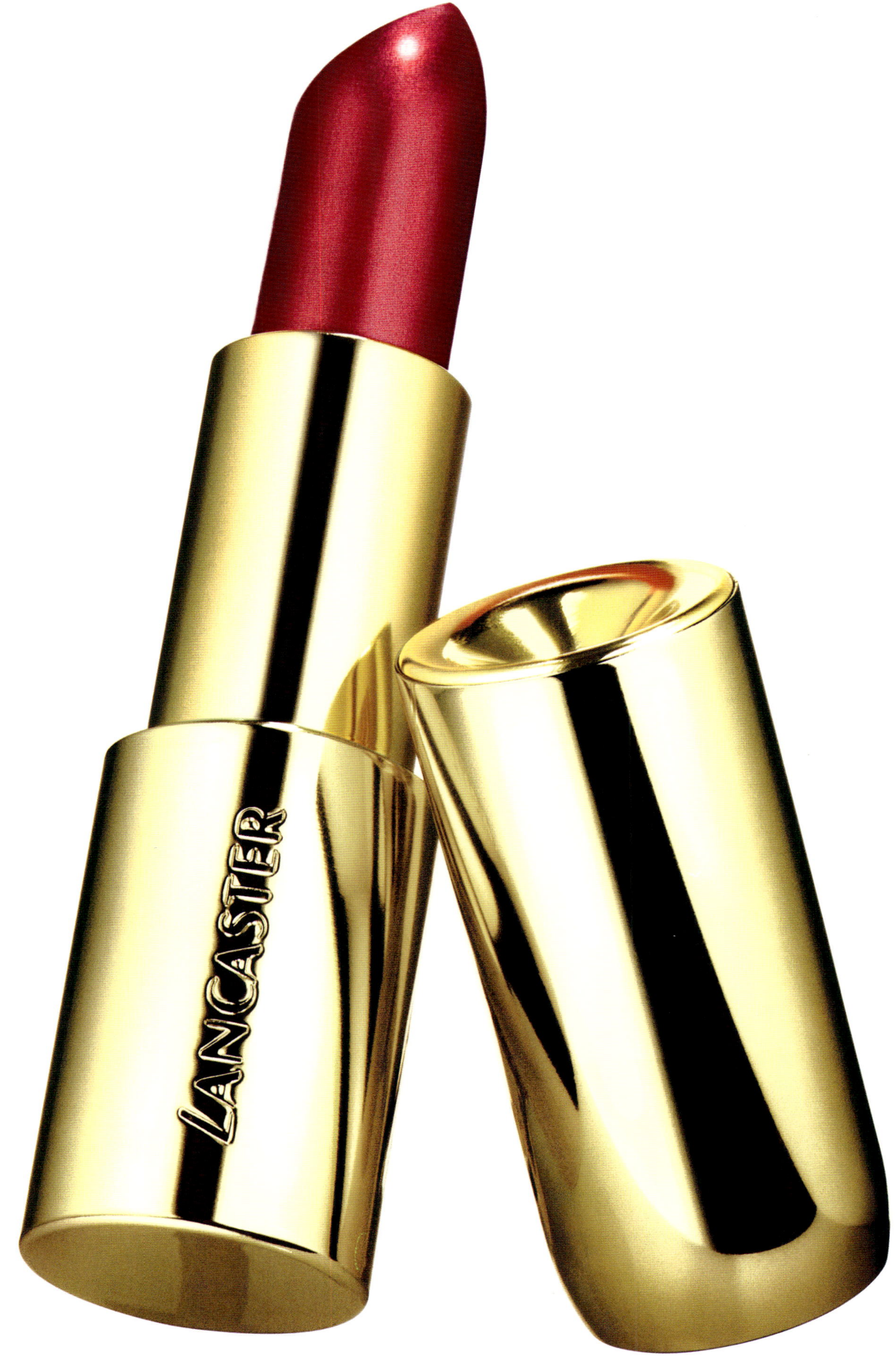

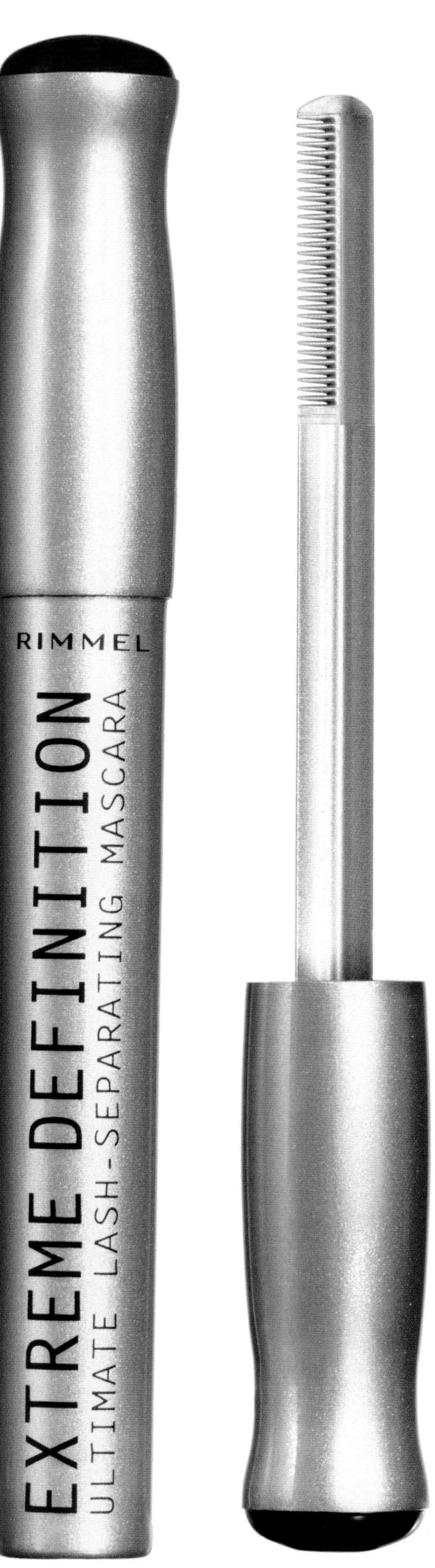

[32] Rimmel *Extreme Definition* mascara launched in 2003.

[33] The Diver Kathy Flicker, 1962.

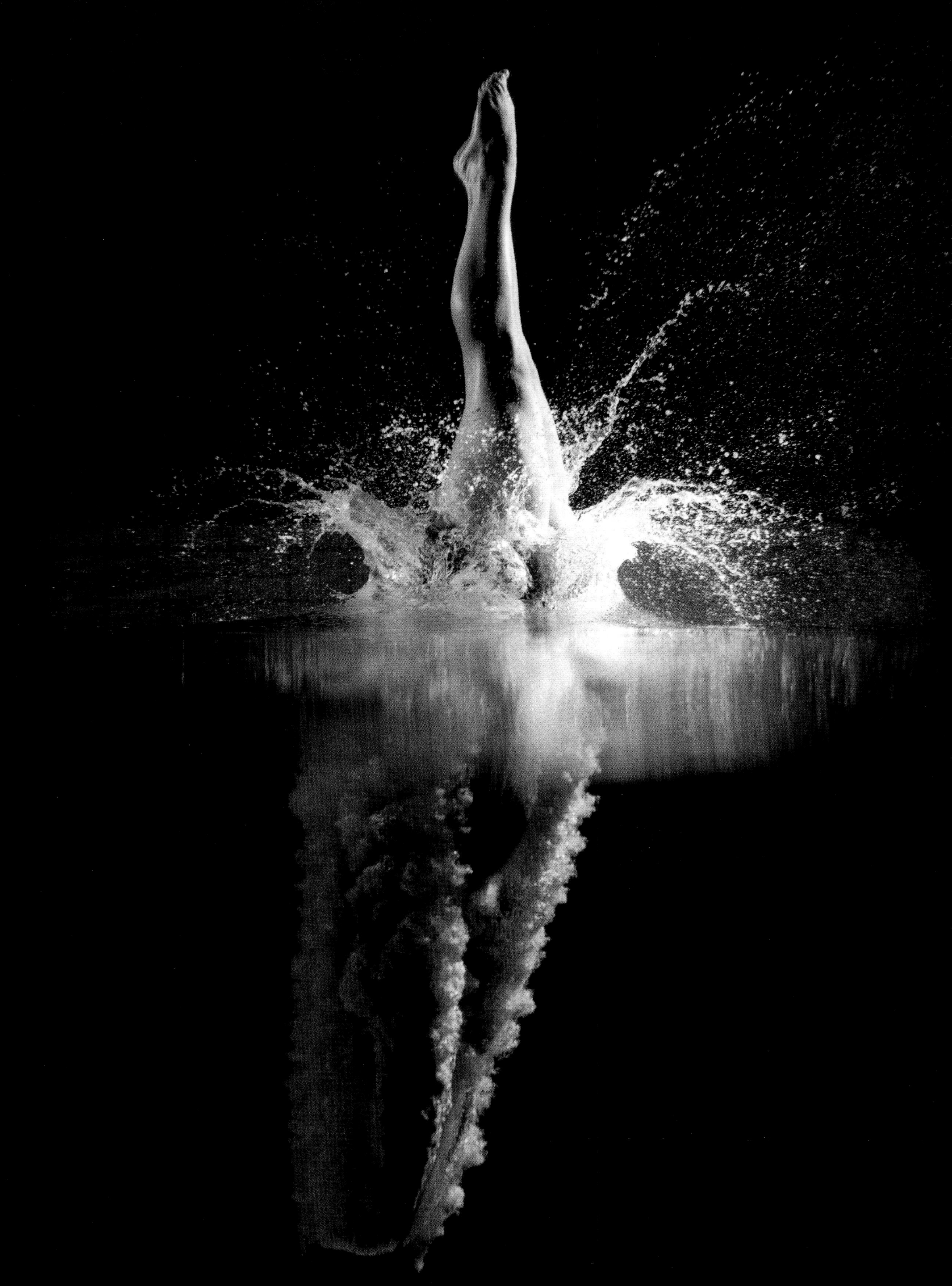

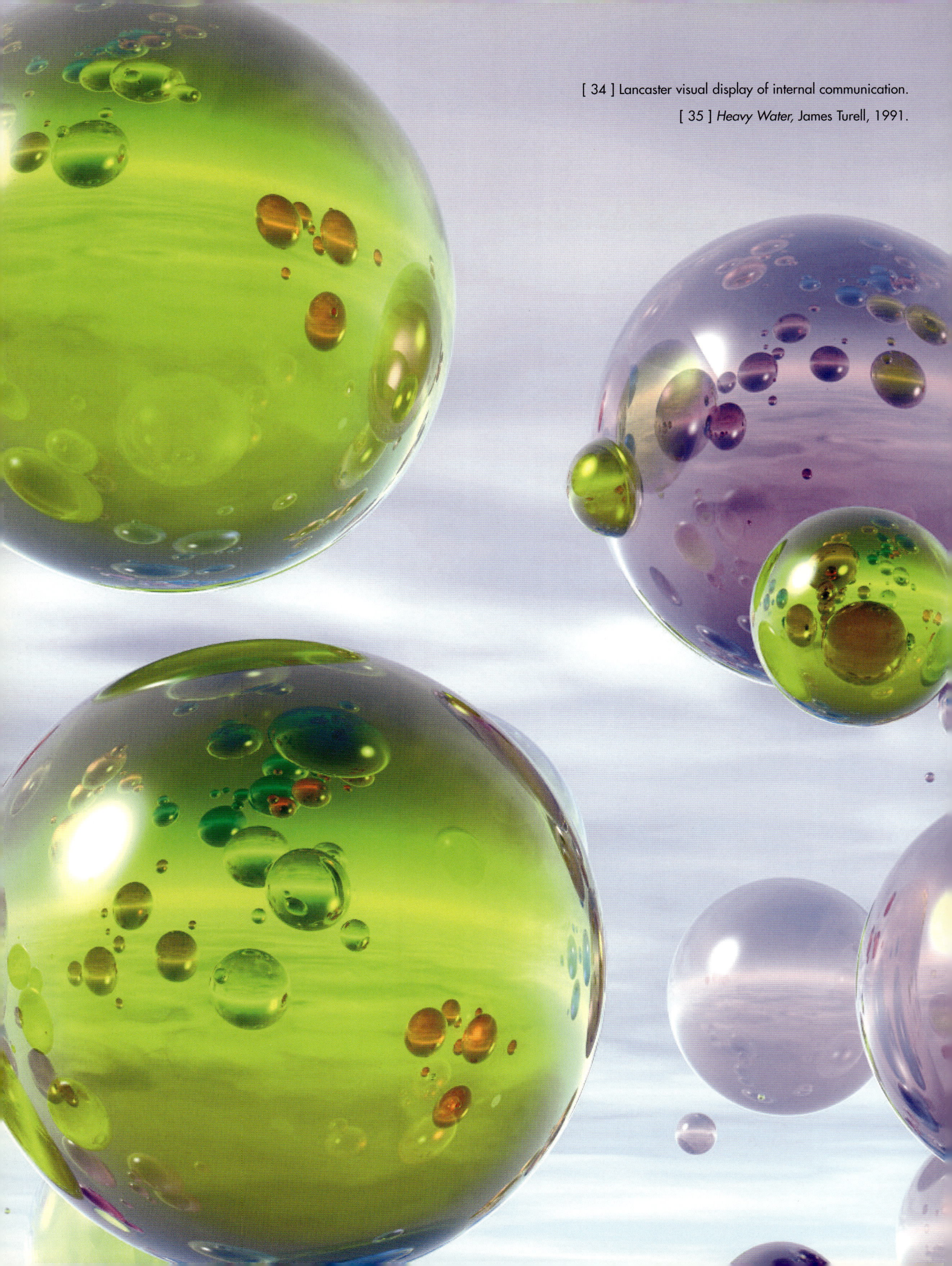

[34] Lancaster visual display of internal communication.

[35] *Heavy Water,* James Turell, 1991.

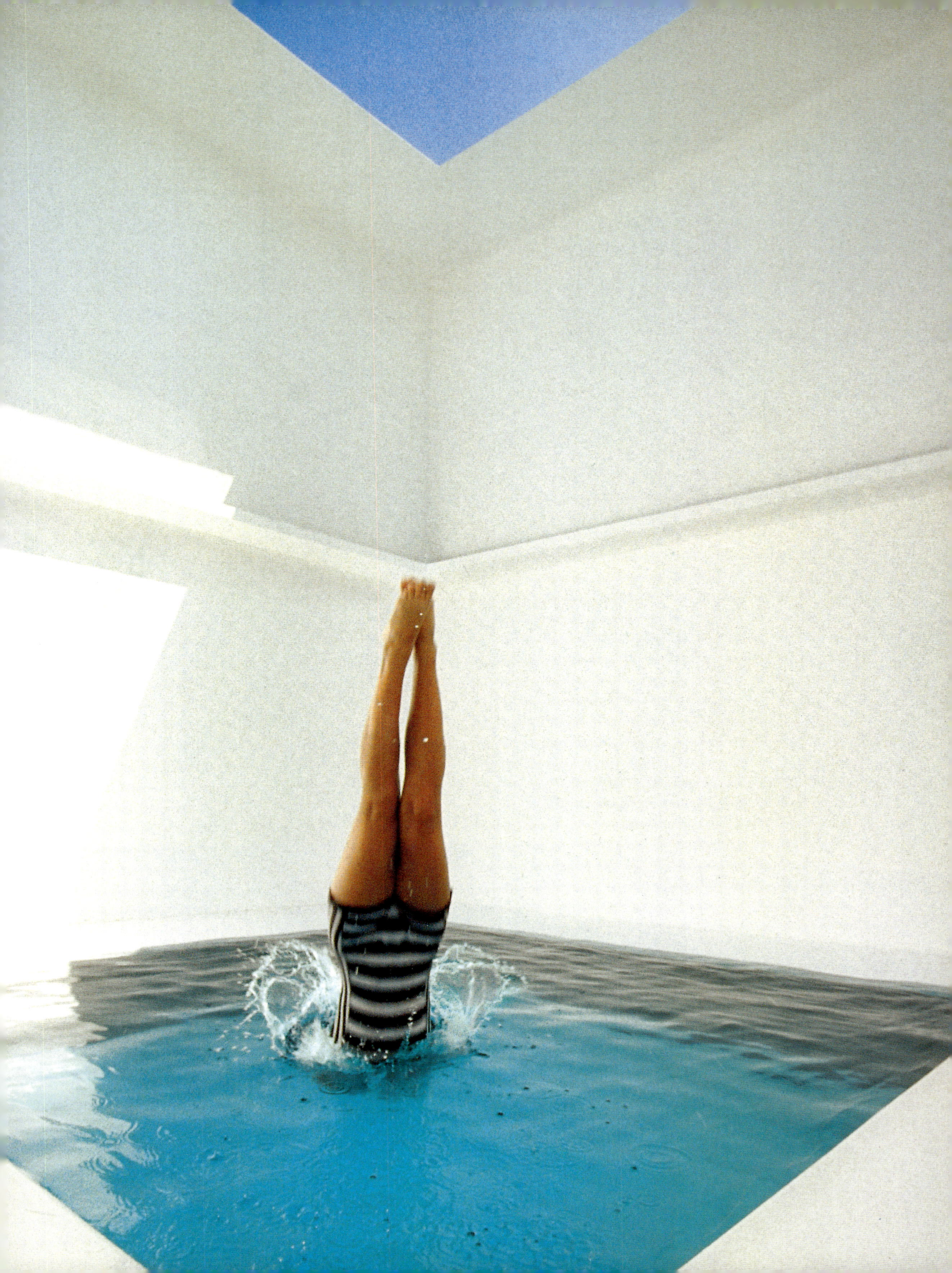

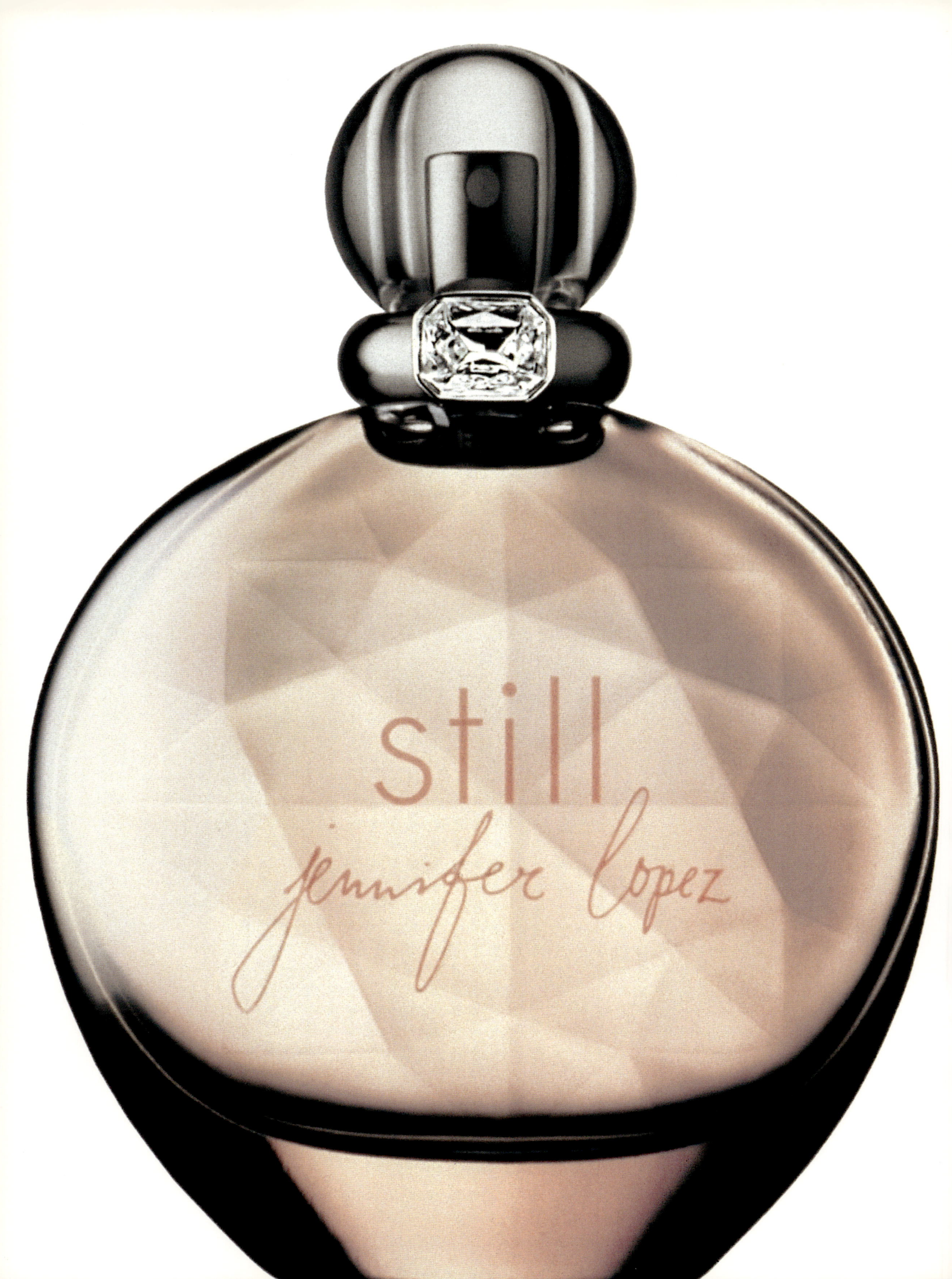
still
jennifer lopez

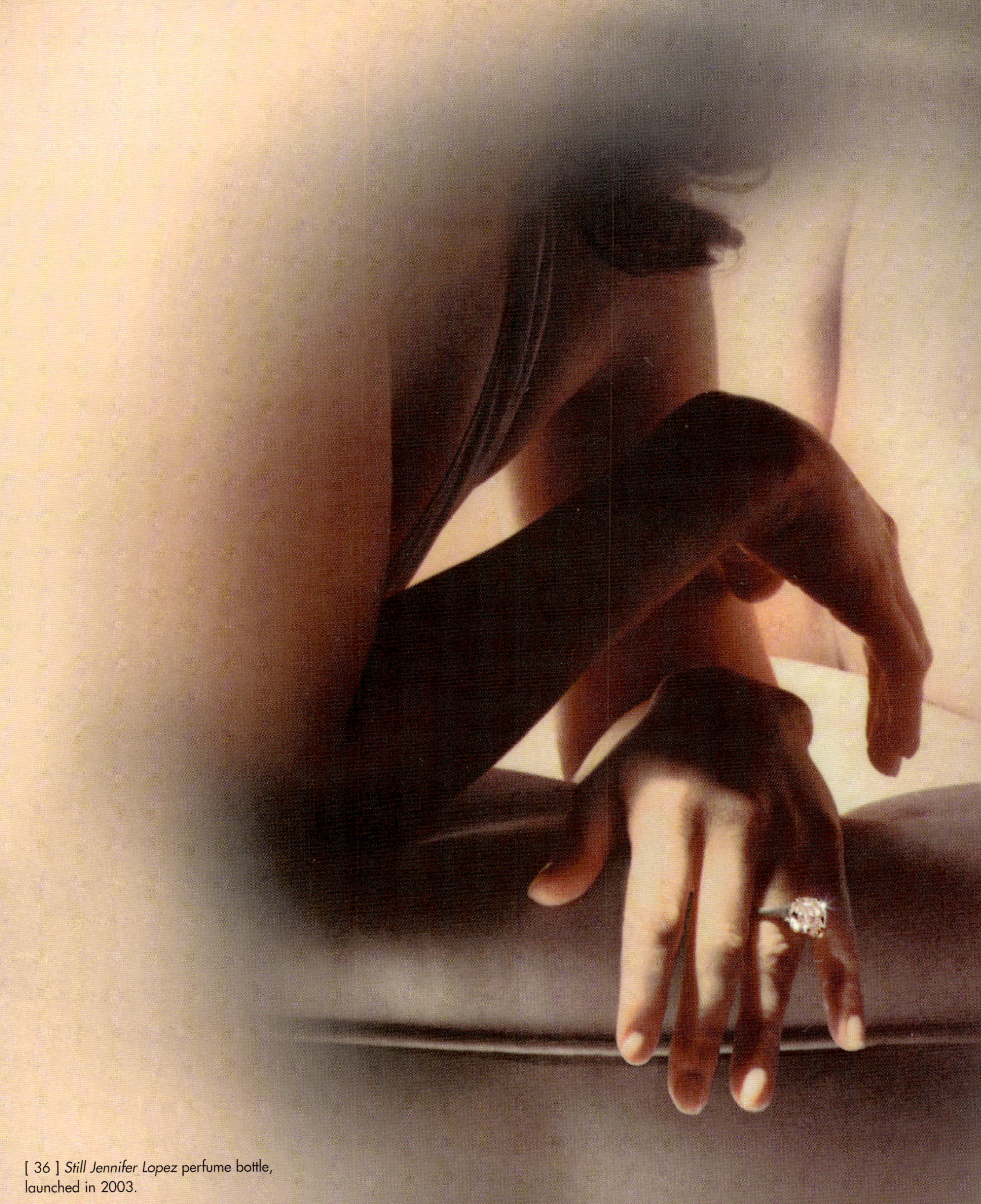

[36] *Still Jennifer Lopez* perfume bottle, launched in 2003.

[37] Portrait of the hands of Jennifer Lopez, by Nick Knight, 2003.

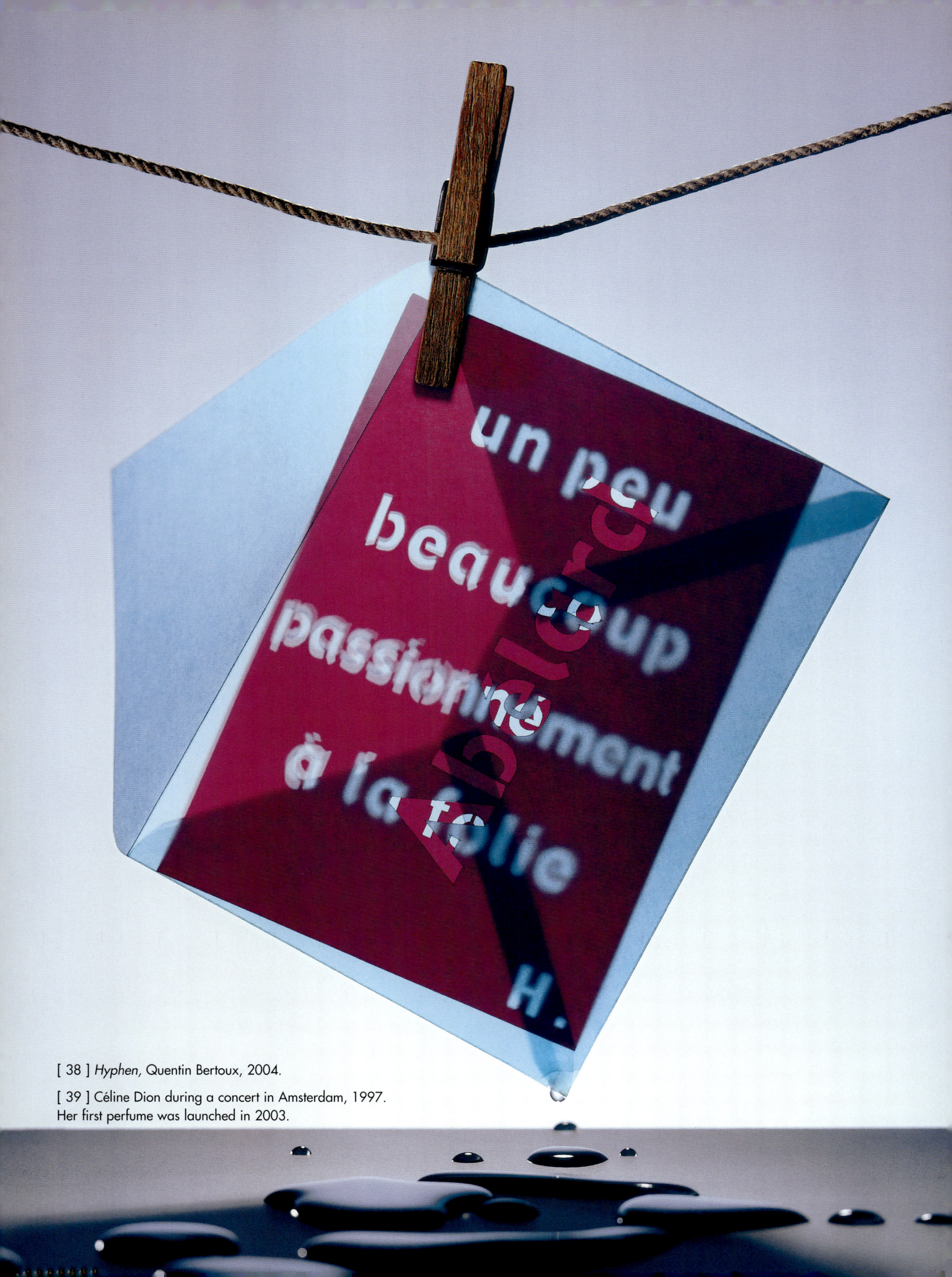

[38] *Hyphen,* Quentin Bertoux, 2004.

[39] Céline Dion during a concert in Amsterdam, 1997. Her first perfume was launched in 2003.

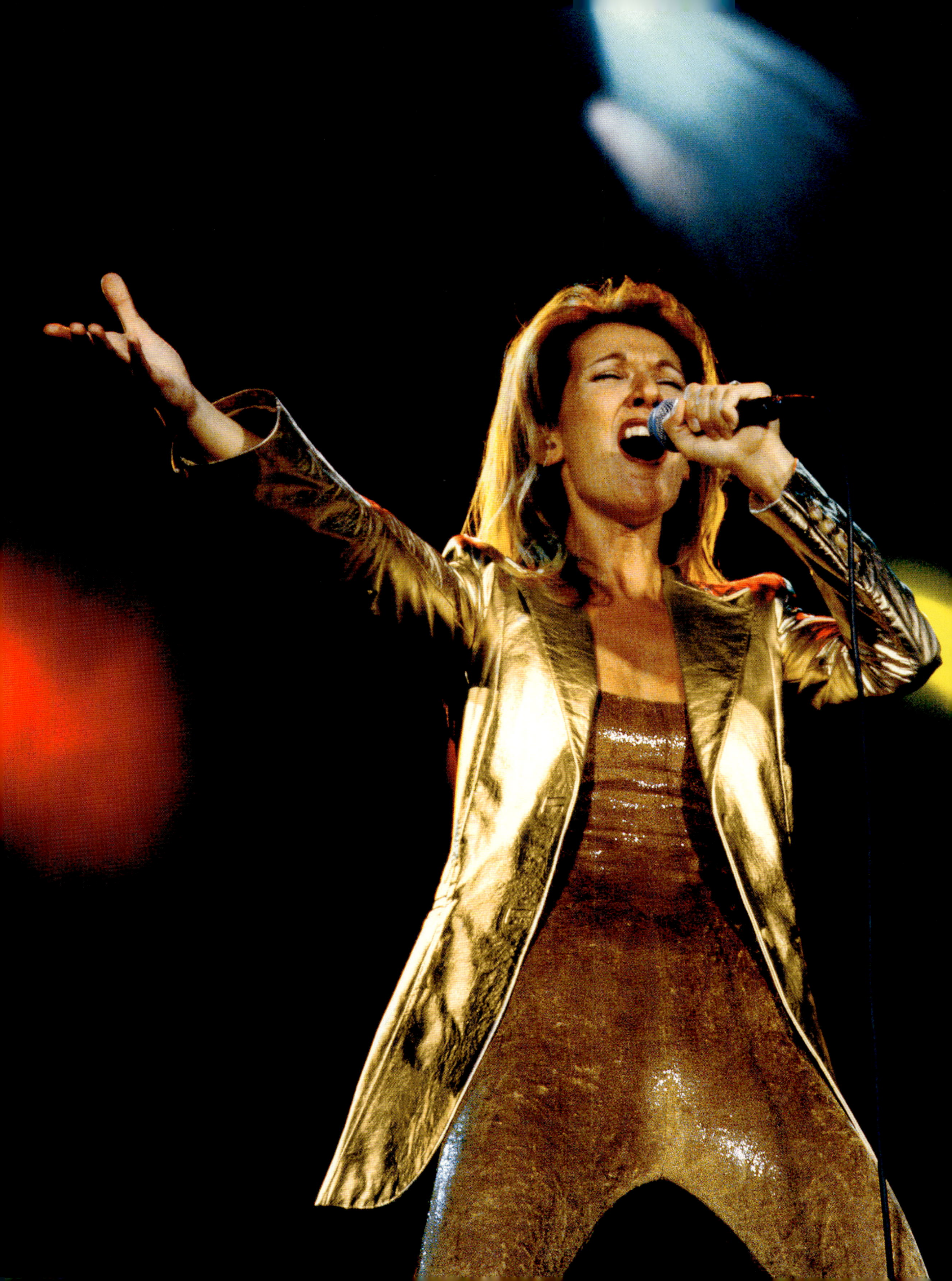

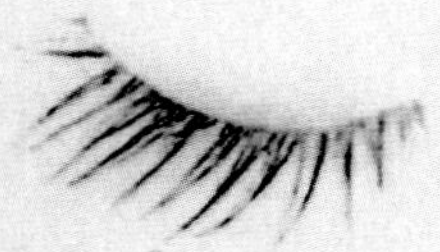

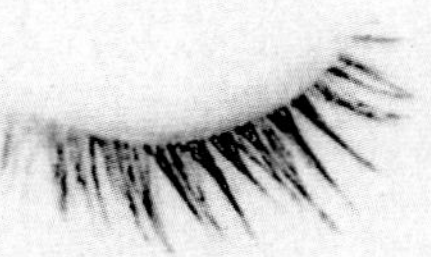

[40] Closed eyelids, Erwin Blumenfeld, 1935.

[41] Kate Moss for Rimmel, of which she has been the face since 2001. Advertising for the *Endless Length & Lift* mascara, launched in 2002.

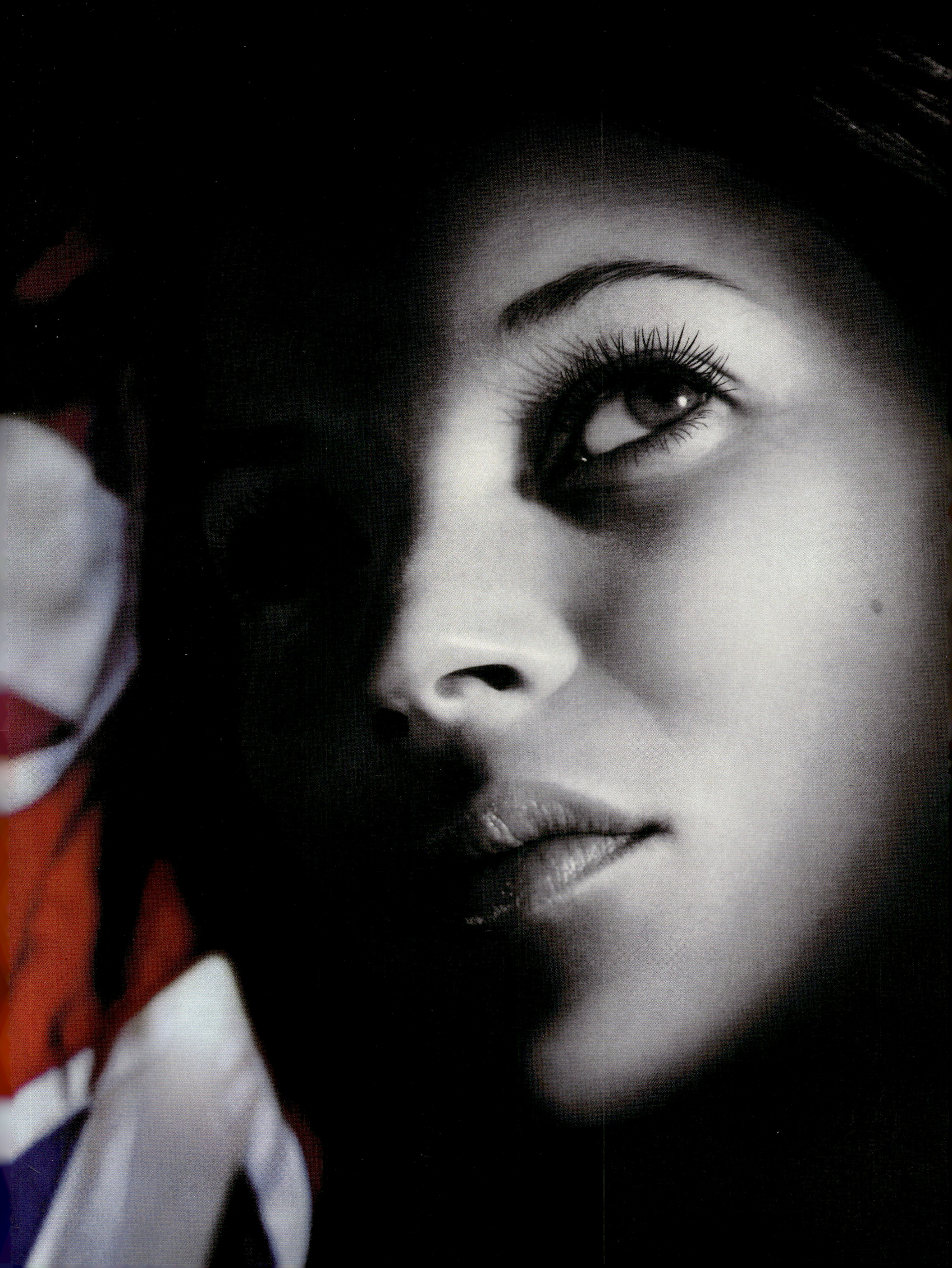

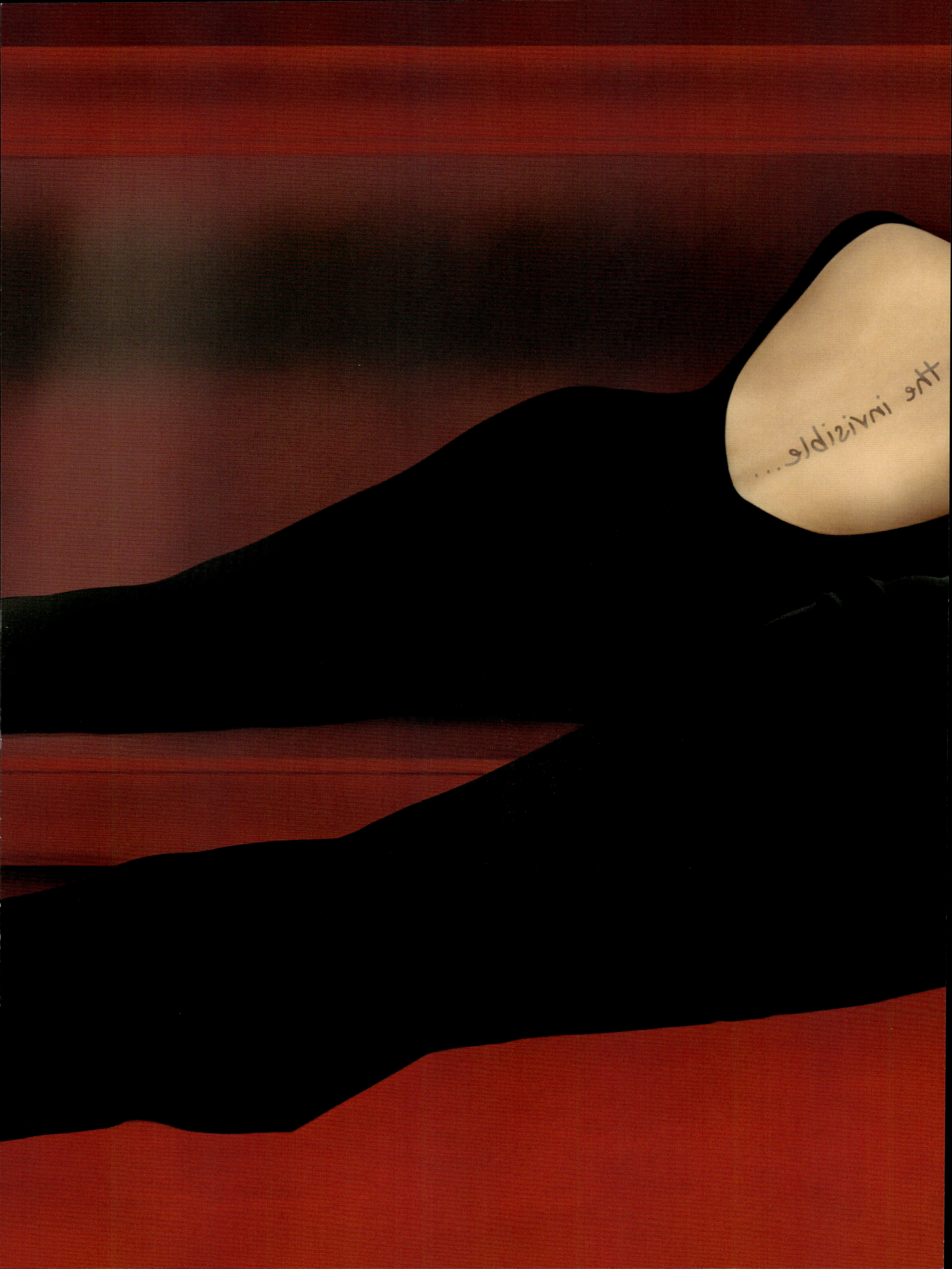
the invisible...

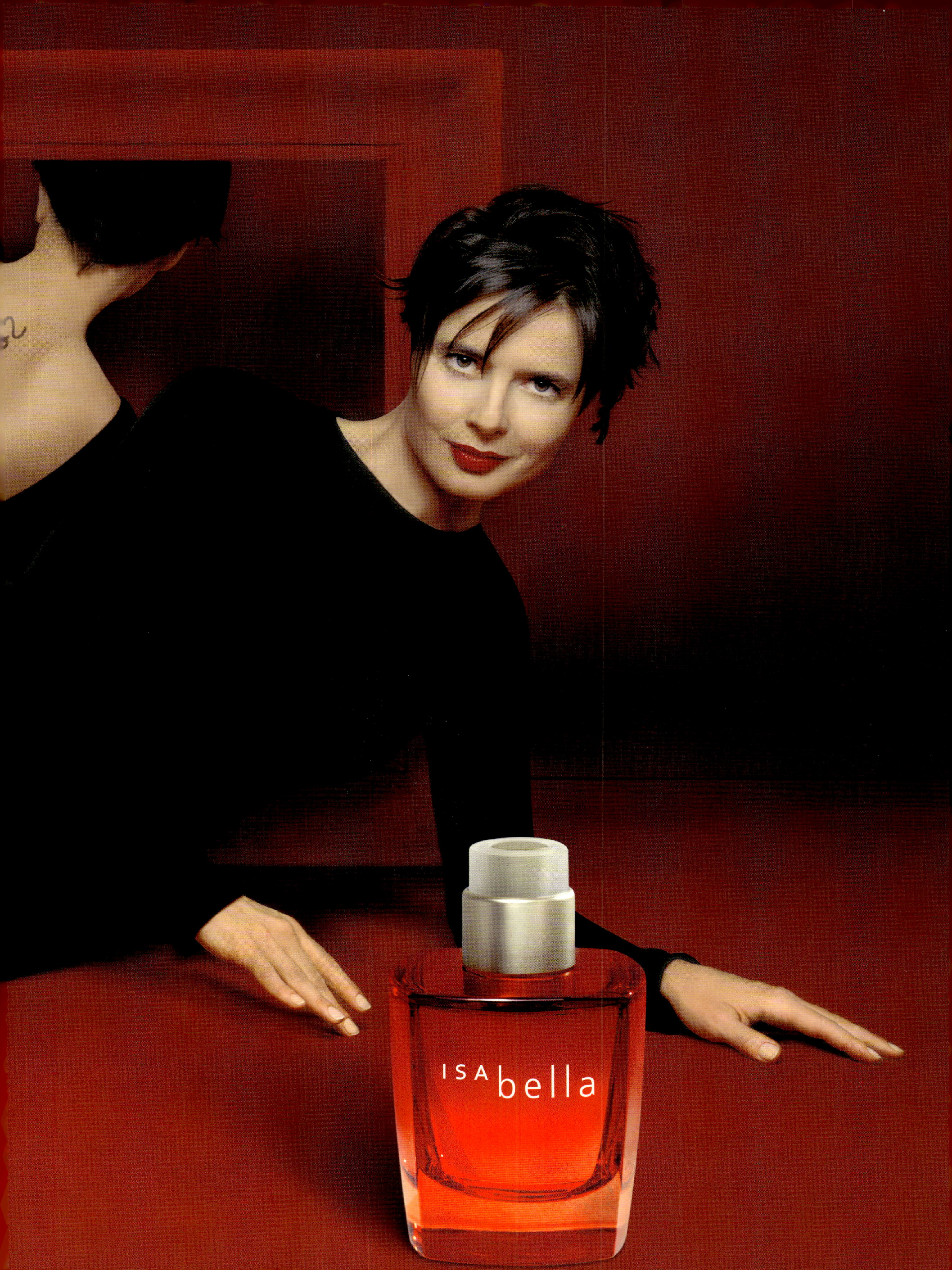
ISA bella

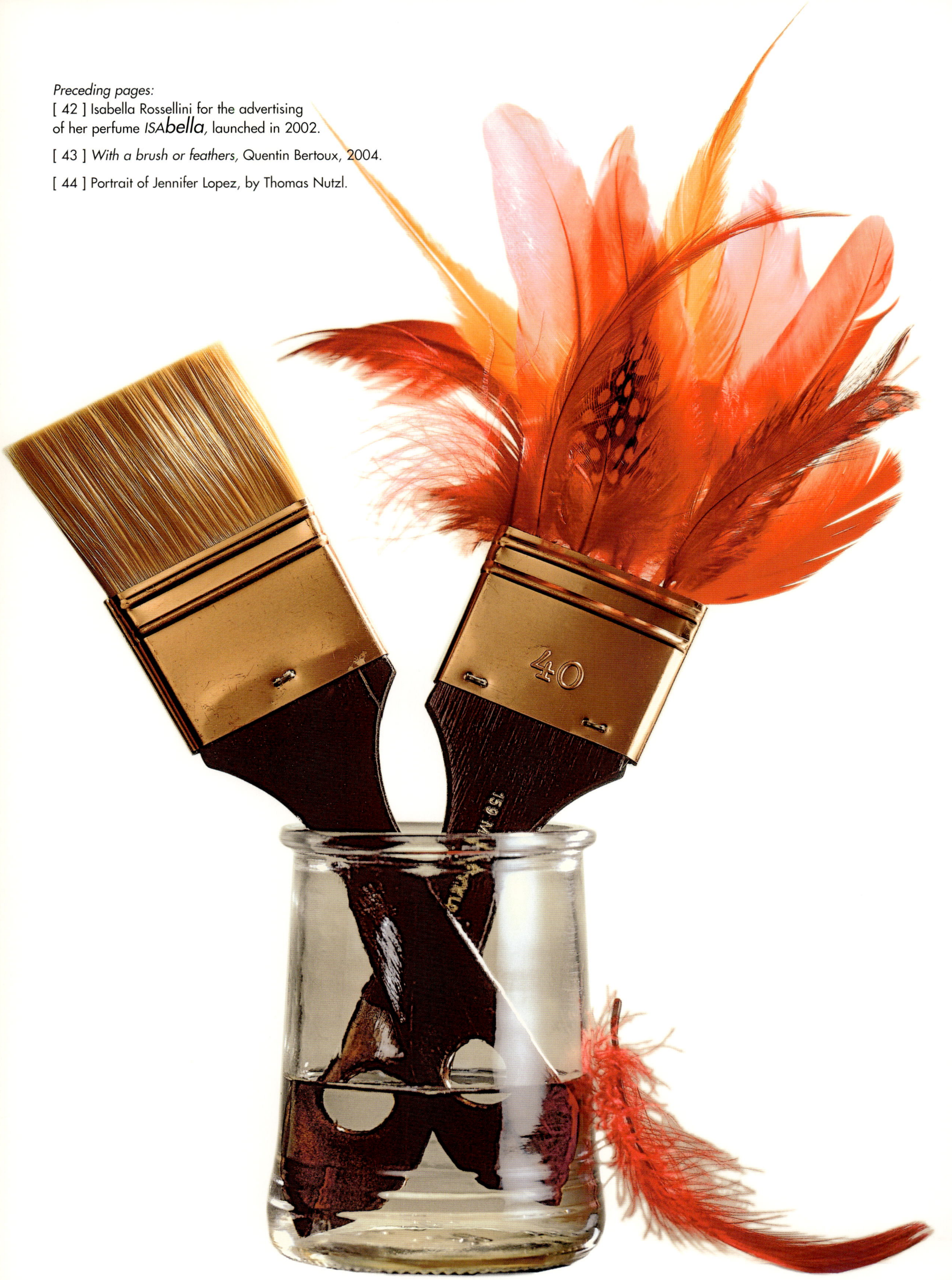

Preceding pages:
[42] Isabella Rossellini for the advertising of her perfume *ISAbella*, launched in 2002.

[43] *With a brush or feathers,* Quentin Bertoux, 2004.

[44] Portrait of Jennifer Lopez, by Thomas Nutzl.

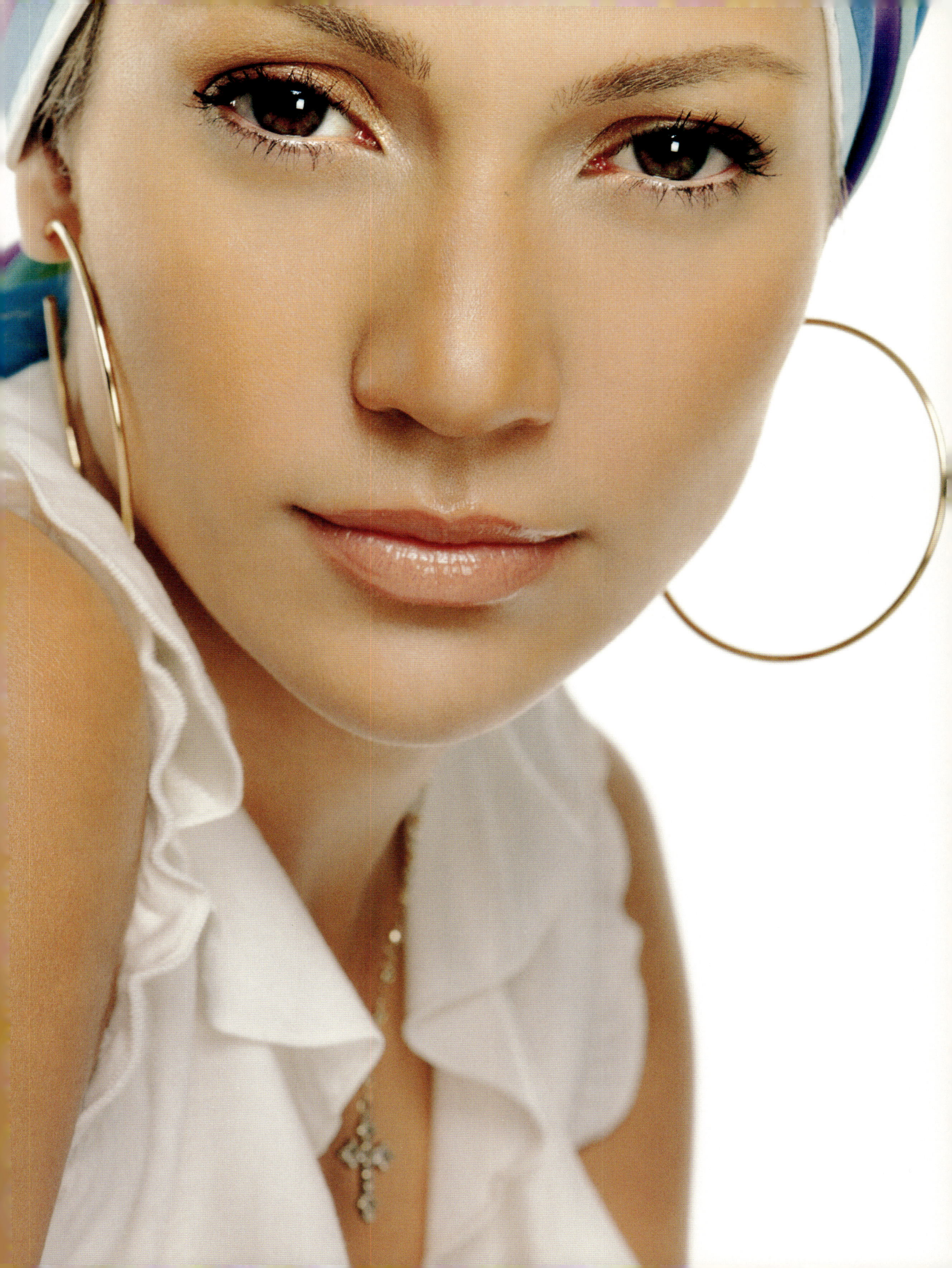

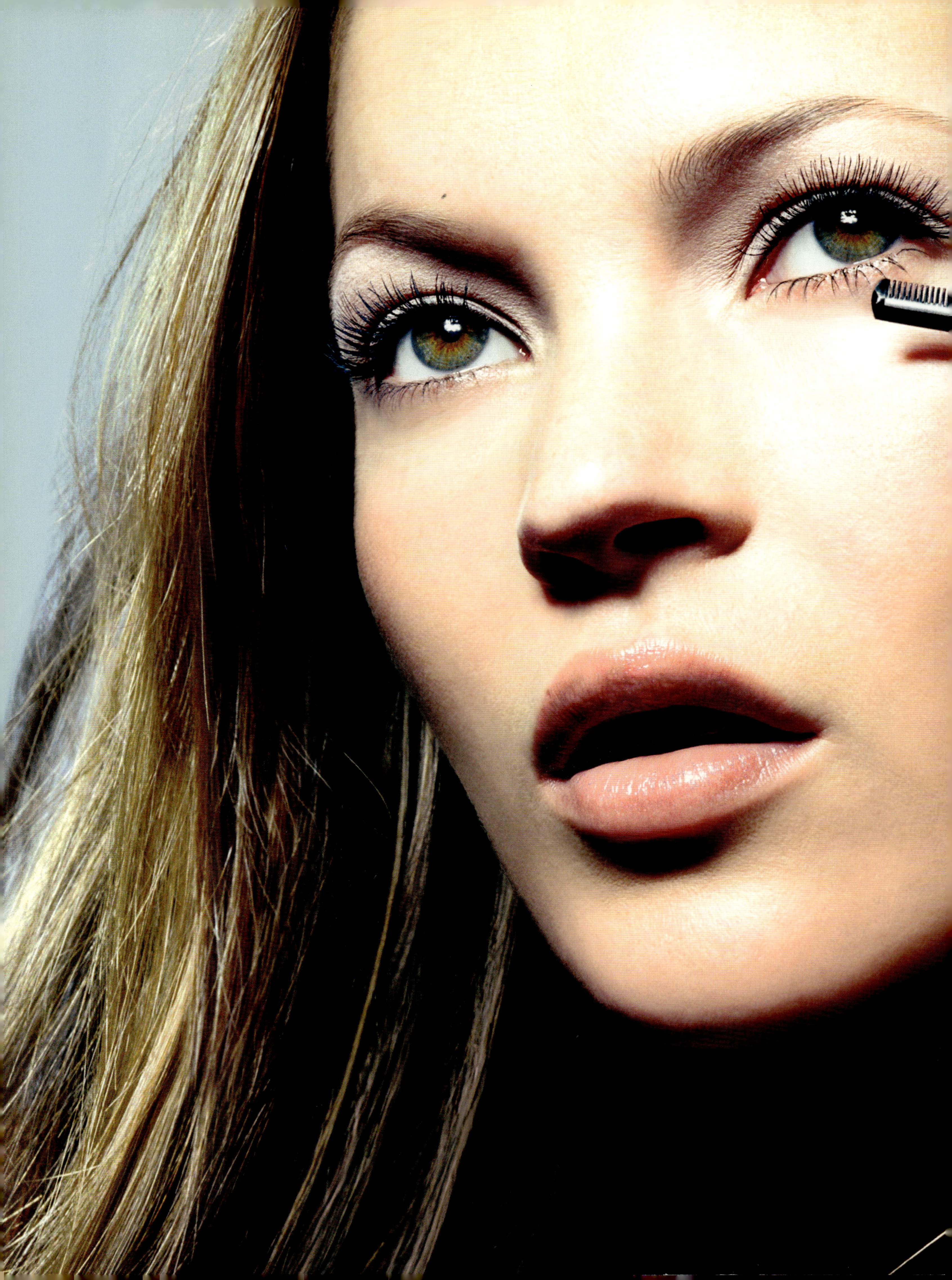

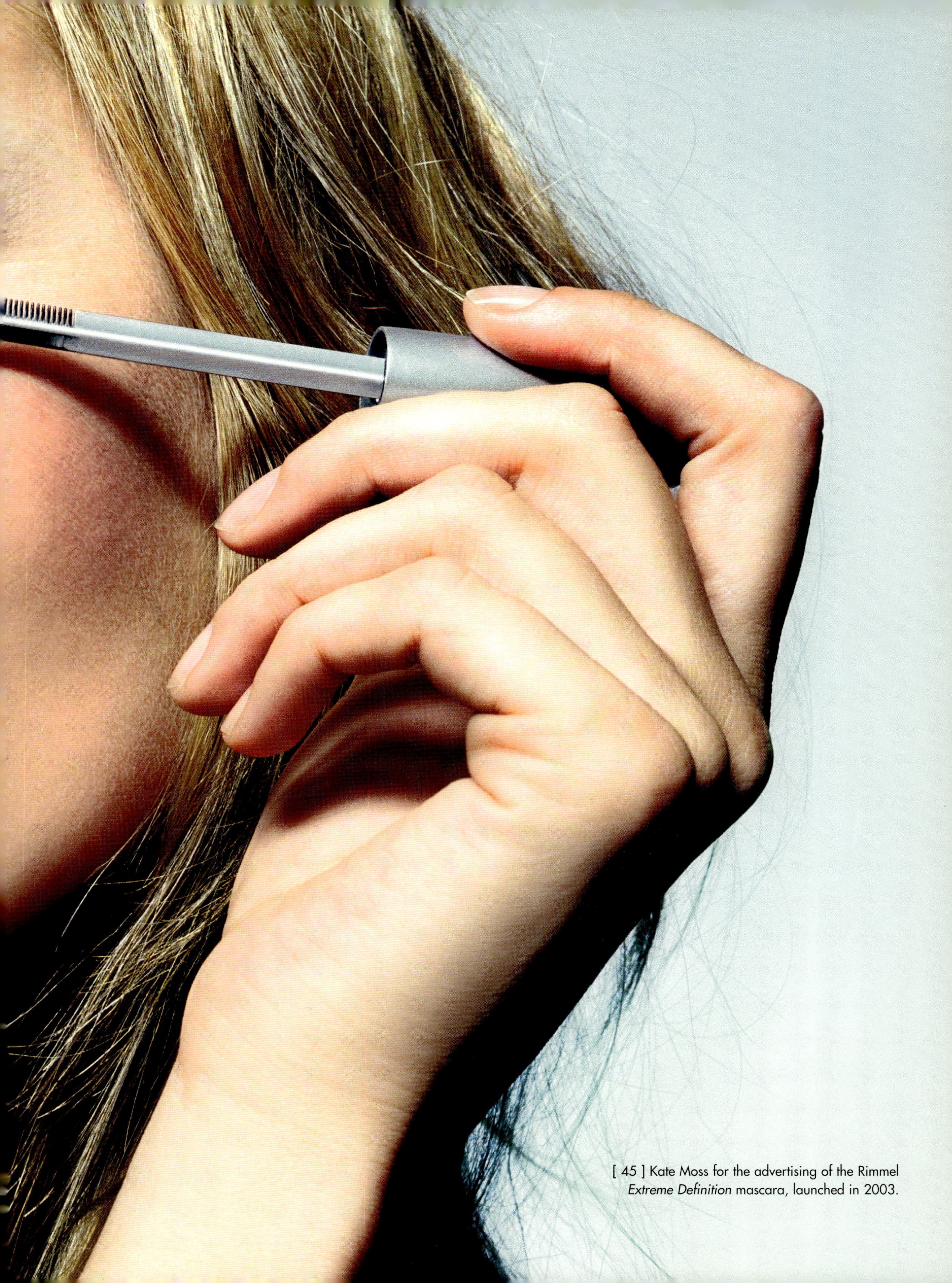

[45] Kate Moss for the advertising of the Rimmel *Extreme Definition* mascara, launched in 2003.

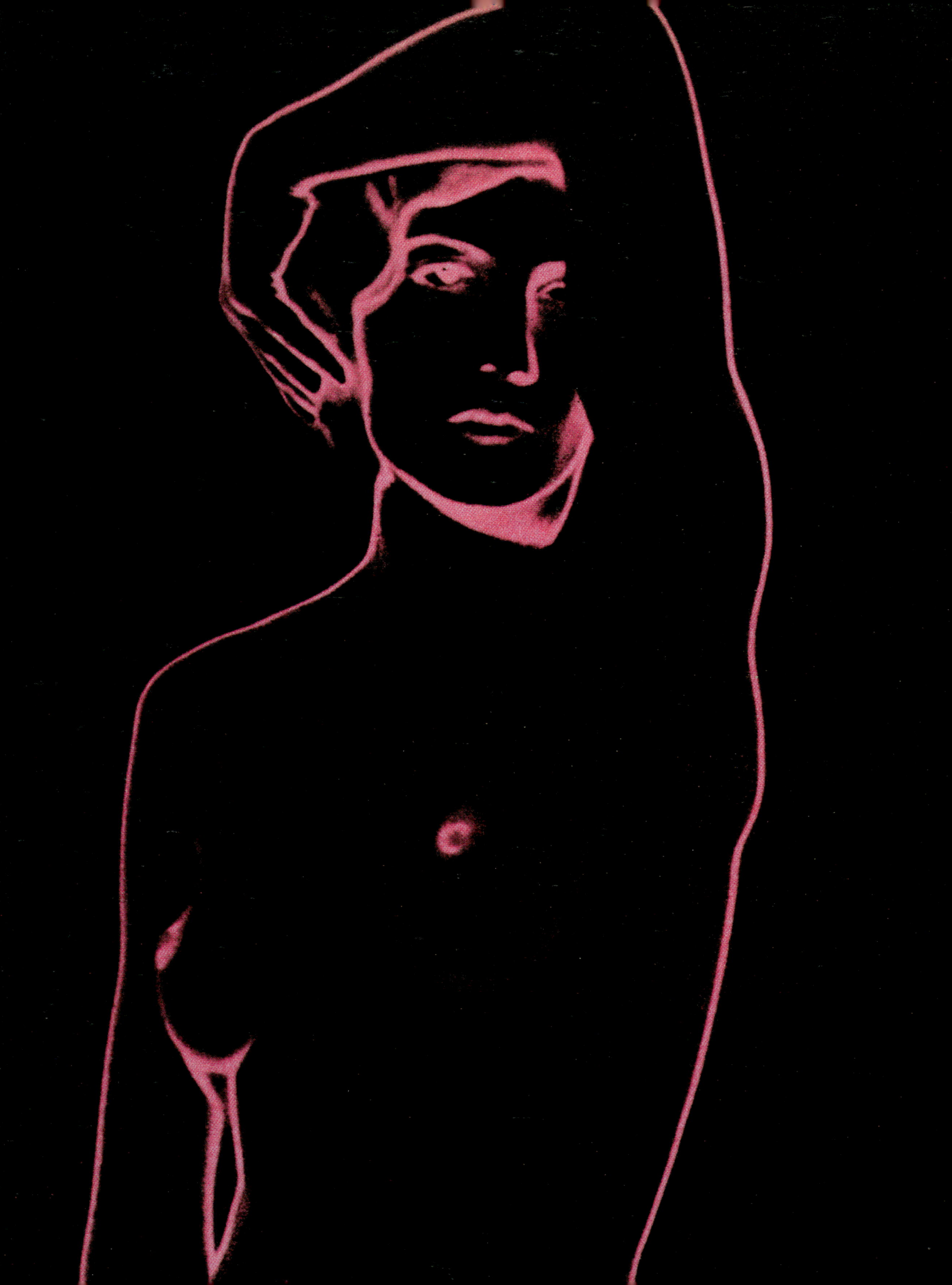

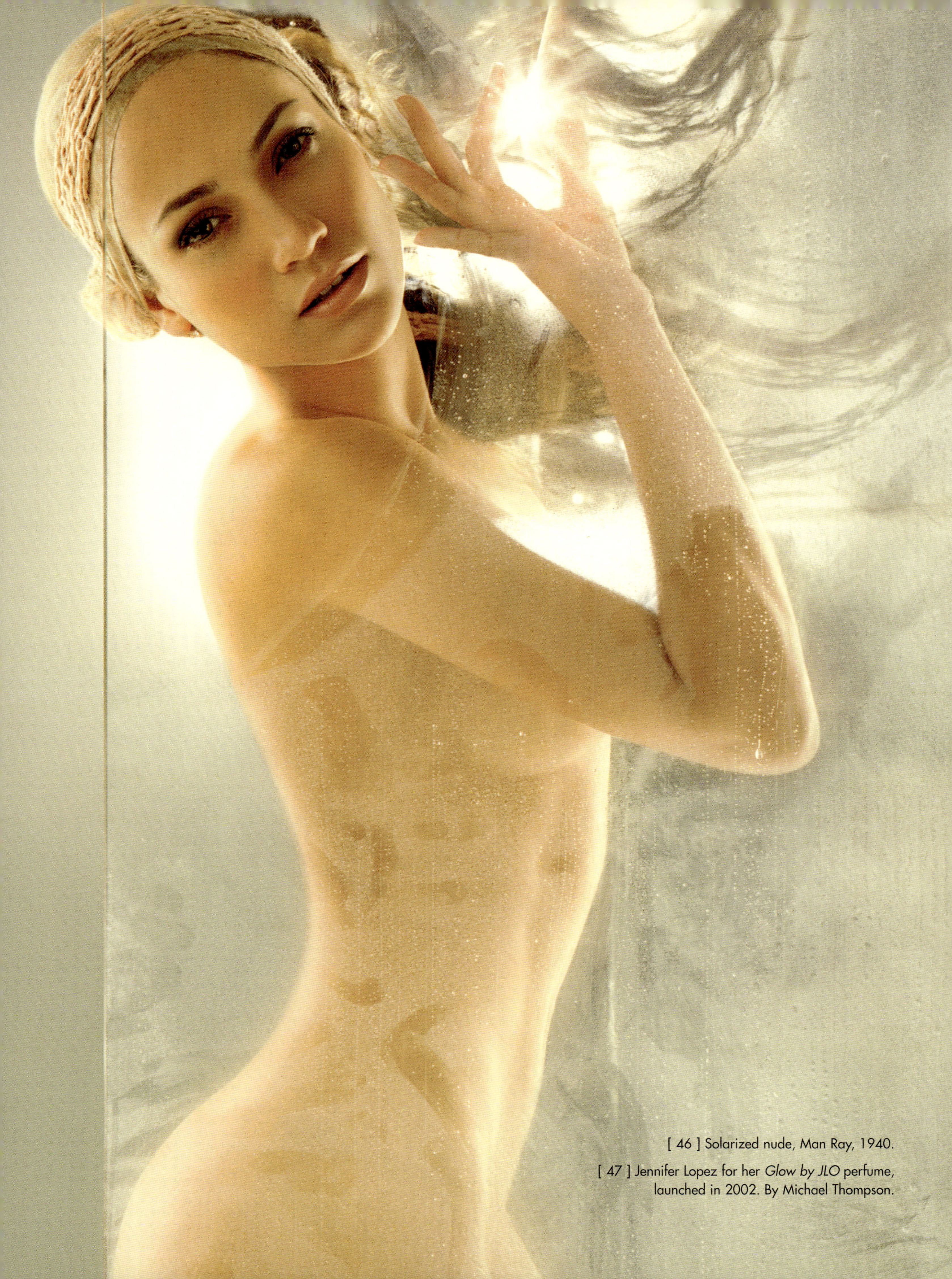

[46] Solarized nude, Man Ray, 1940.

[47] Jennifer Lopez for her *Glow by JLO* perfume, launched in 2002. By Michael Thompson.

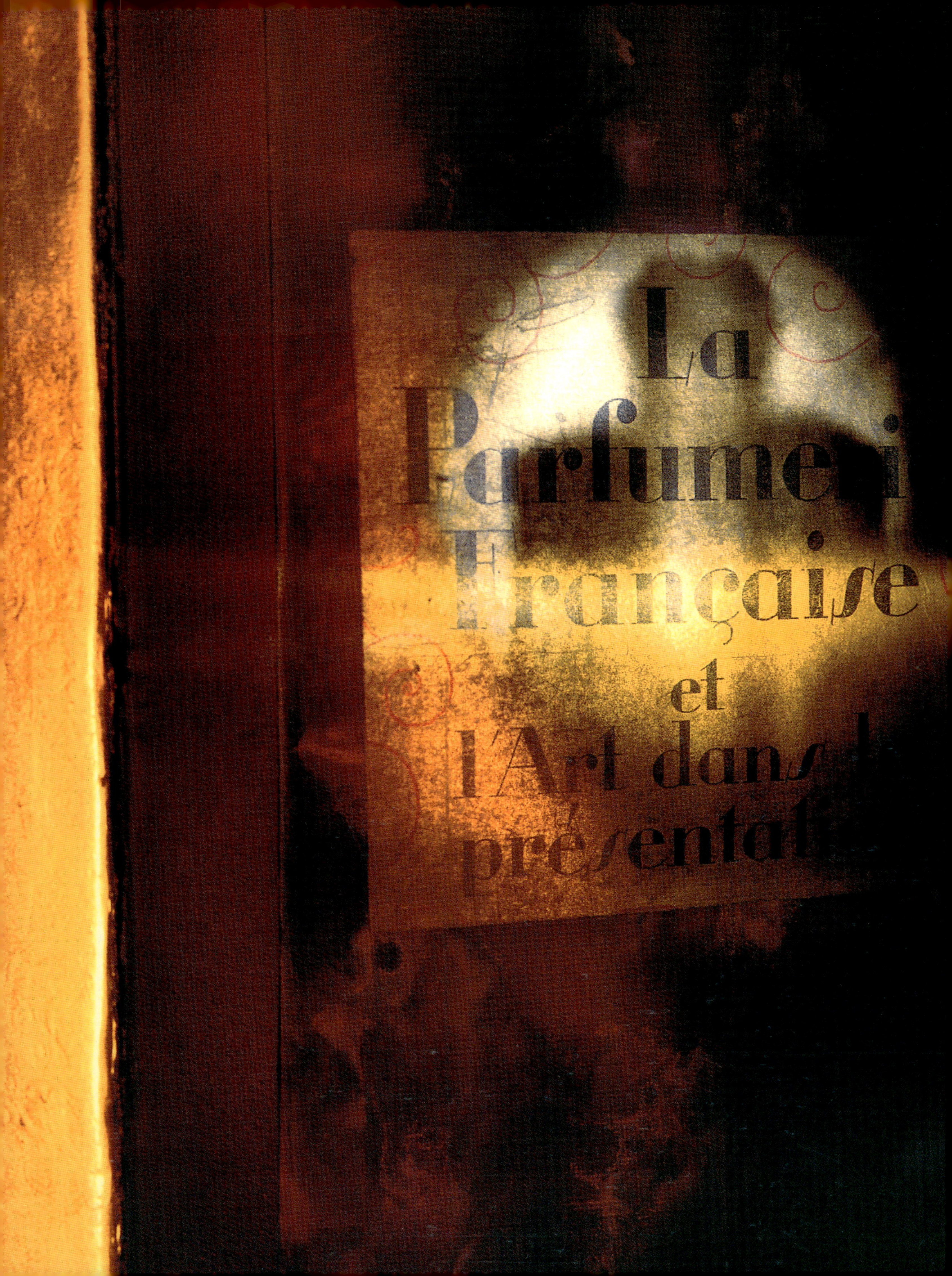

La
Parfumeri
Française
et
l'Art dans
présentat

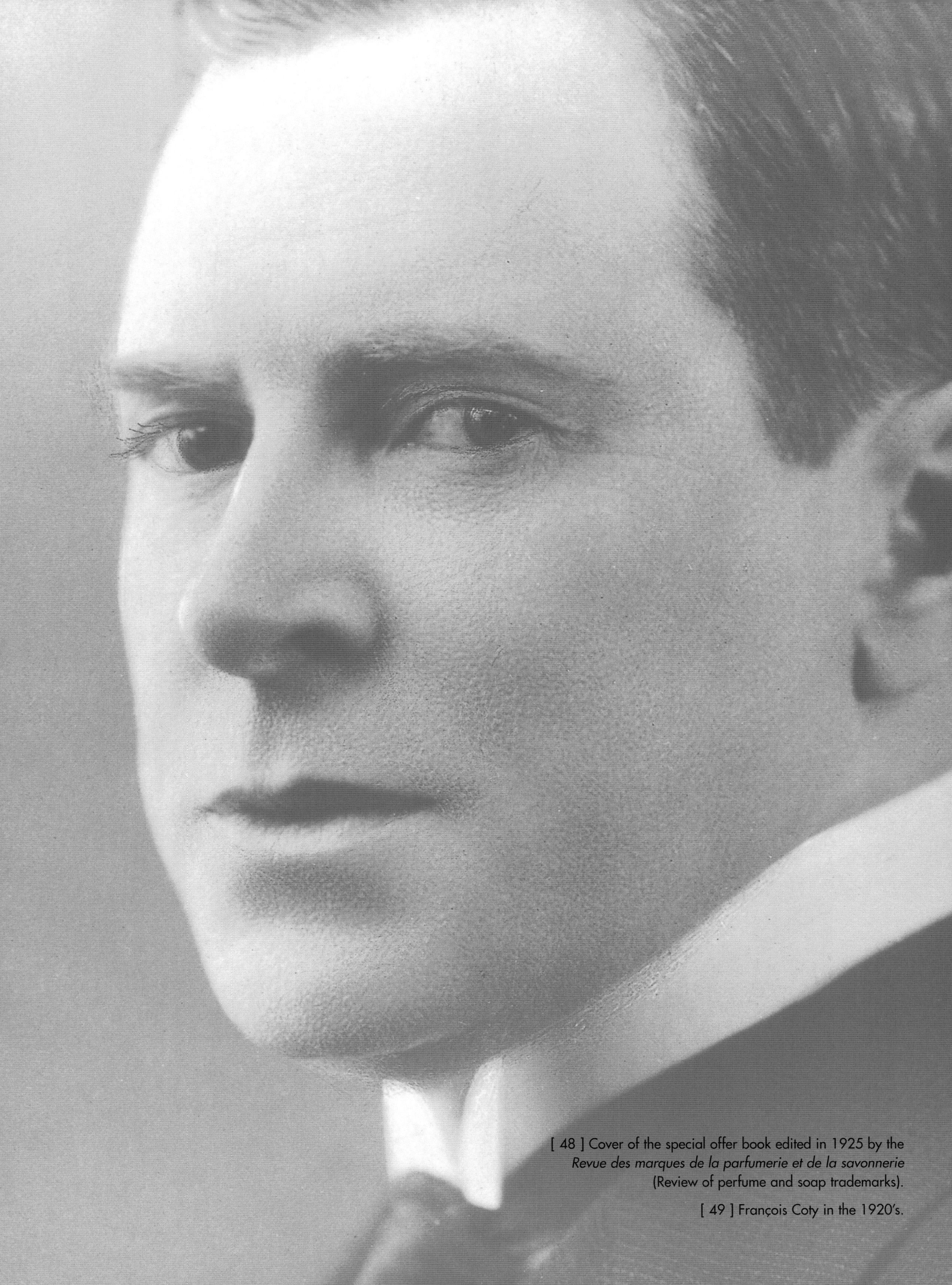

[48] Cover of the special offer book edited in 1925 by the *Revue des marques de la parfumerie et de la savonnerie* (Review of perfume and soap trademarks).

[49] François Coty in the 1920's.

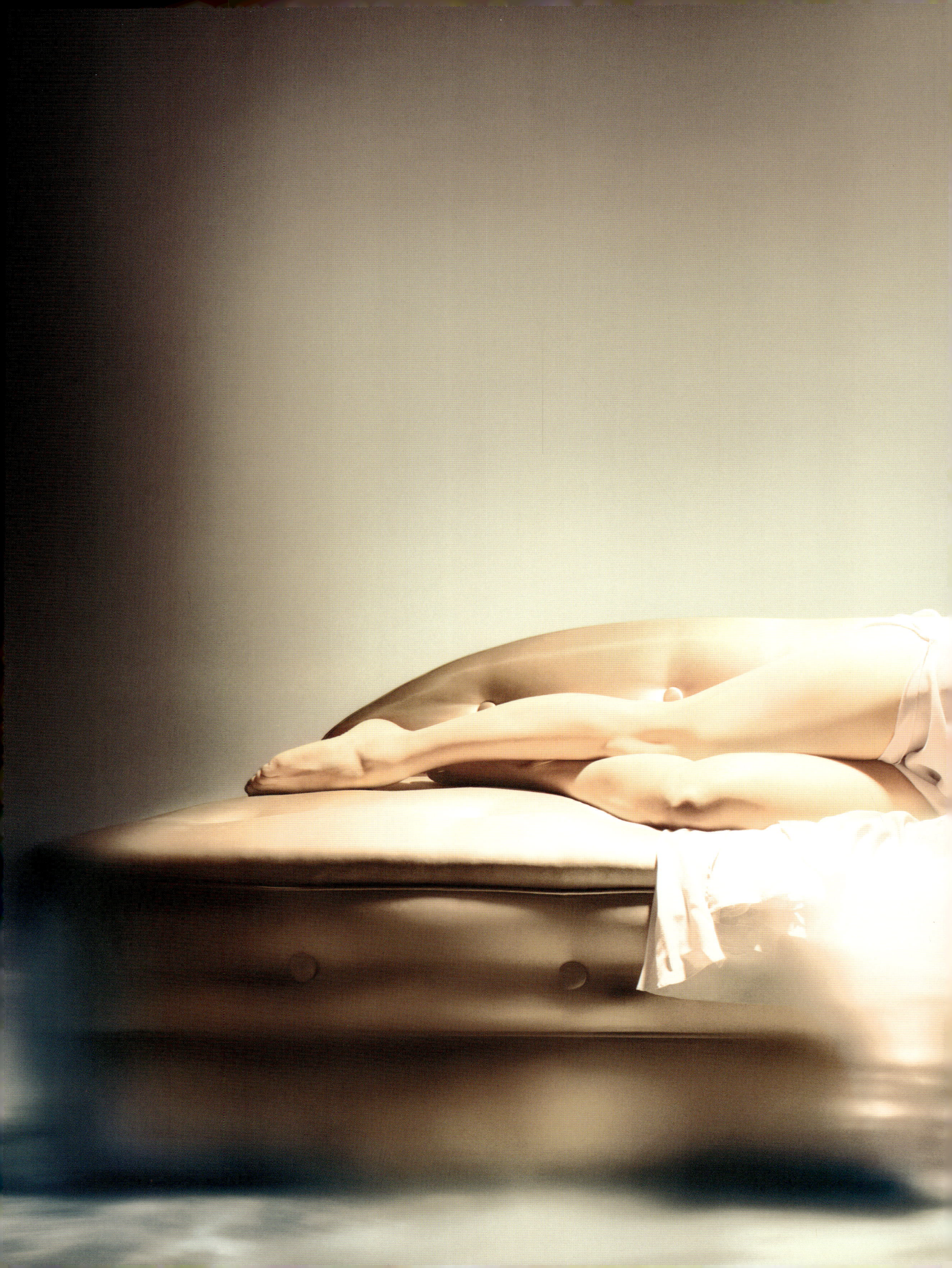

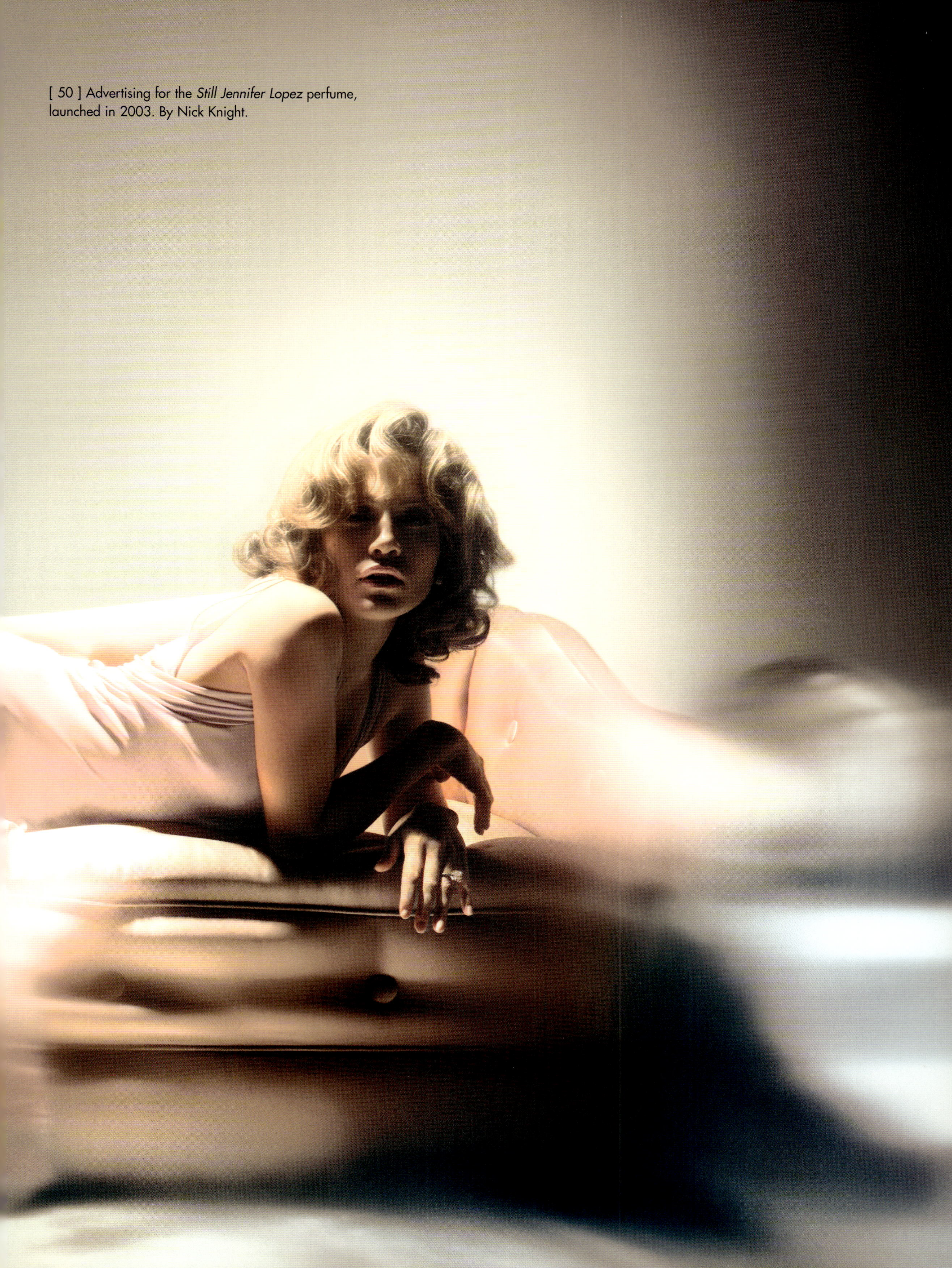

[50] Advertising for the *Still Jennifer Lopez* perfume, launched in 2003. By Nick Knight.

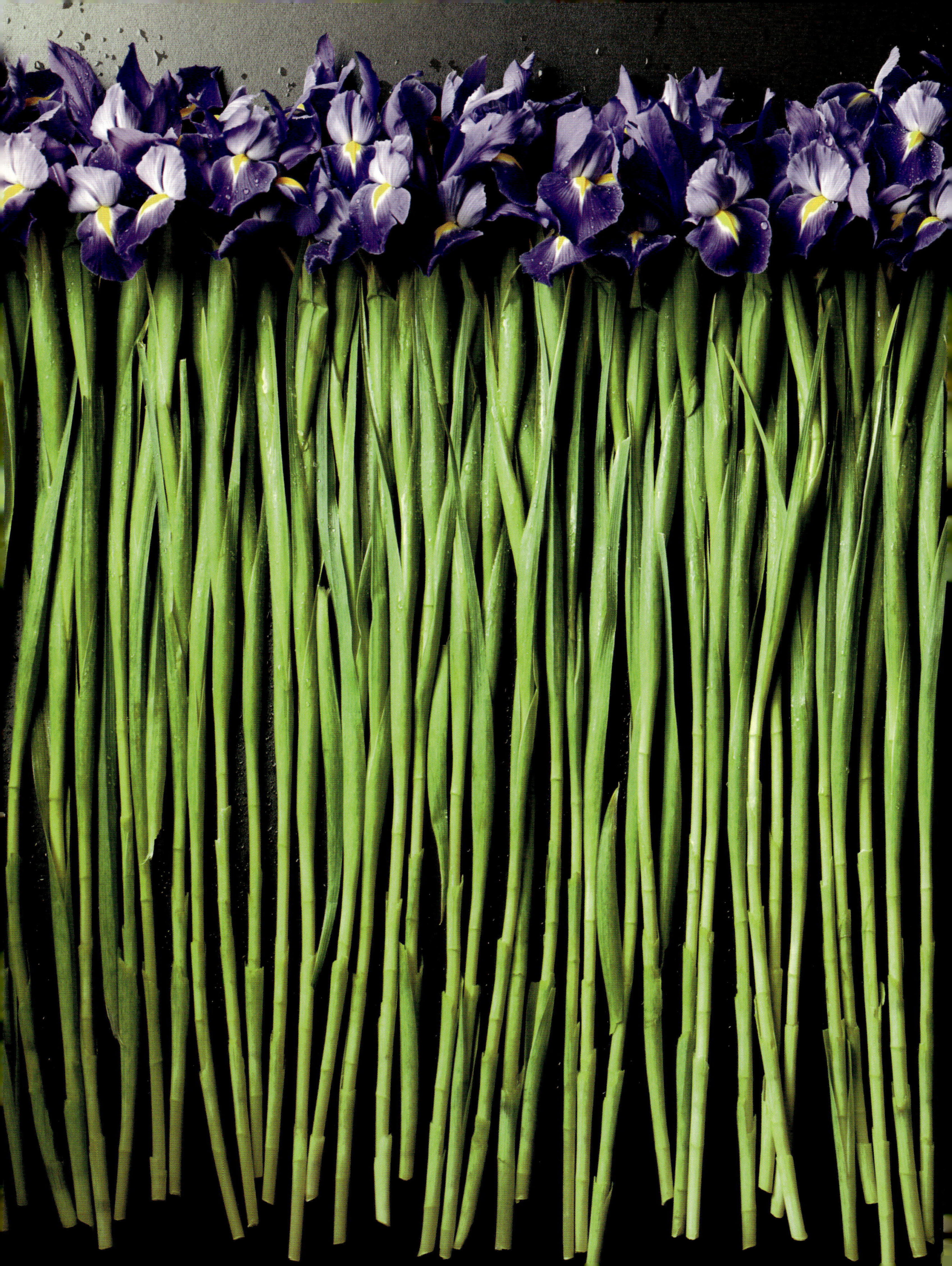

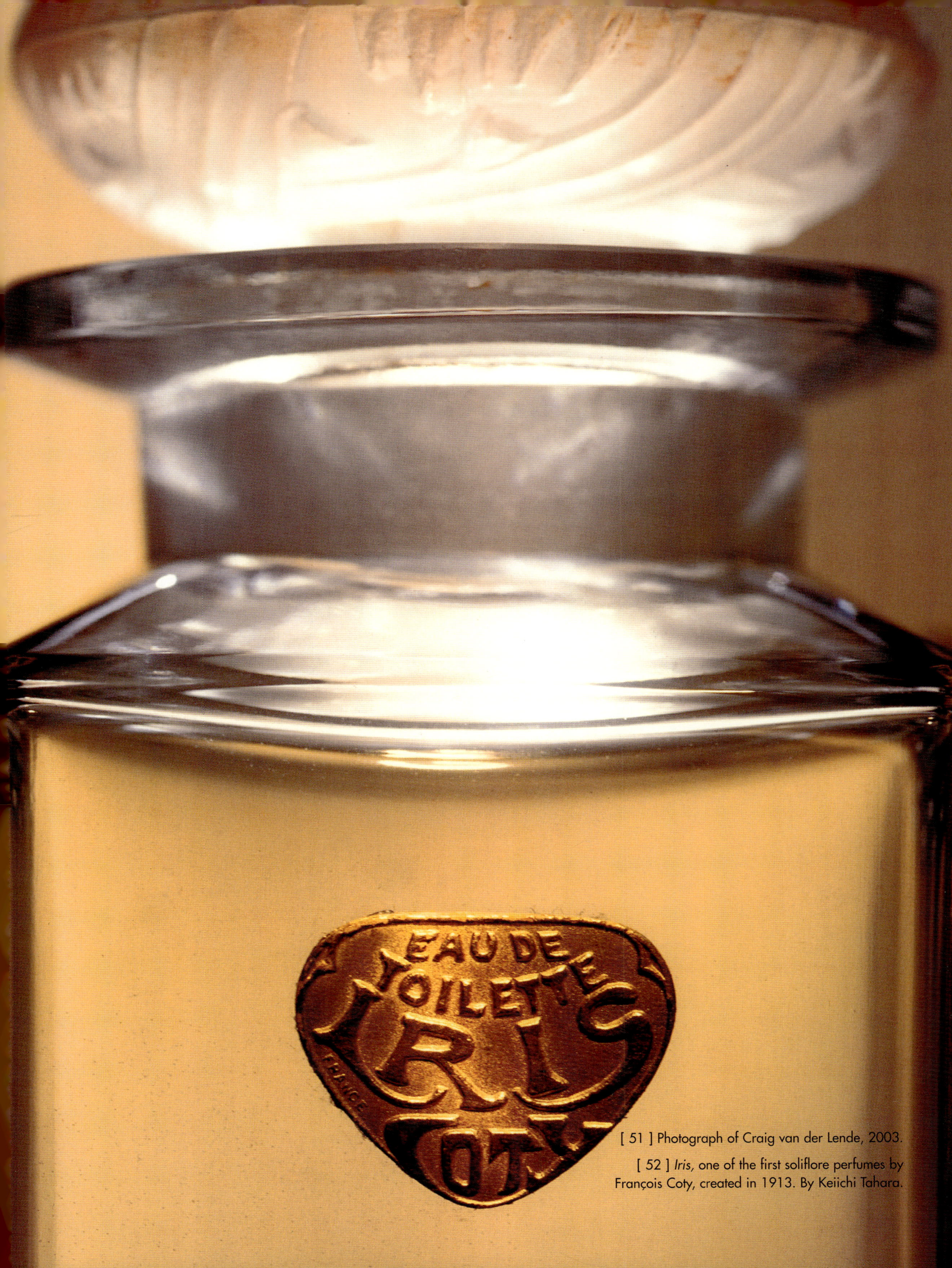

[51] Photograph of Craig van der Lende, 2003.

[52] *Iris*, one of the first soliflore perfumes by François Coty, created in 1913. By Keiichi Tahara.

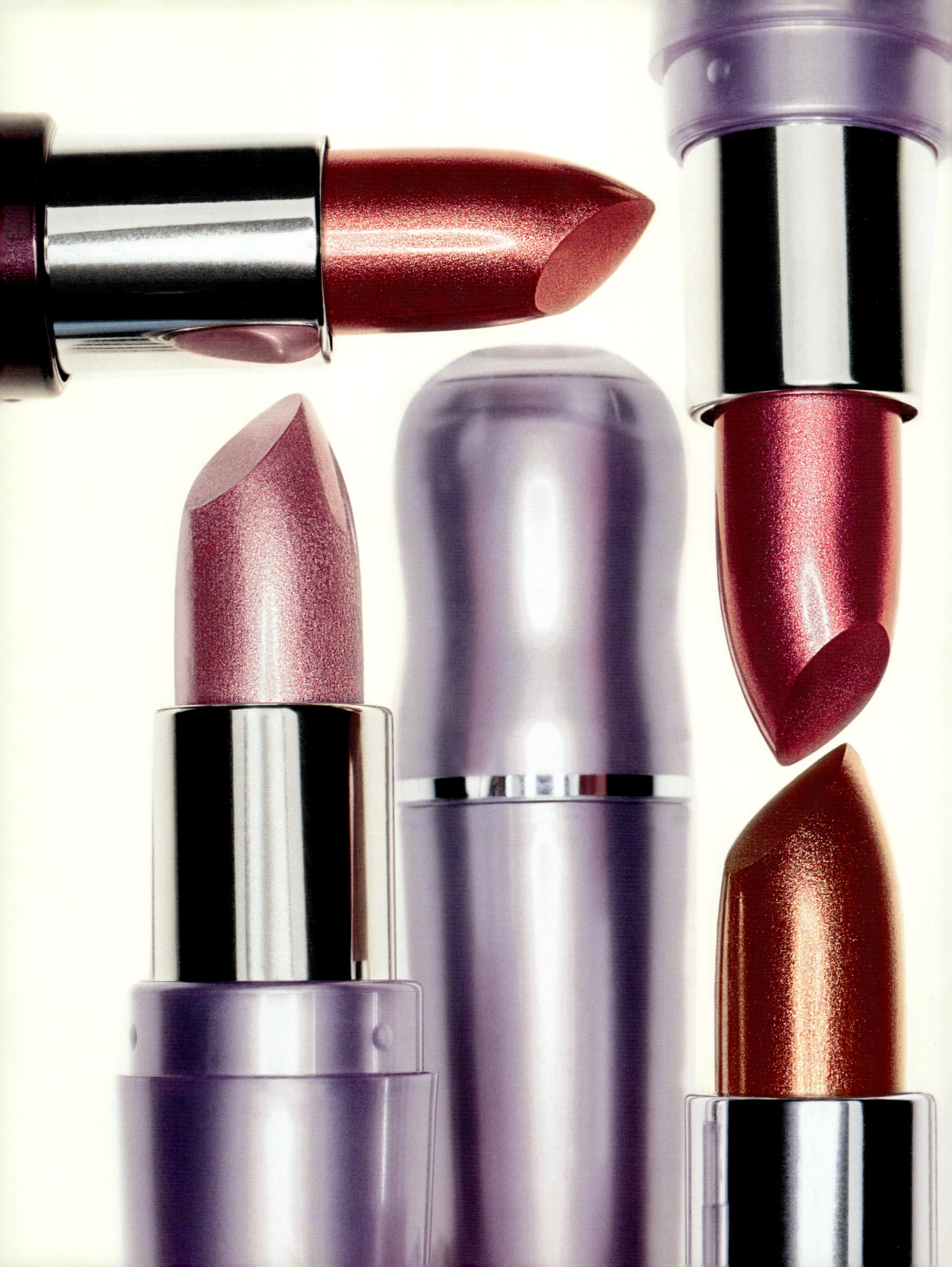

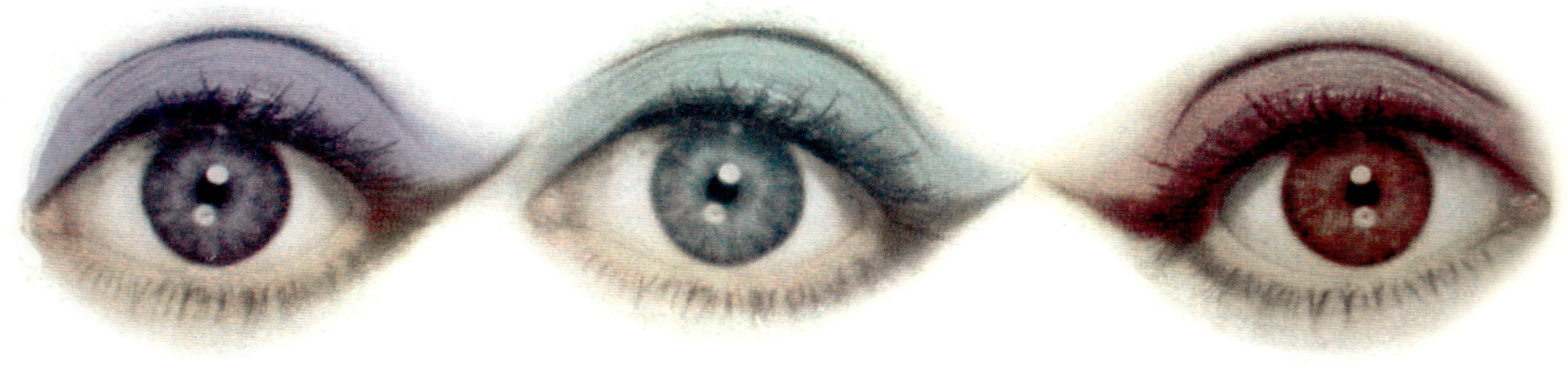

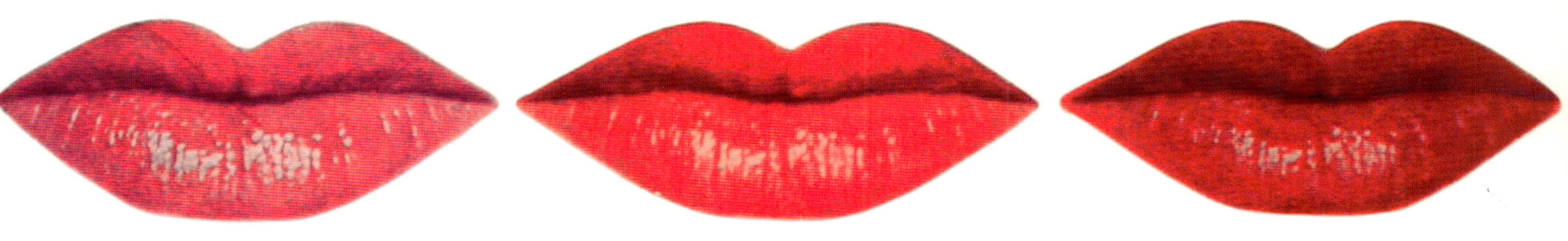

[53] Lipsticks Astor *Shine Extreme,* trademark created in 1952.

[54] *Vogue,* "special beauty", 1952.

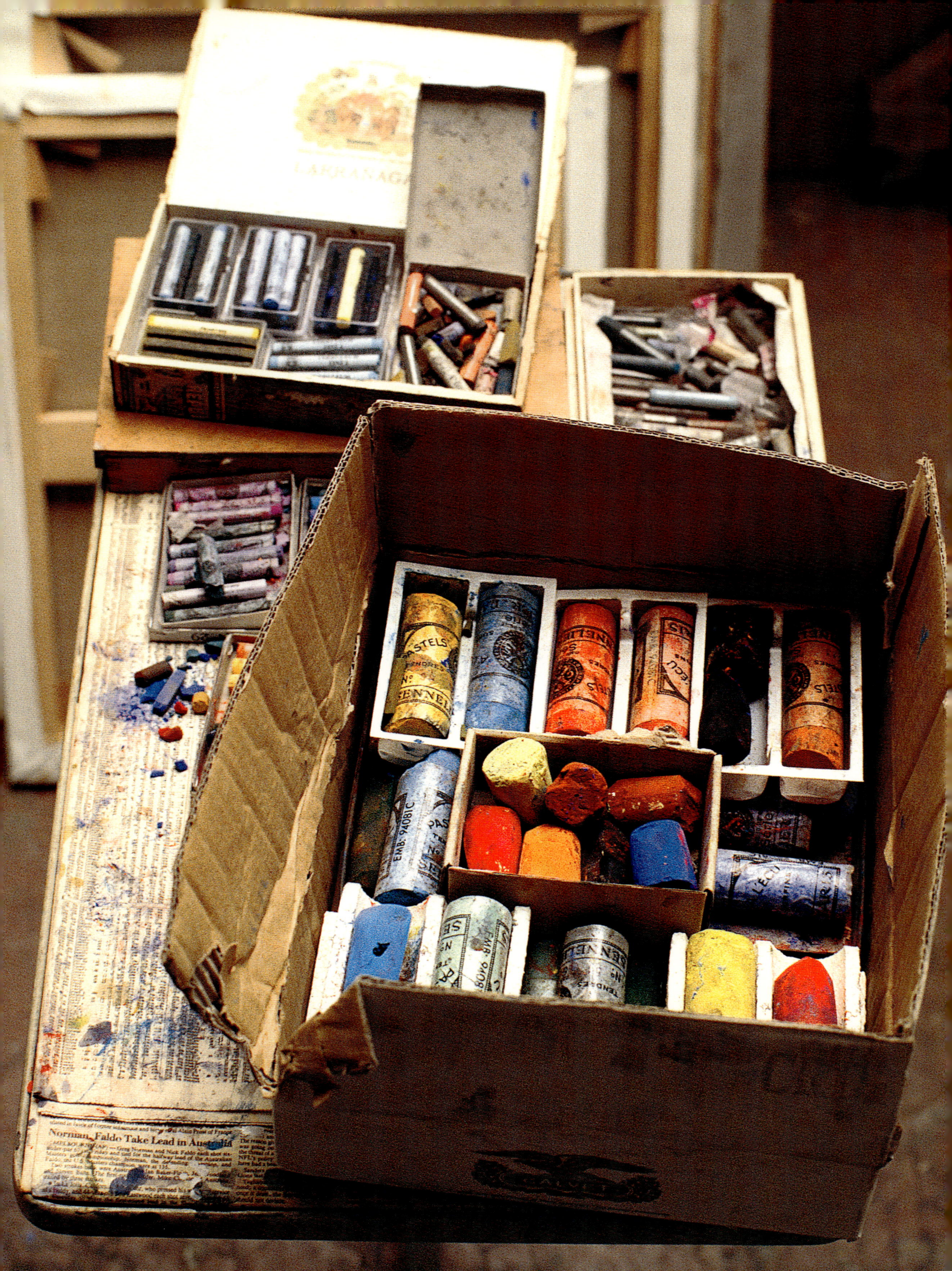
Norman, Faldo Take Lead in Australia

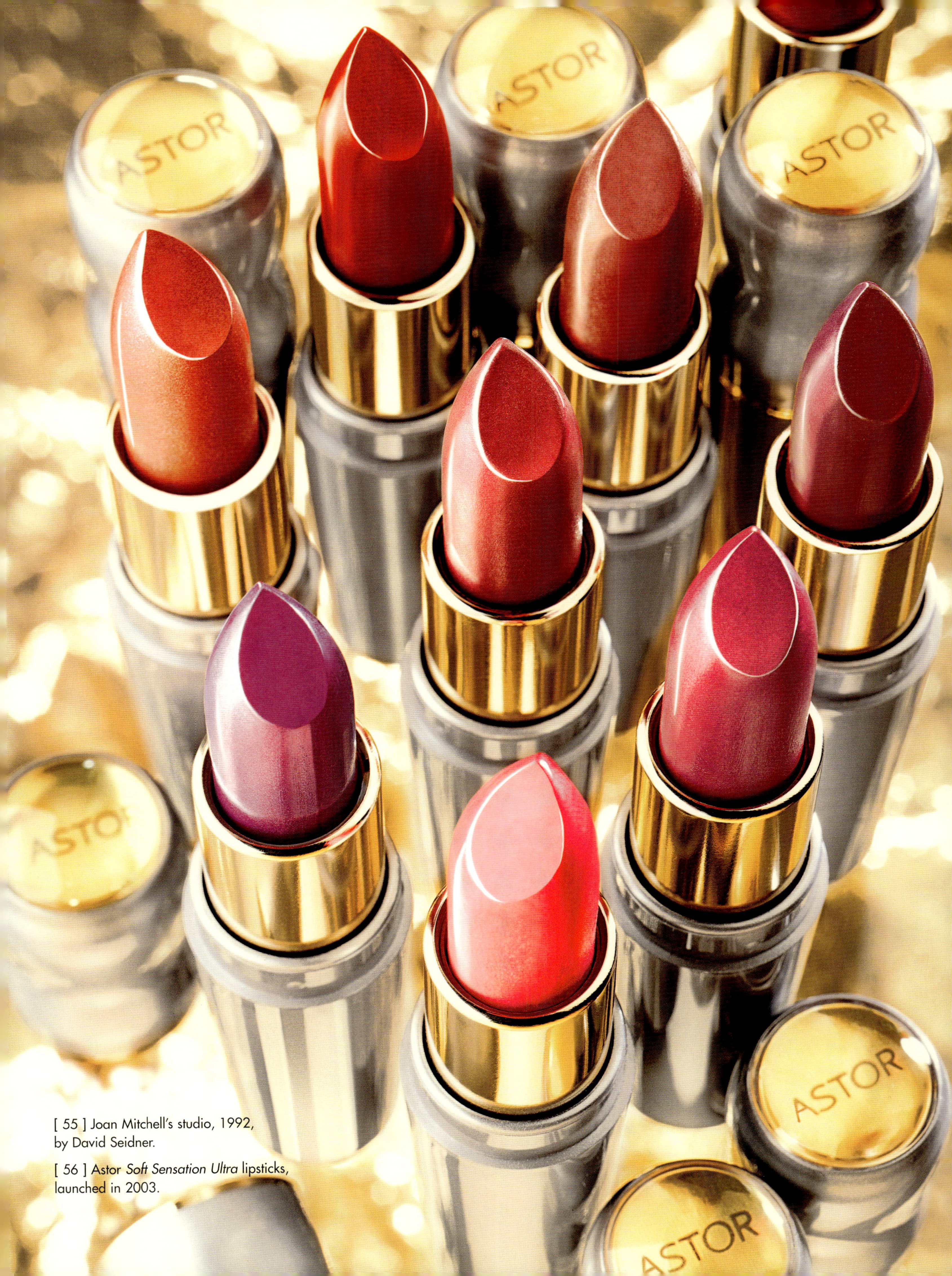

[55] Joan Mitchell's studio, 1992, by David Seidner.

[56] Astor *Soft Sensation Ultra* lipsticks, launched in 2003.

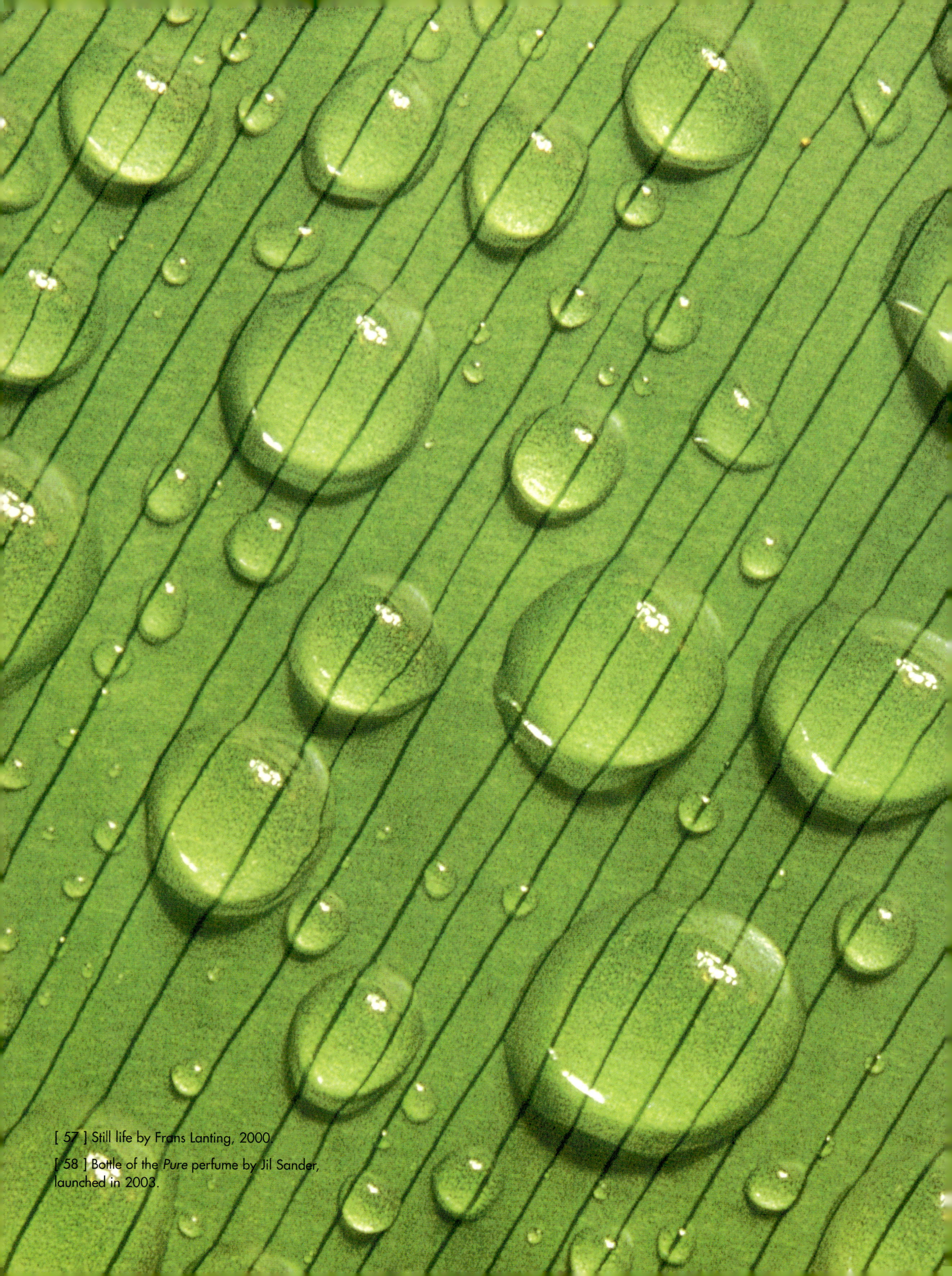

[57] Still life by Frans Lanting, 2000.

[58] Bottle of the *Pure* perfume by Jil Sander, launched in 2003.

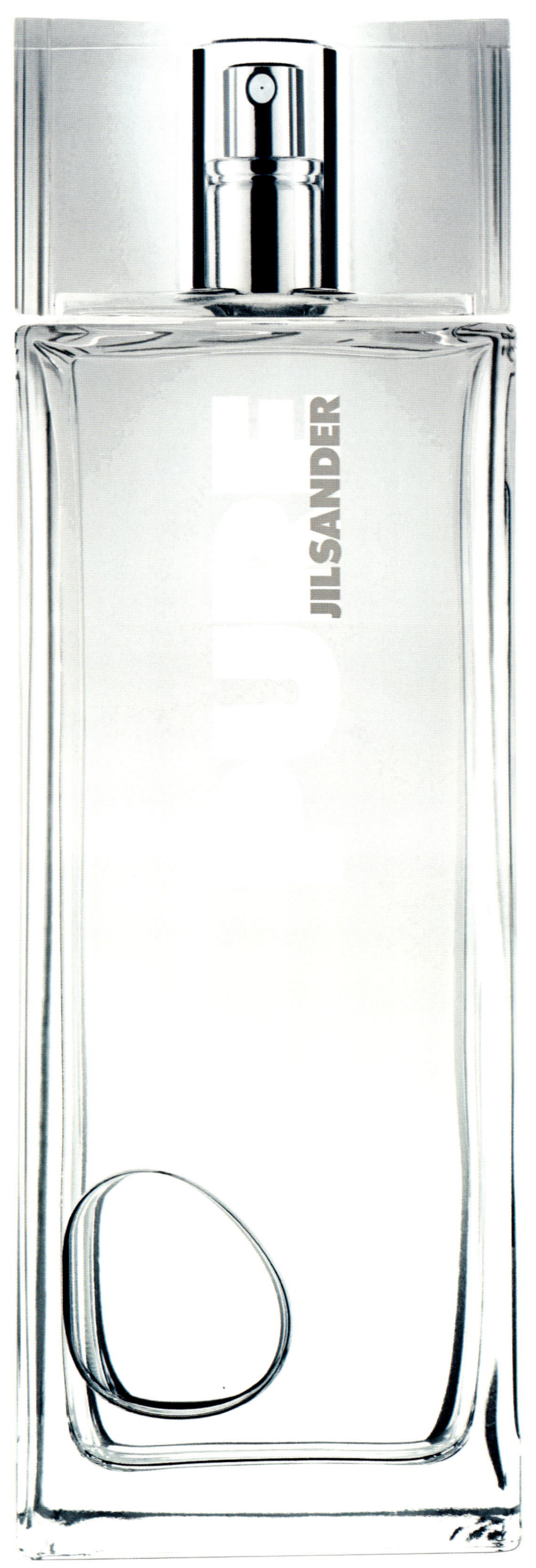
JILSANDER

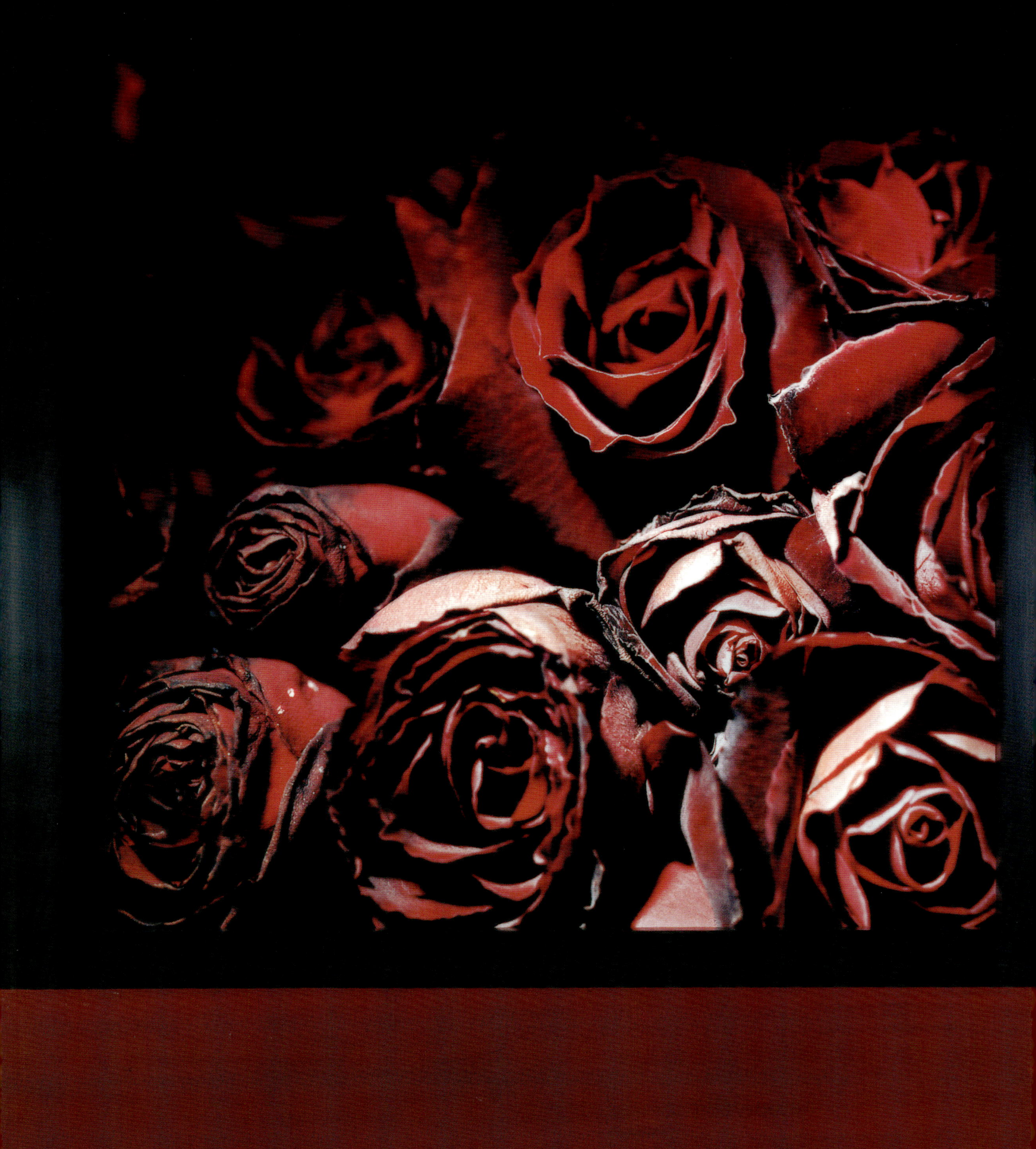

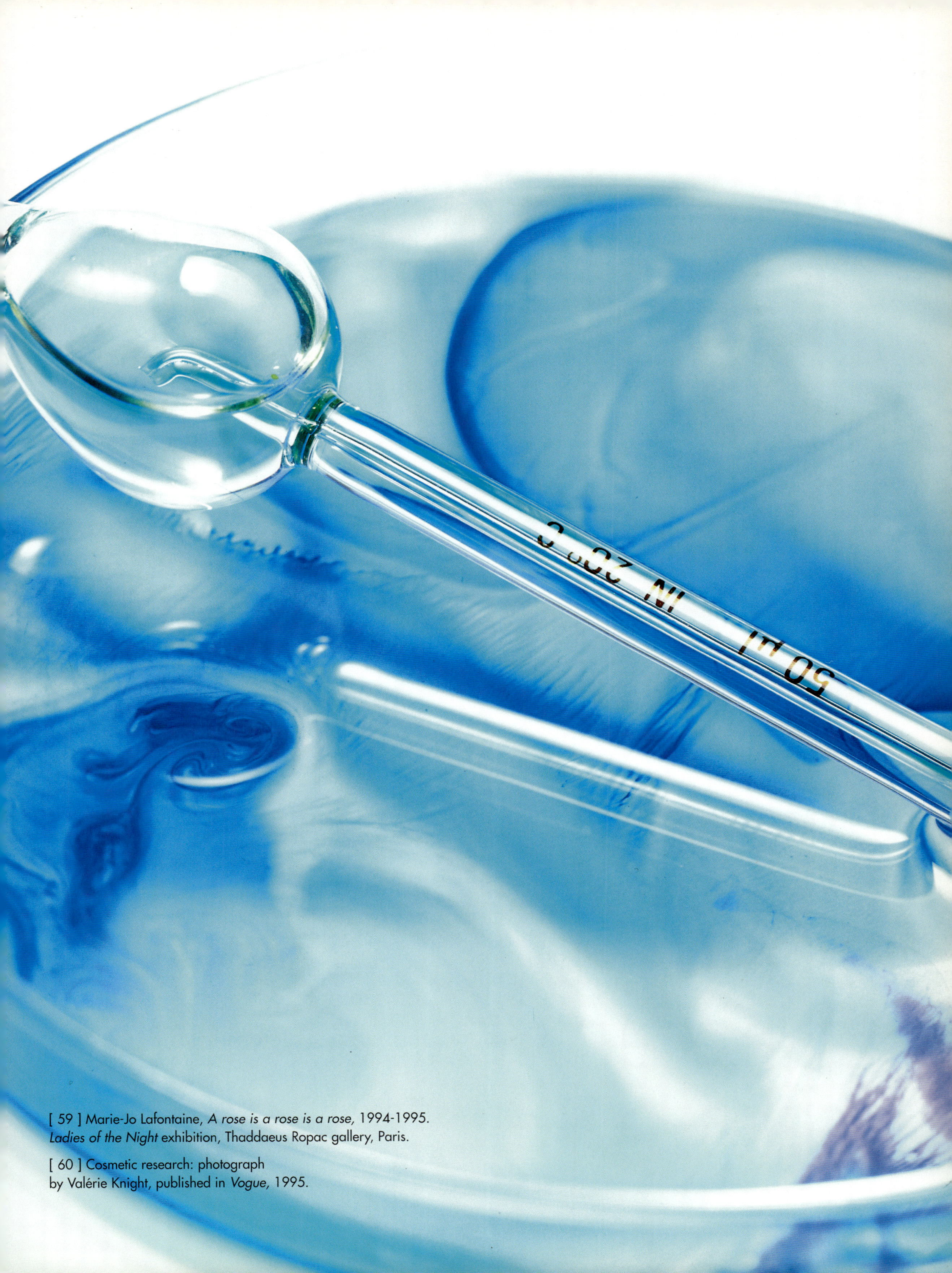

[59] Marie-Jo Lafontaine, *A rose is a rose is a rose,* 1994-1995.
Ladies of the Night exhibition, Thaddaeus Ropac gallery, Paris.

[60] Cosmetic research: photograph
by Valérie Knight, published in *Vogue*, 1995.

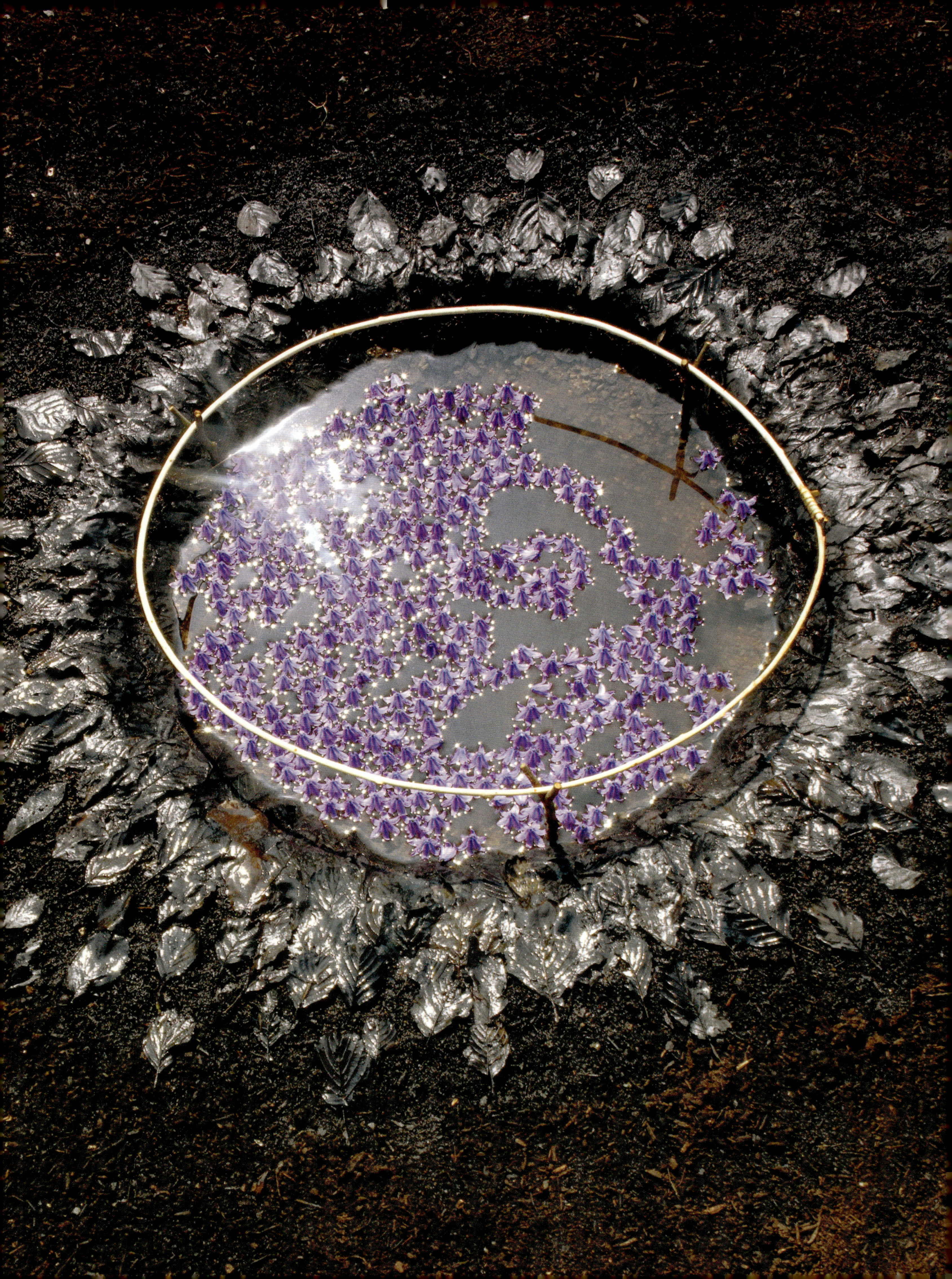

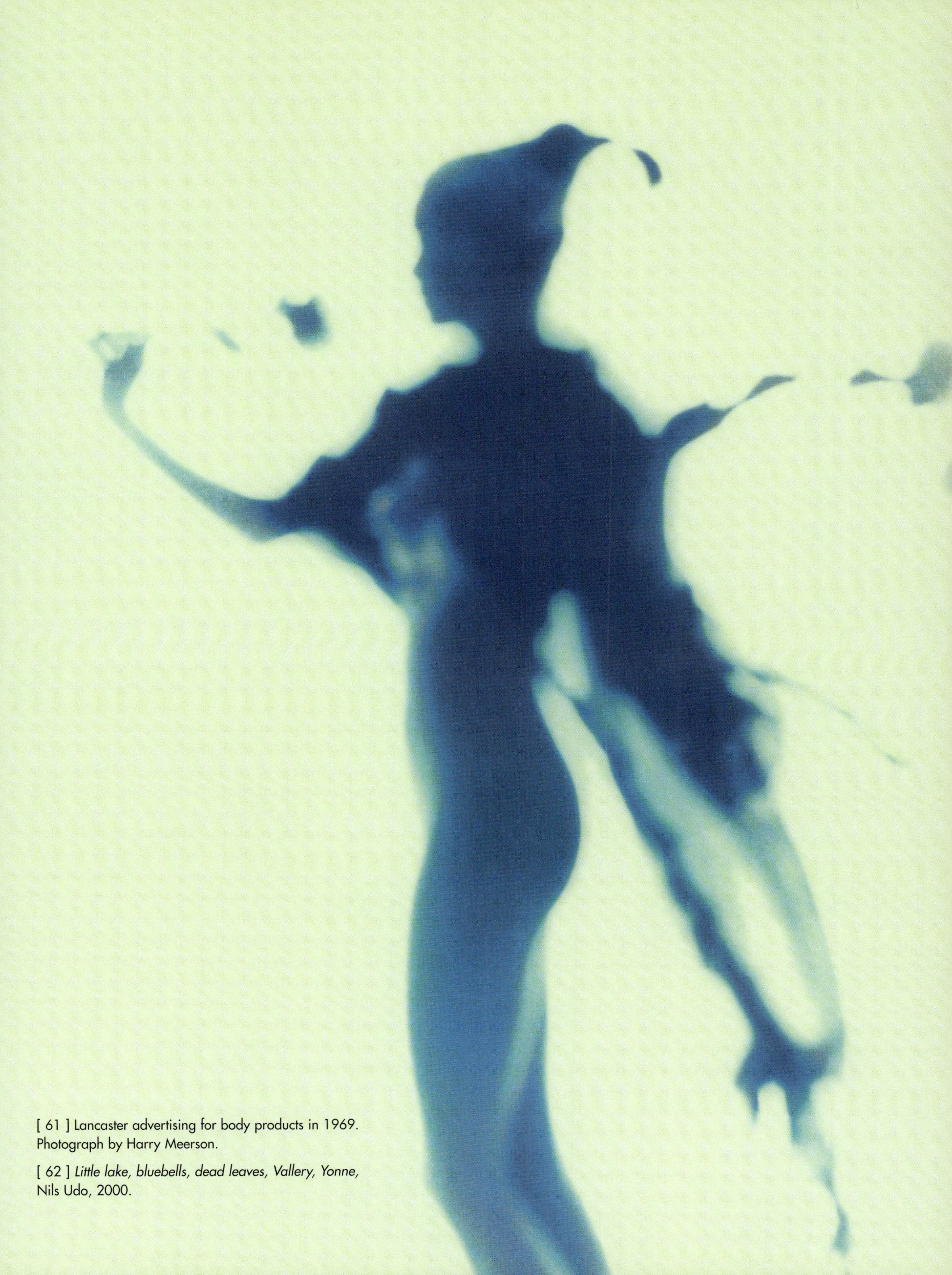

[61] Lancaster advertising for body products in 1969. Photograph by Harry Meerson.

[62] *Little lake, bluebells, dead leaves, Vallery, Yonne,* Nils Udo, 2000.

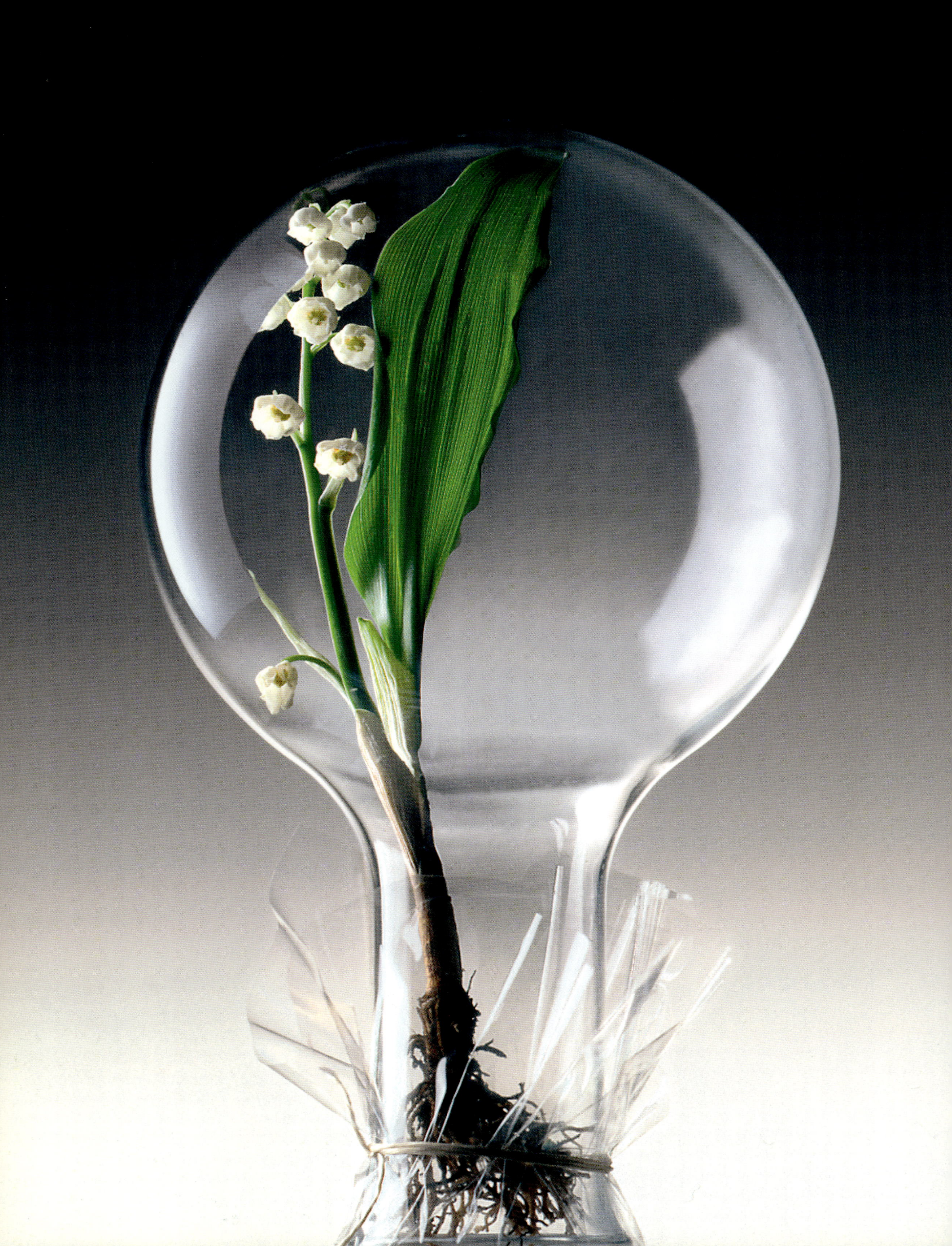

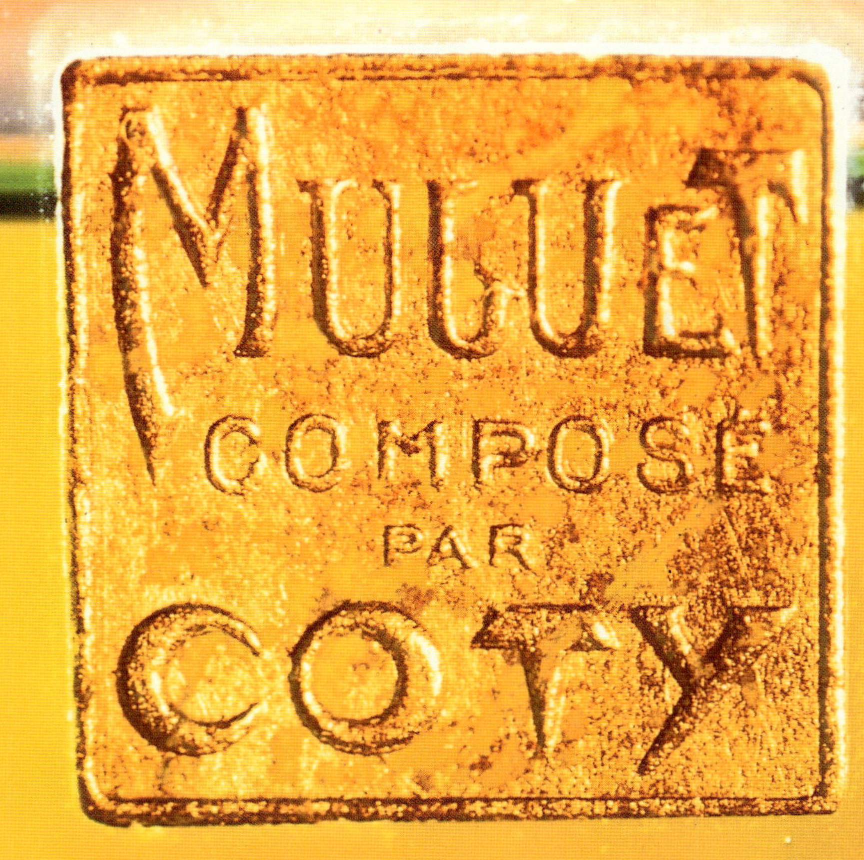

[63] Still life by Peter Knaup, 1988.

[64] *Muguet* perfume by Coty with the label designed in 1908 by René Lalique. By Keiichi Tahara.

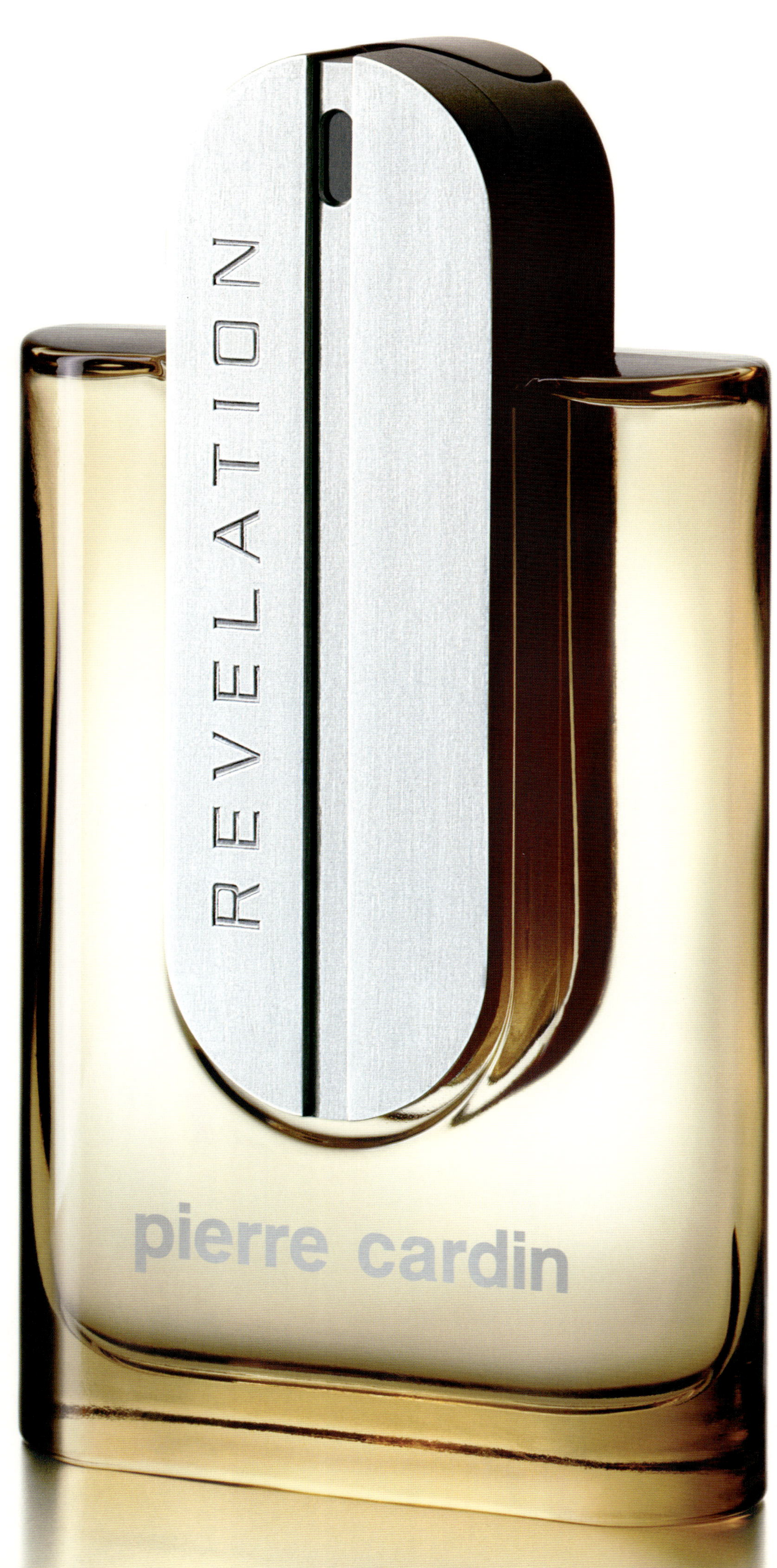
REVELATION
pierre cardin

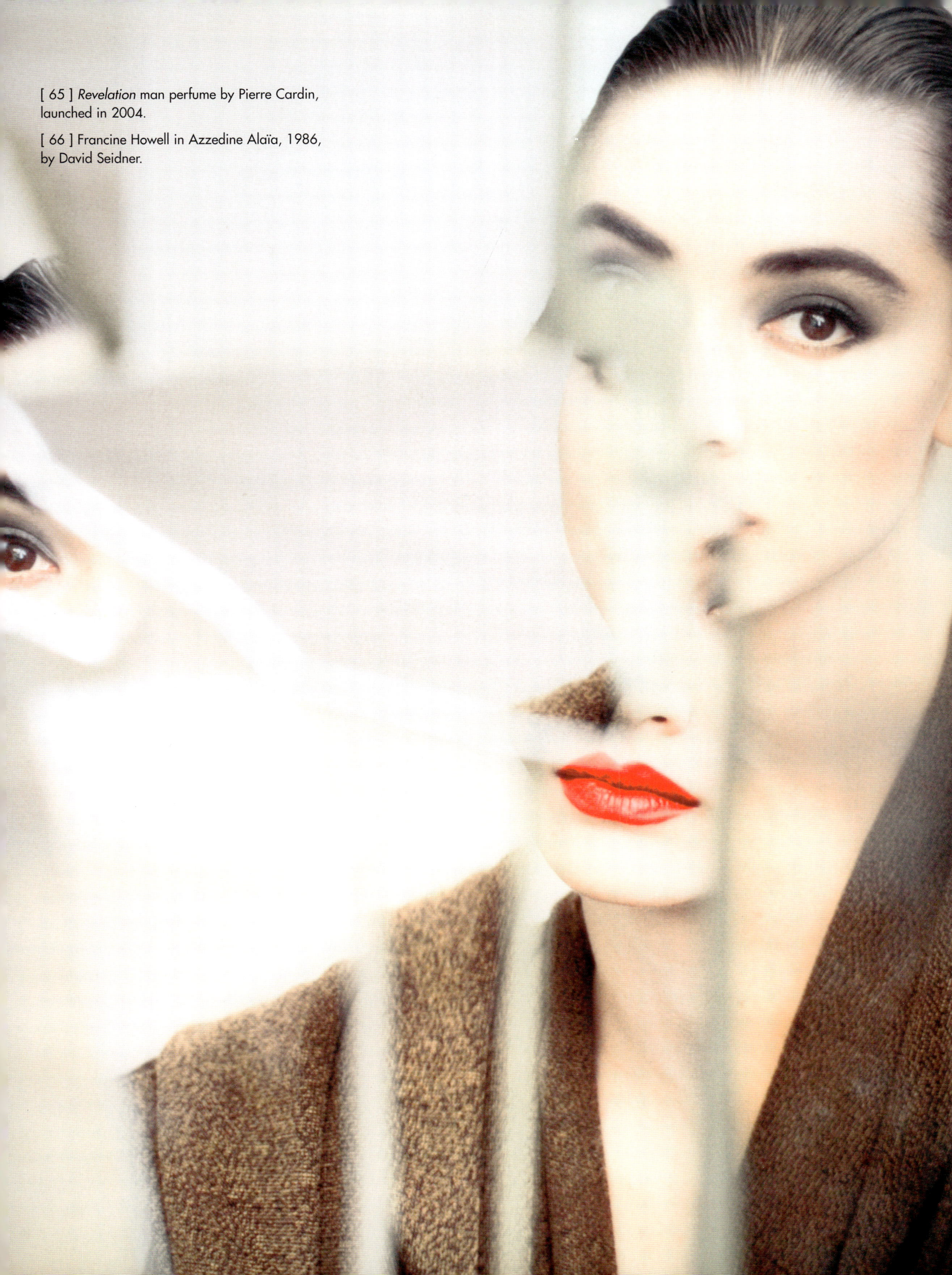

[65] *Revelation* man perfume by Pierre Cardin, launched in 2004.

[66] Francine Howell in Azzedine Alaïa, 1986, by David Seidner.

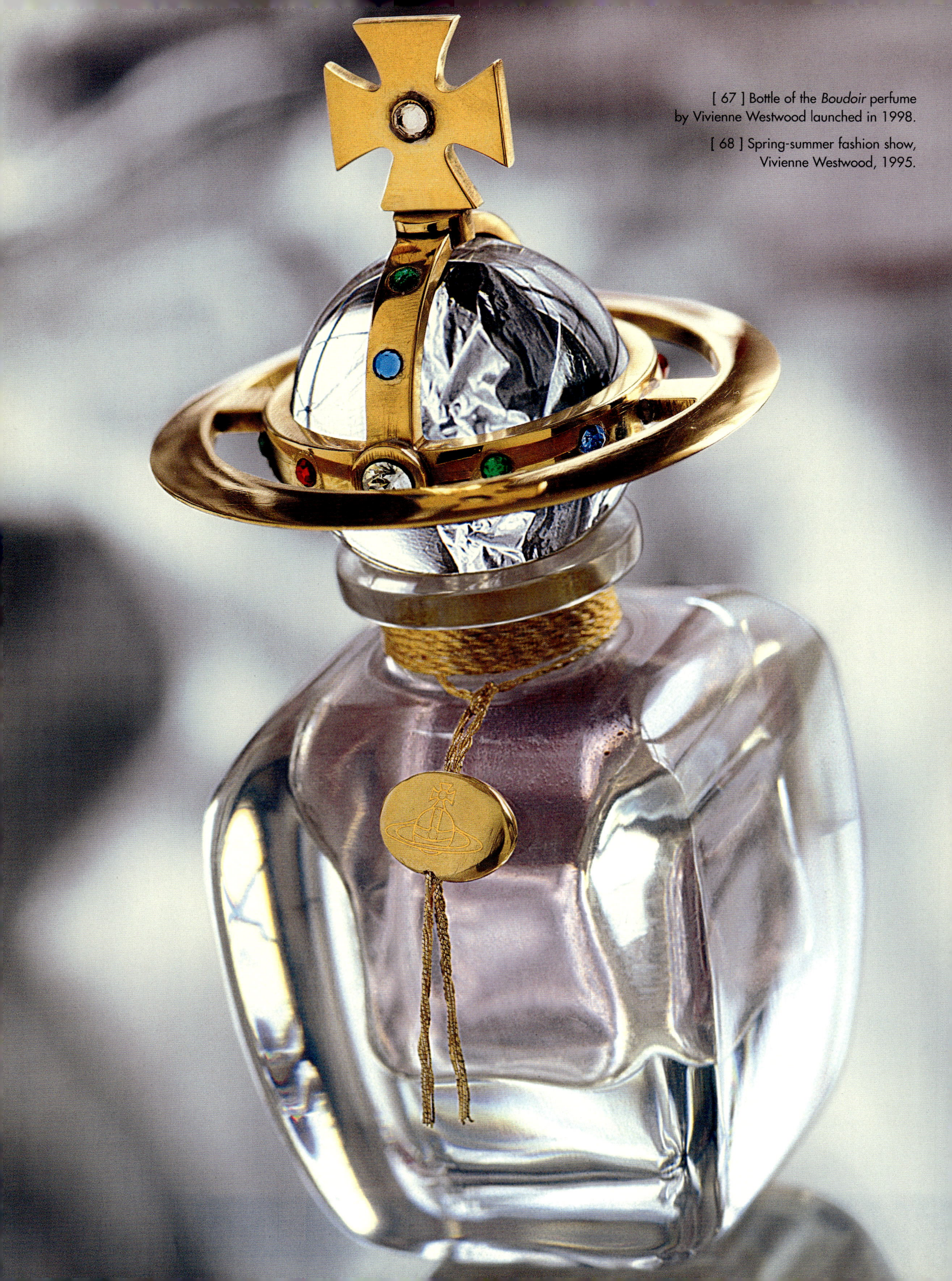

[67] Bottle of the *Boudoir* perfume by Vivienne Westwood launched in 1998.

[68] Spring-summer fashion show, Vivienne Westwood, 1995.

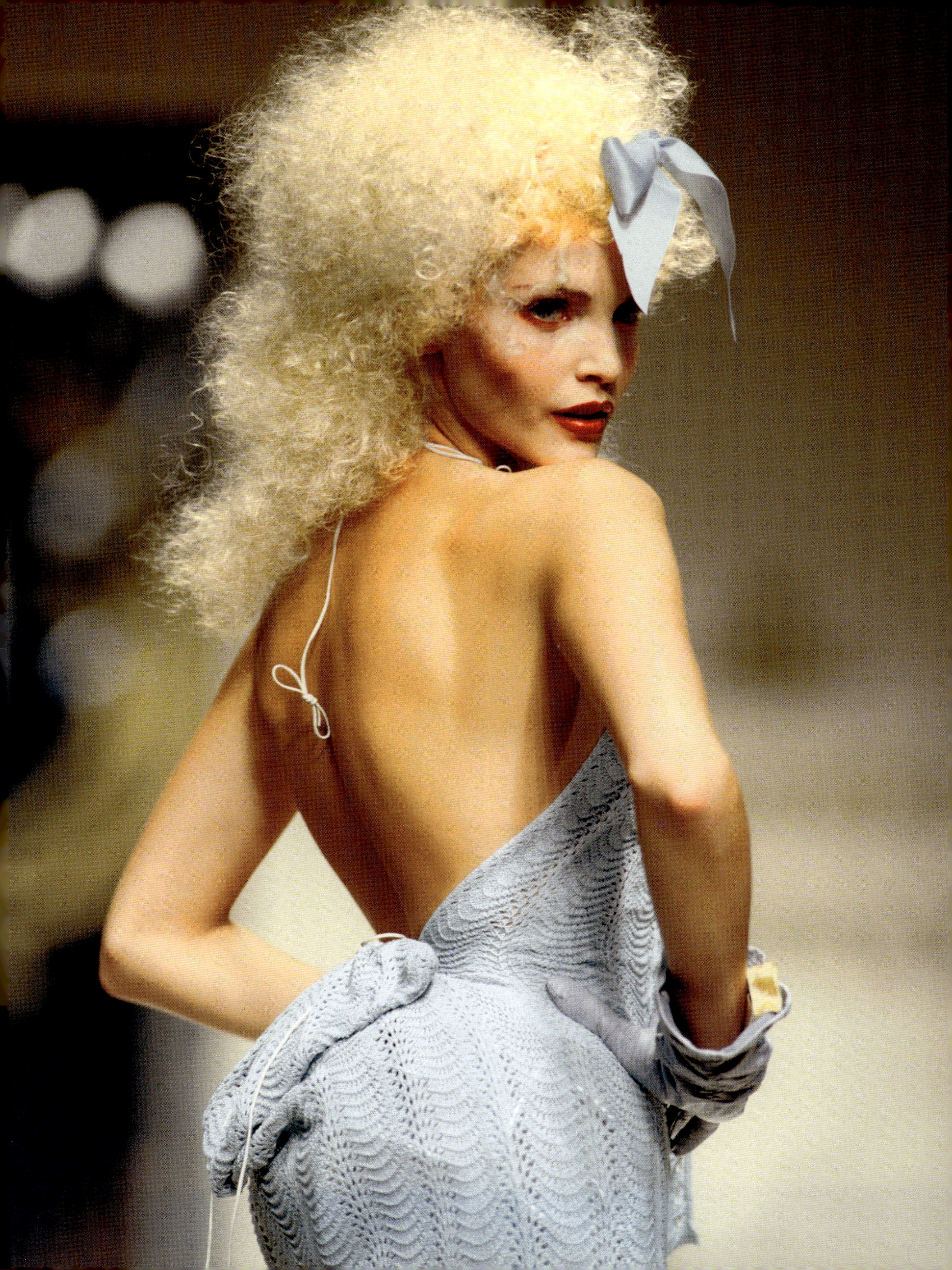

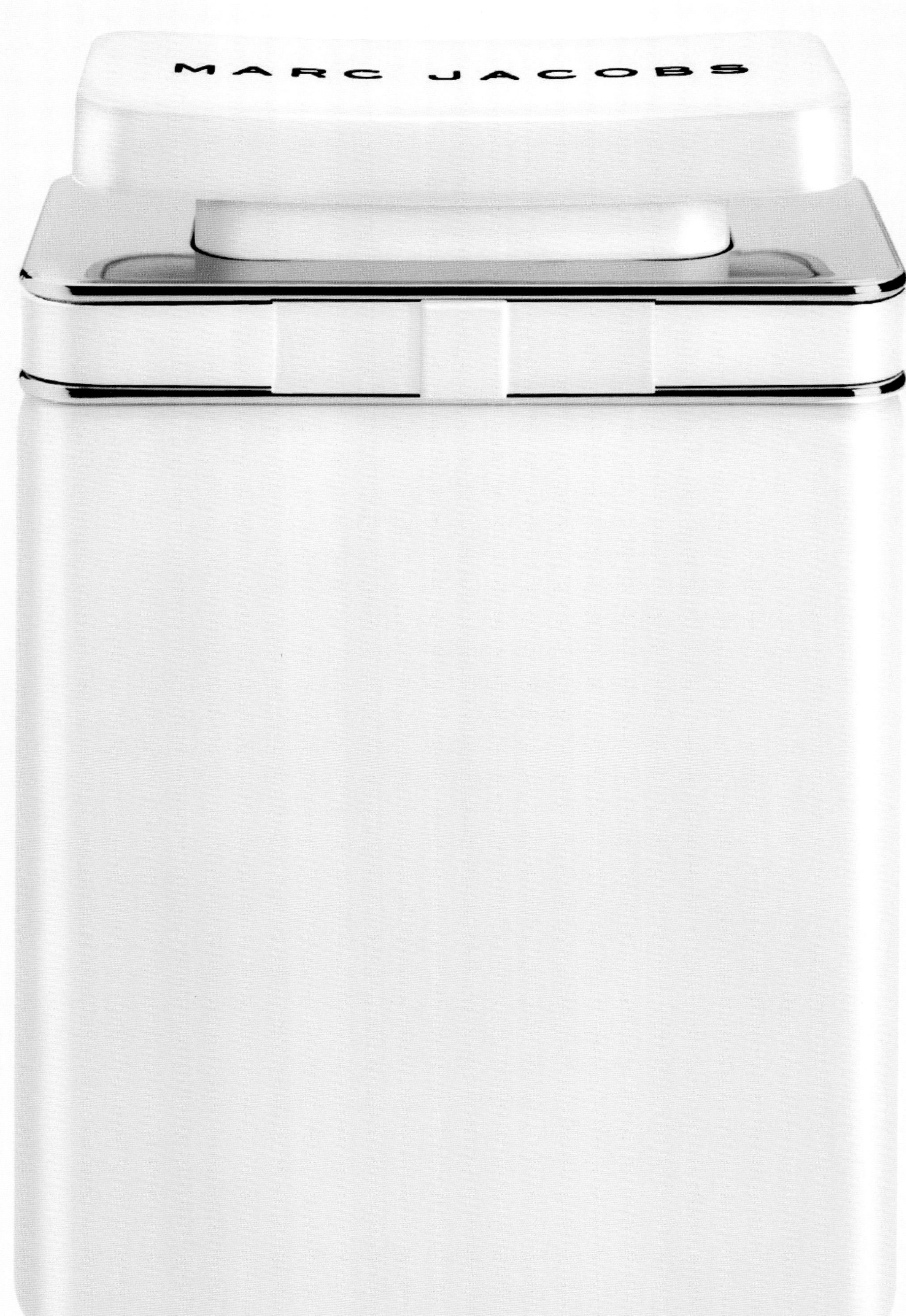
MARC JACOBS

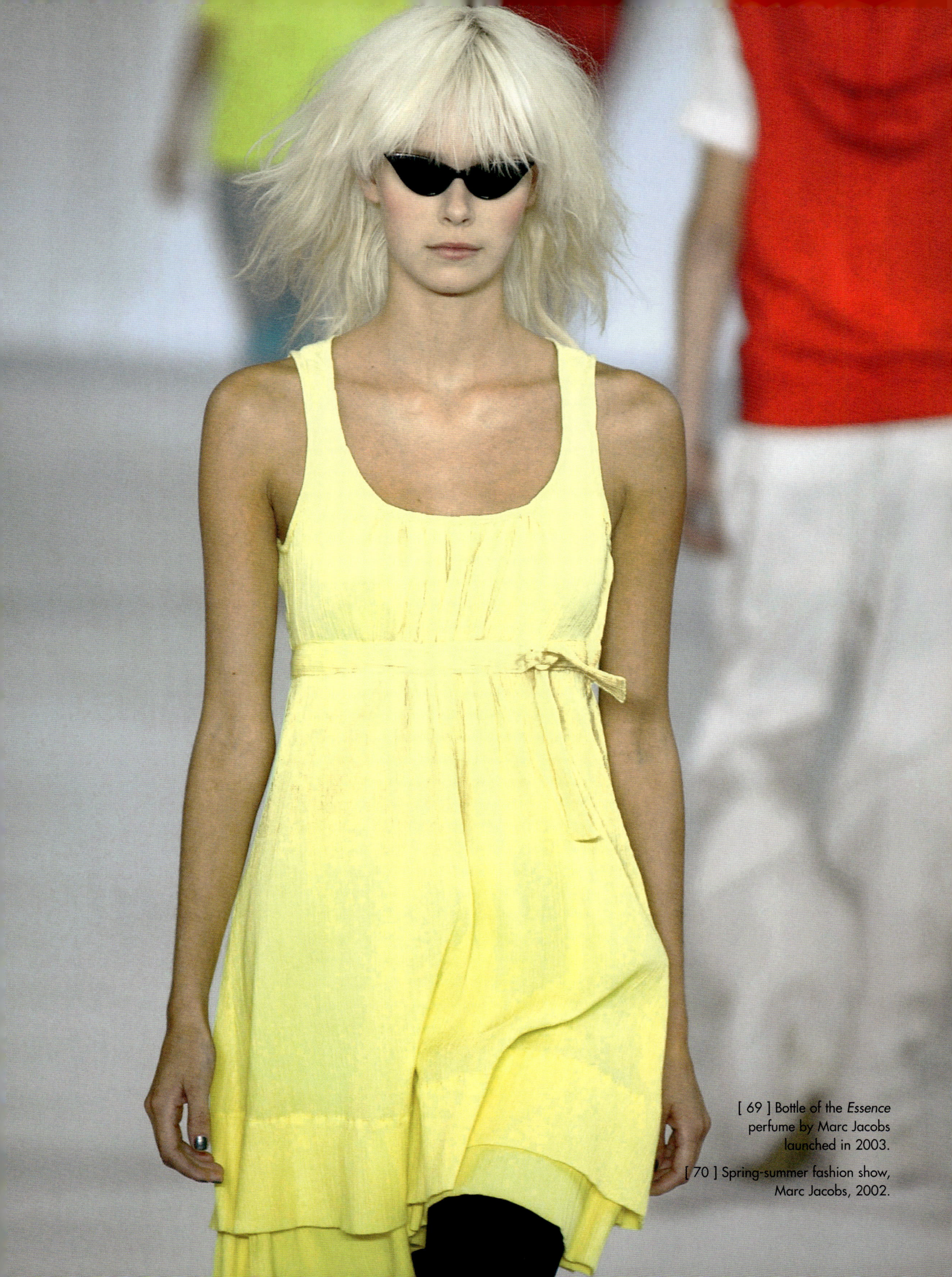

[69] Bottle of the *Essence* perfume by Marc Jacobs launched in 2003.

[70] Spring-summer fashion show, Marc Jacobs, 2002.

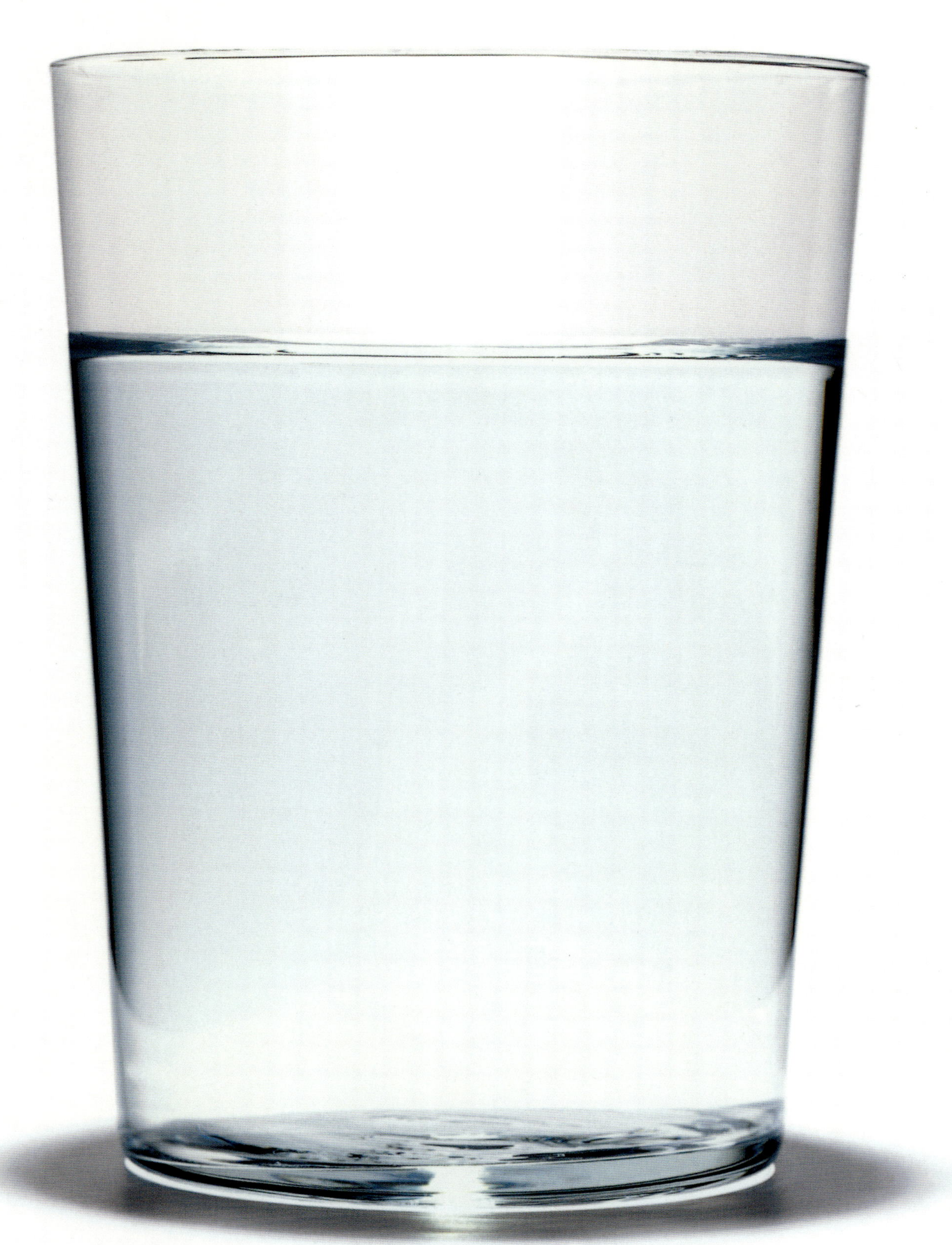

[71] Still life by Laziz Hamani, 2000.

[72] Advertising for the *Echo* perfume by Davidoff, launched in 2003.

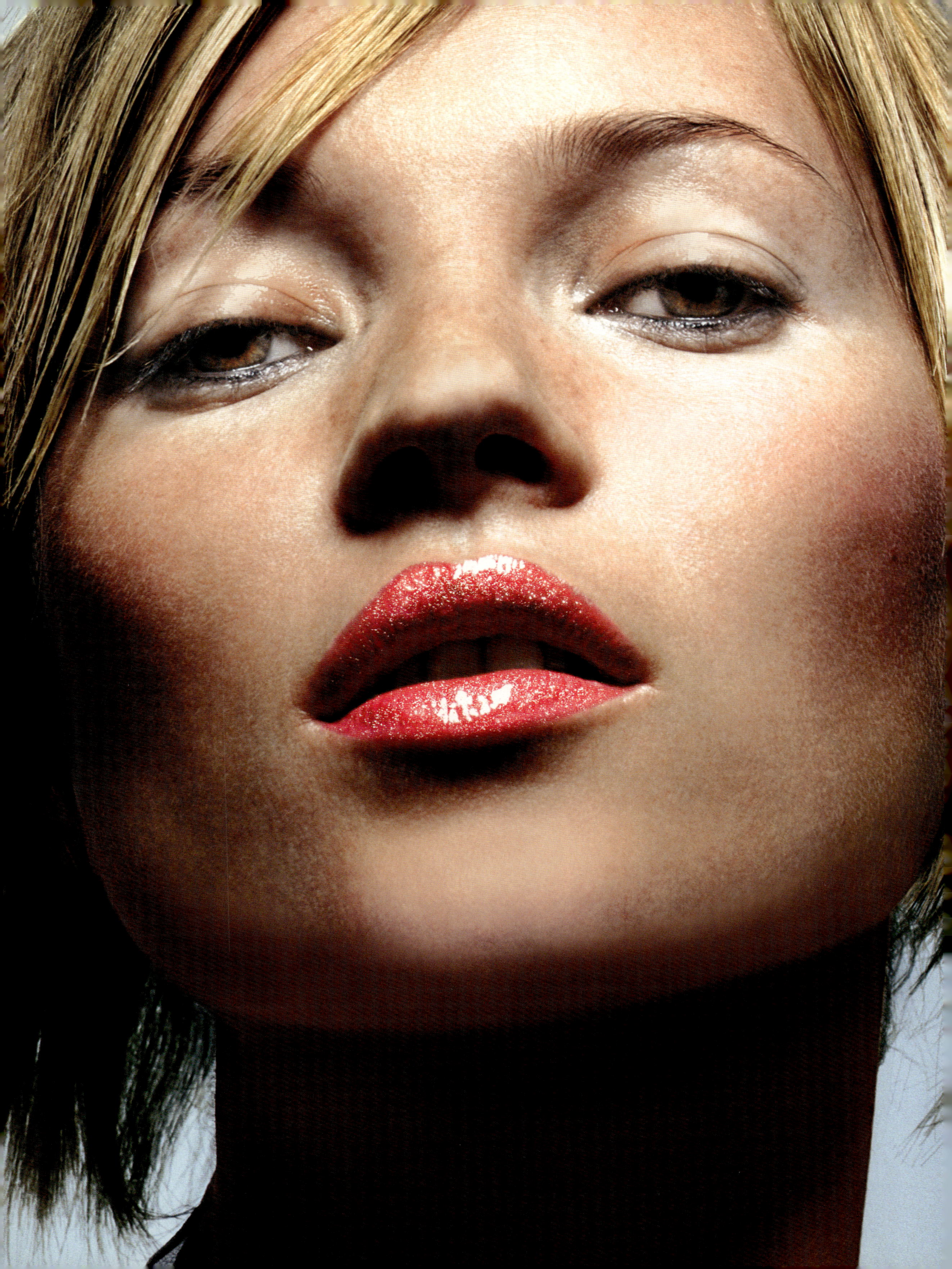

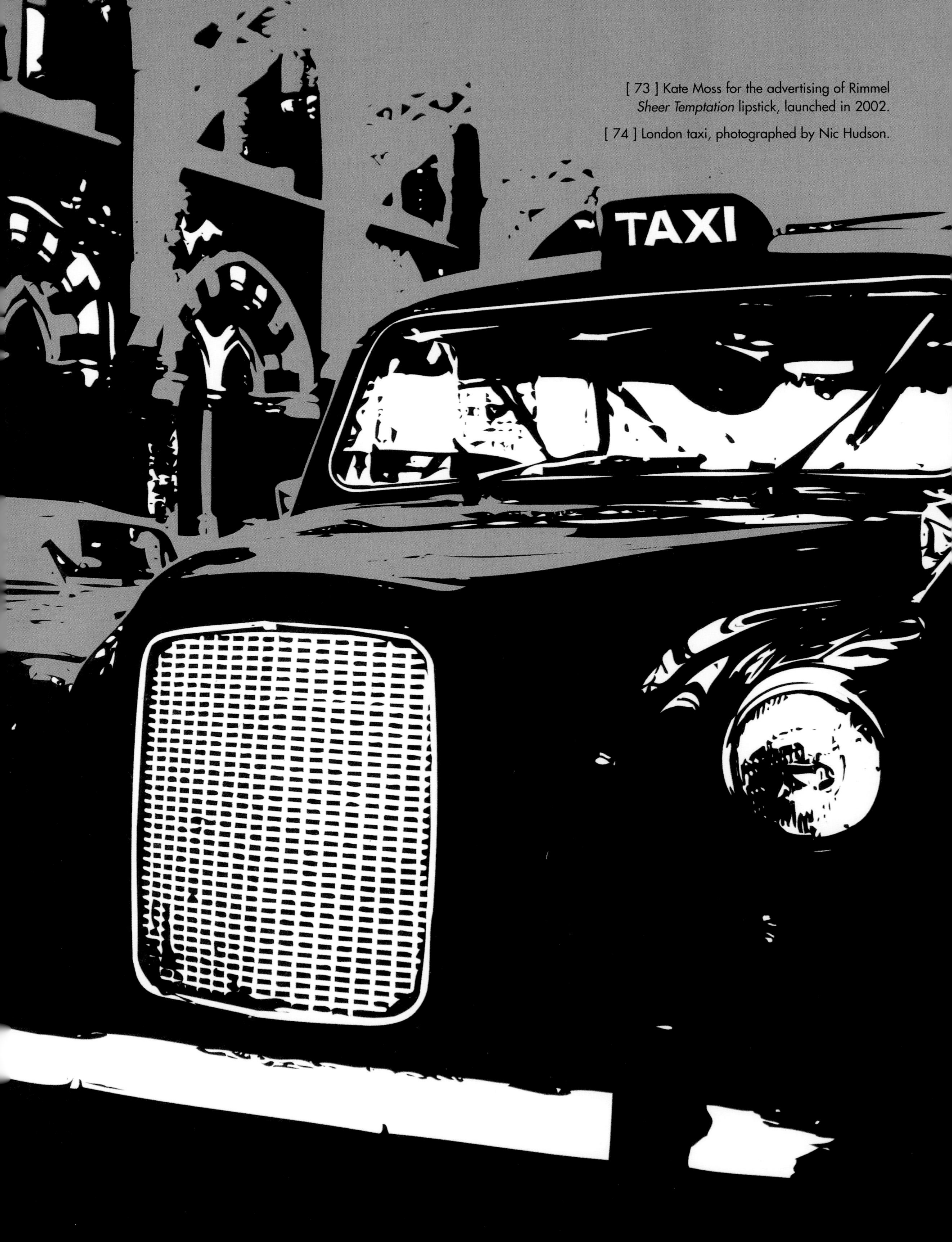

[73] Kate Moss for the advertising of Rimmel *Sheer Temptation* lipstick, launched in 2002.

[74] London taxi, photographed by Nic Hudson.

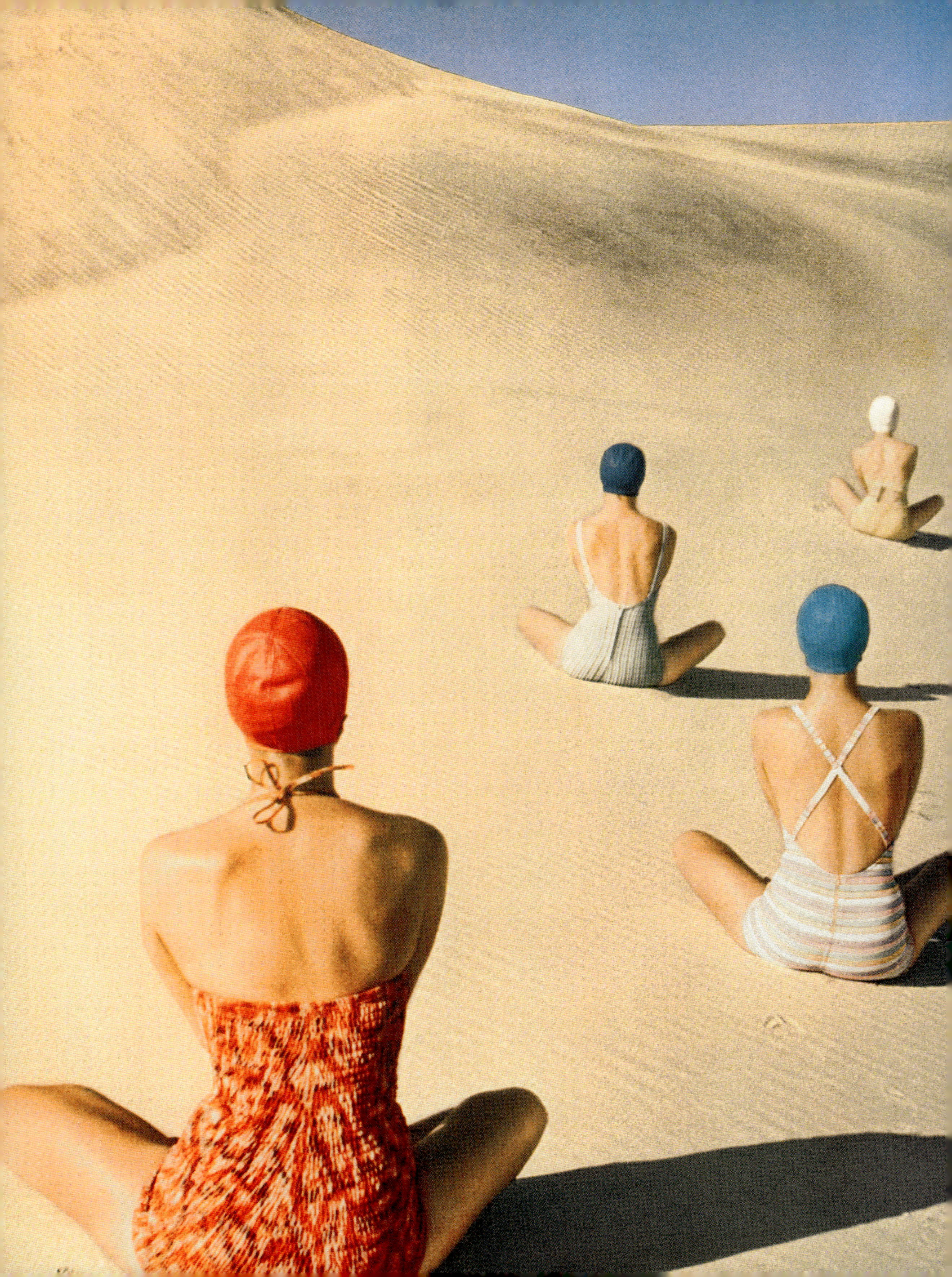

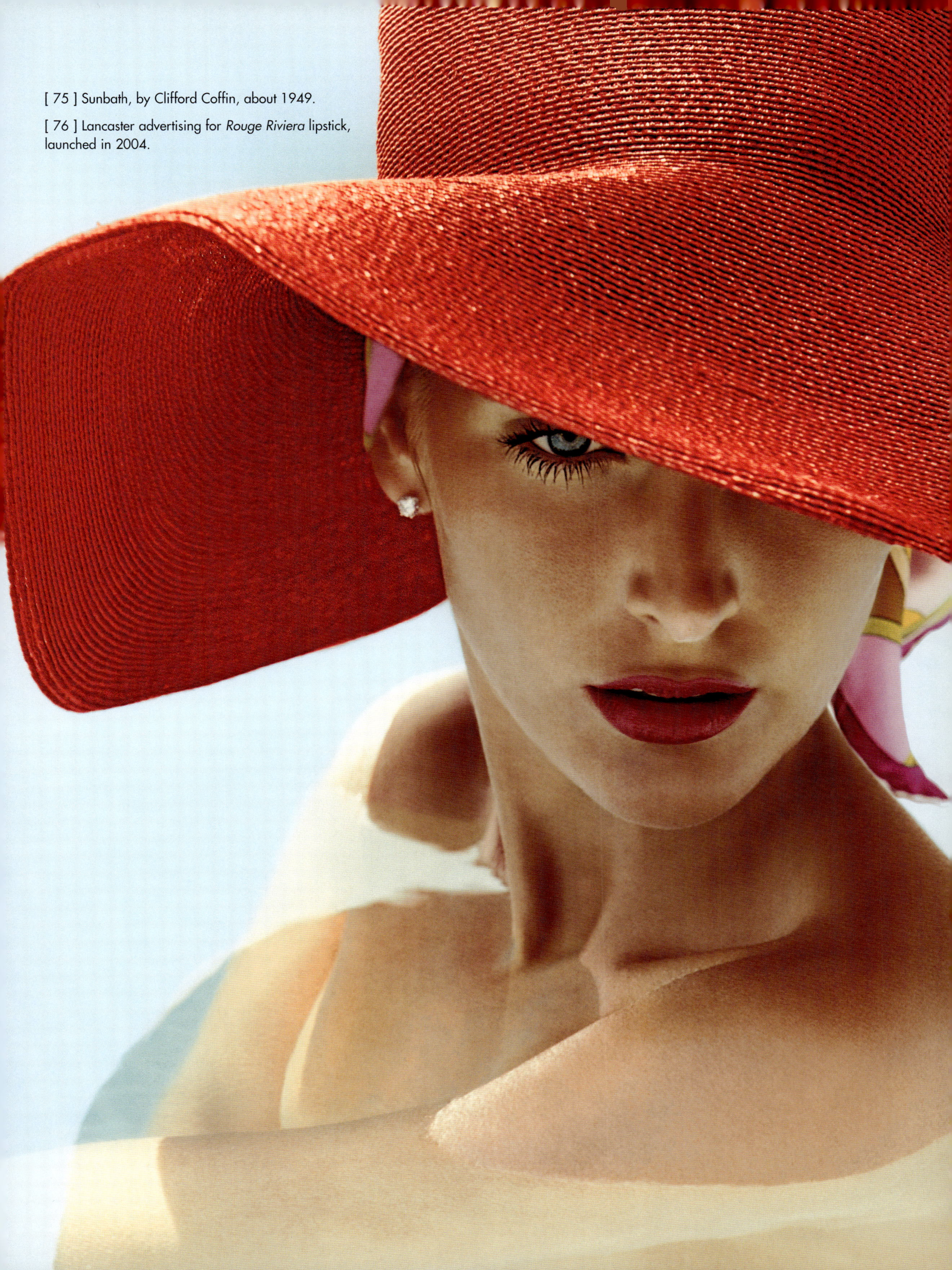

[75] Sunbath, by Clifford Coffin, about 1949.

[76] Lancaster advertising for *Rouge Riviera* lipstick, launched in 2004.

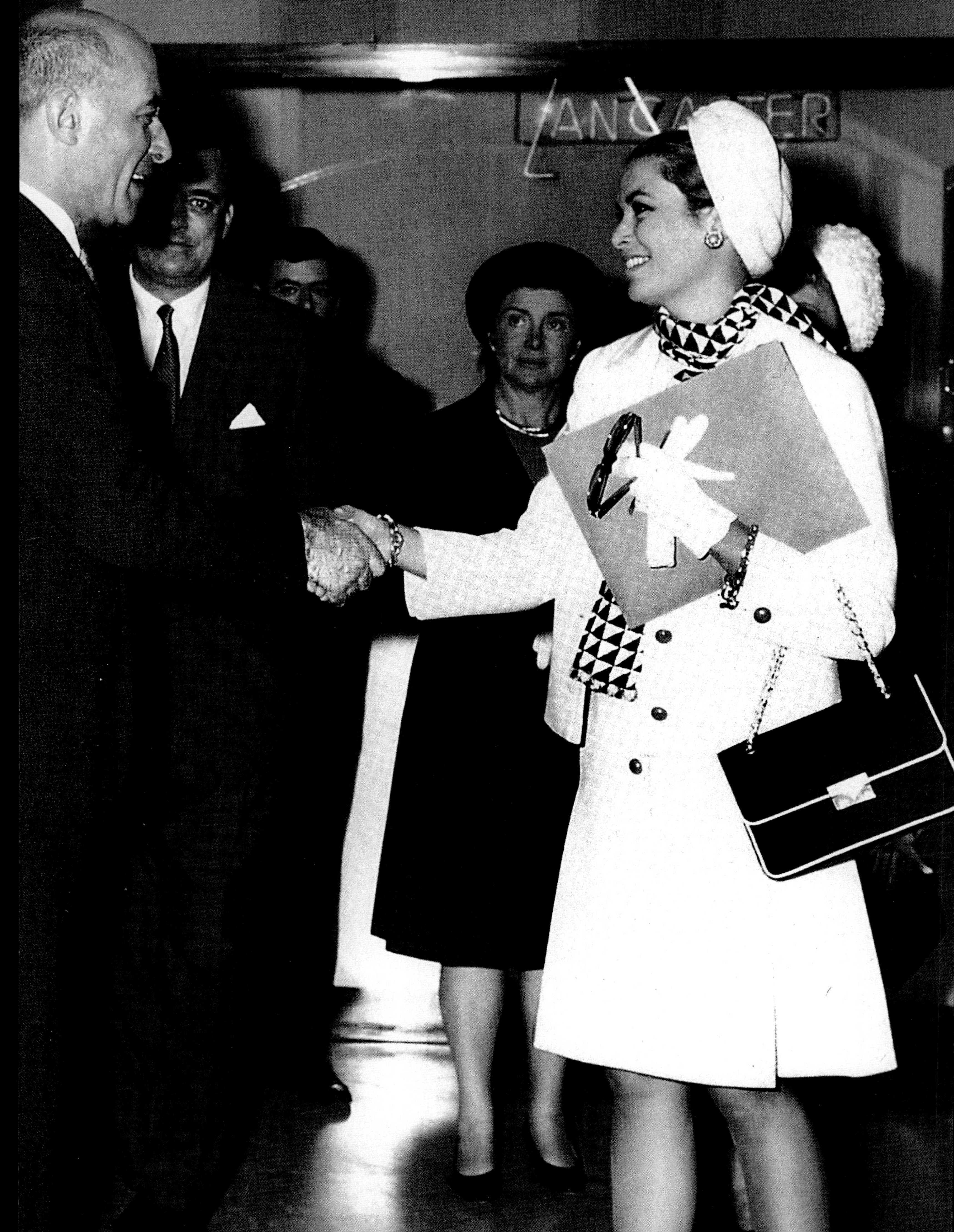

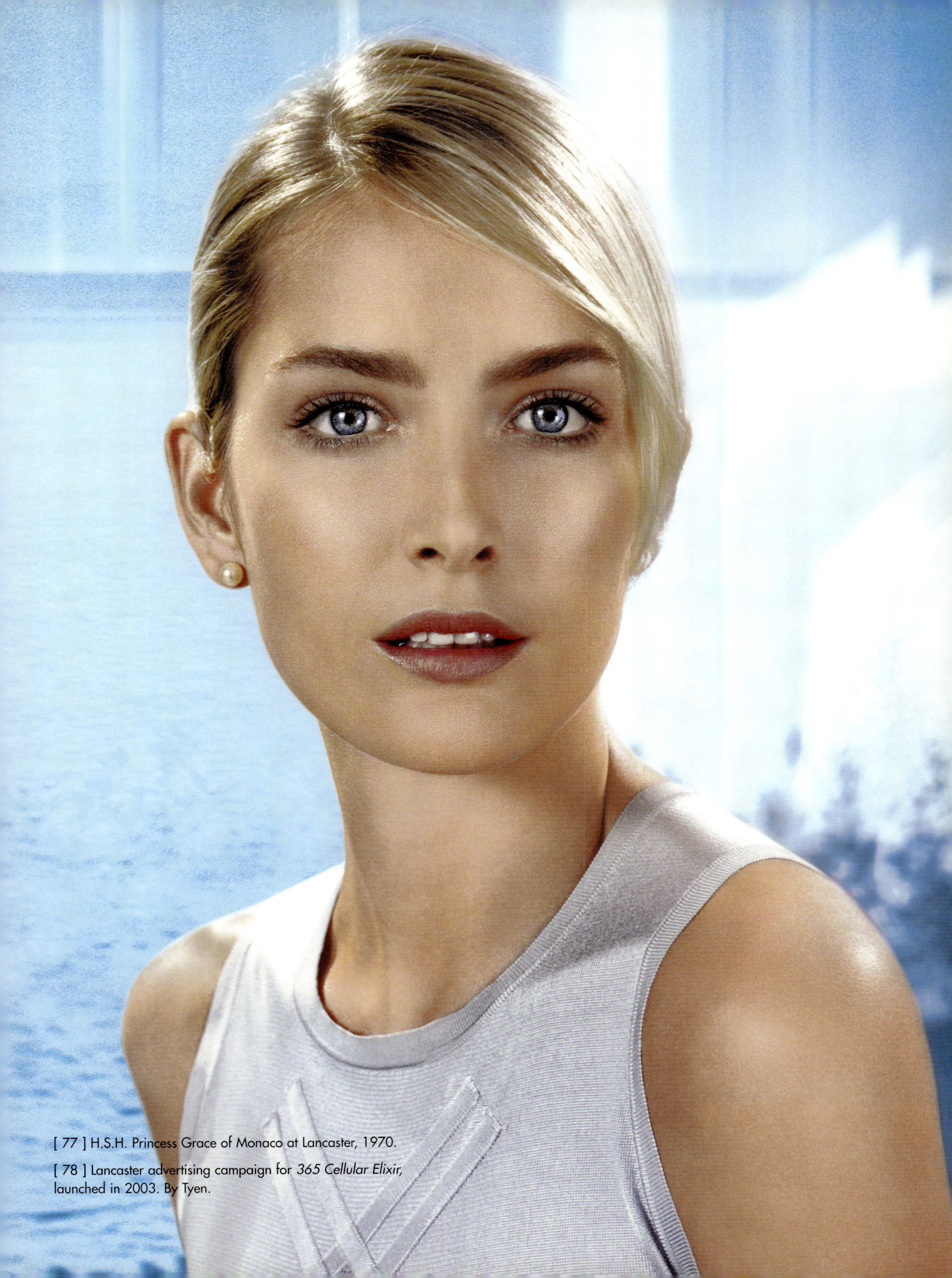

[77] H.S.H. Princess Grace of Monaco at Lancaster, 1970.

[78] Lancaster advertising campaign for *365 Cellular Elixir*, launched in 2003. By Tyen.

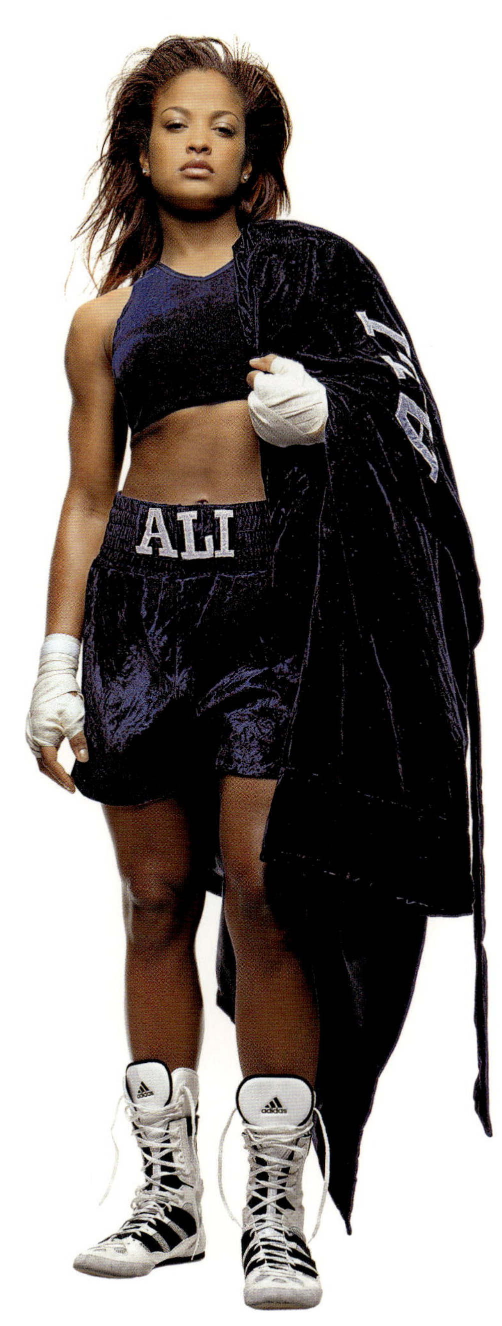

[79] Laïla Ali, Mohammed Ali's daughter, in adidas, photographed by Gilles Bensimon, 2000.

[80] Advertising for the *Active Skincare for Men* care line of adidas, launched in 2003.

Following pages:
[81] Photograph by Guy Bourdin for *Vogue,* 1970.

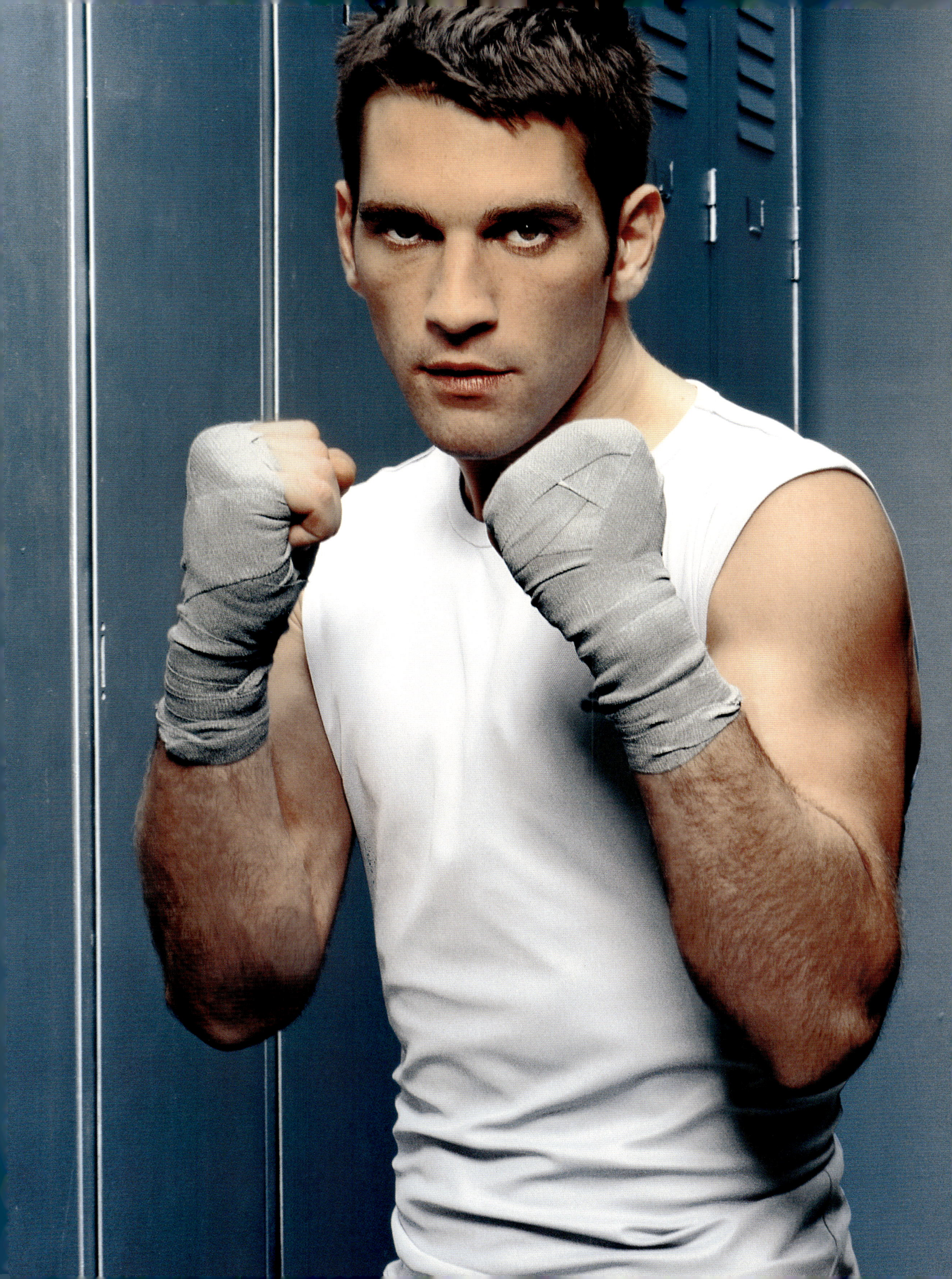

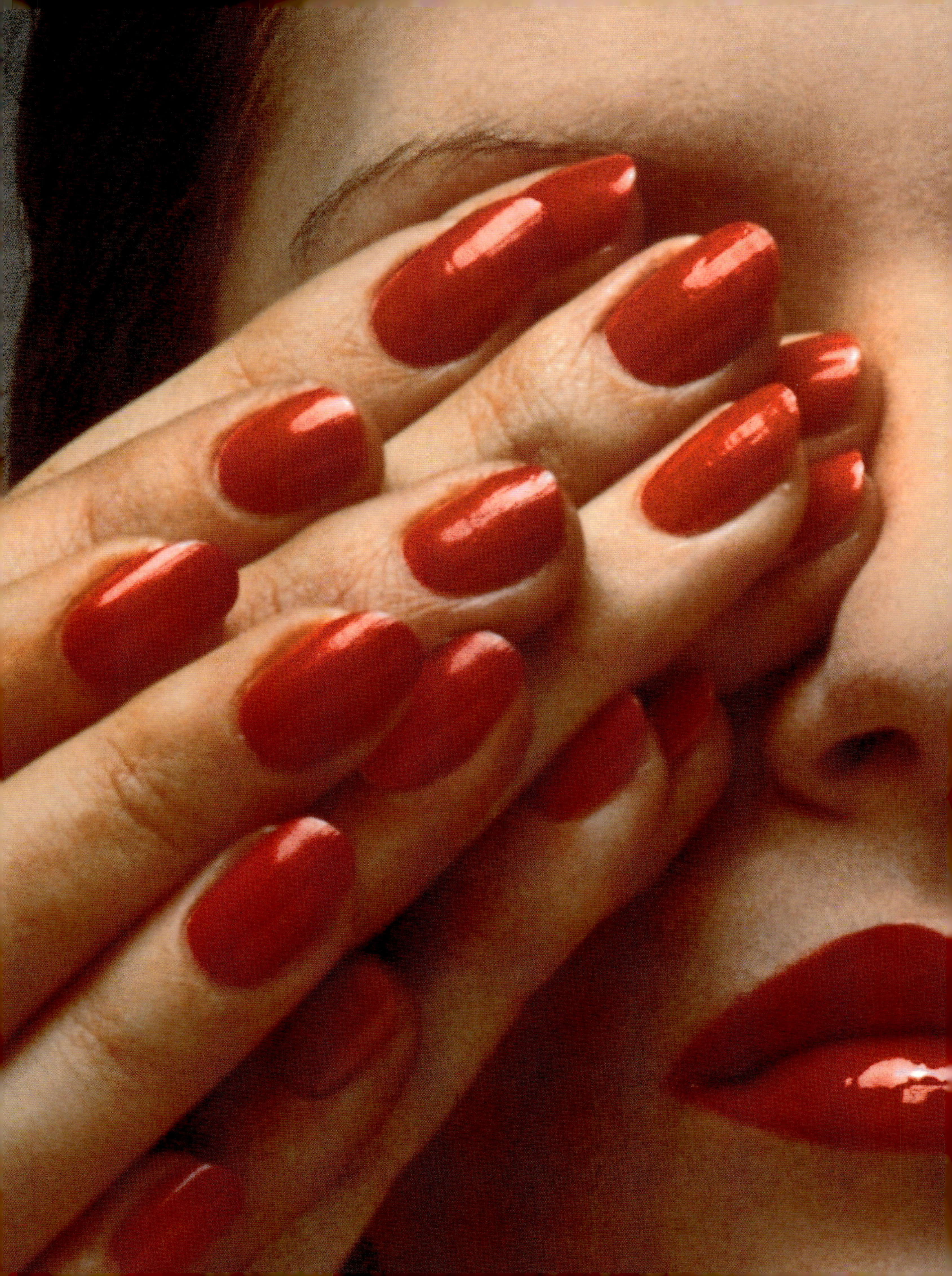

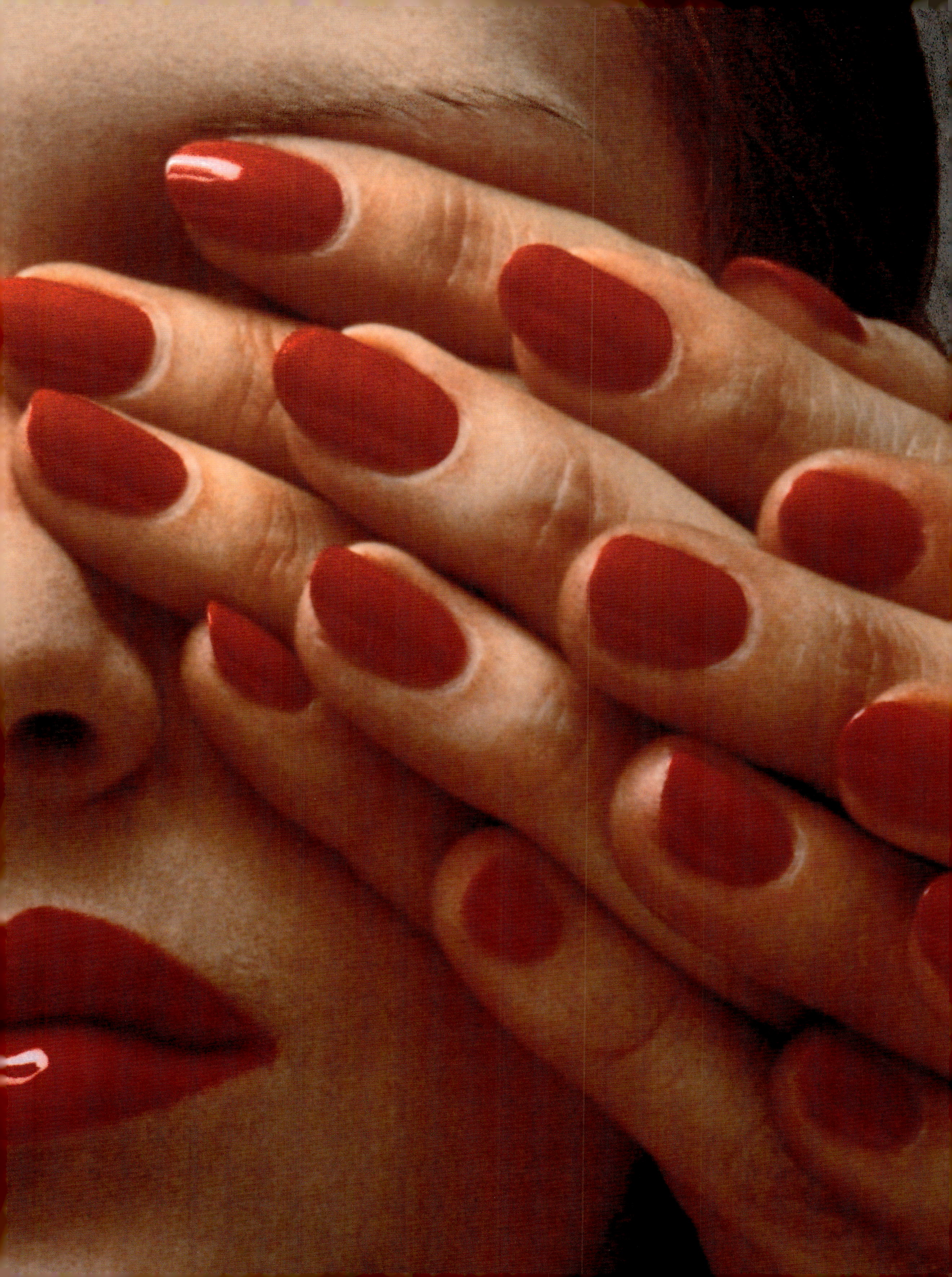

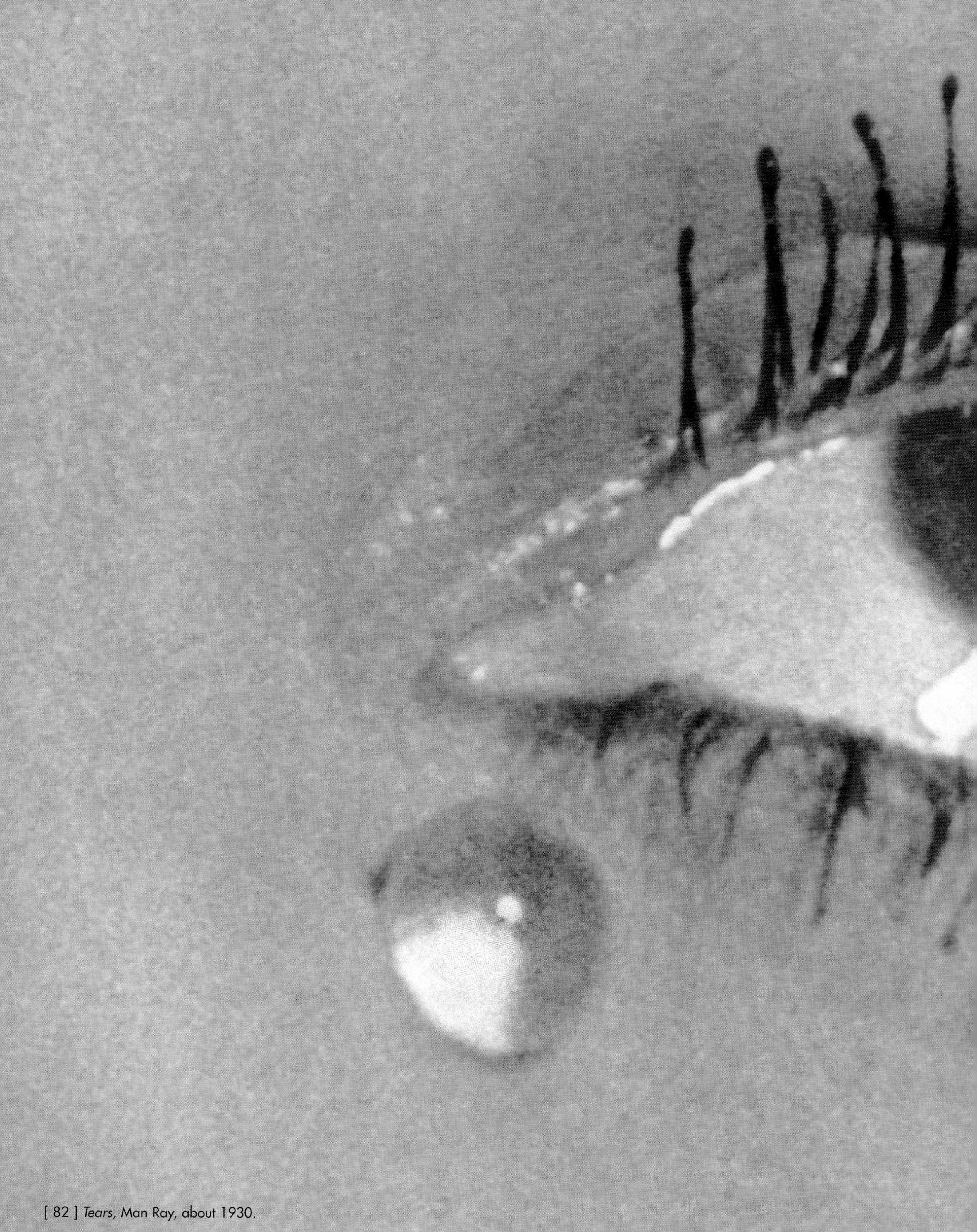

[82] *Tears,* Man Ray, about 1930.

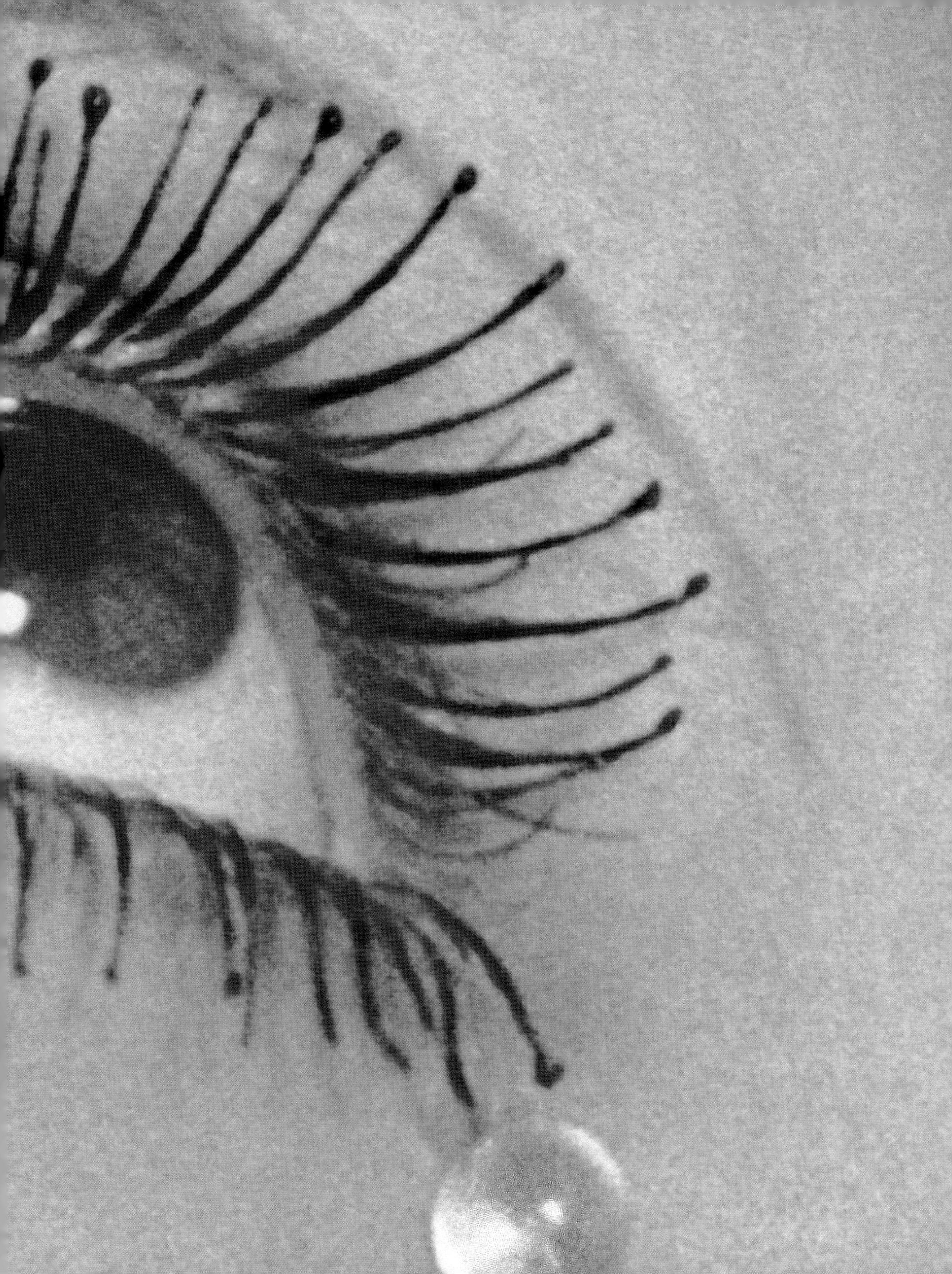

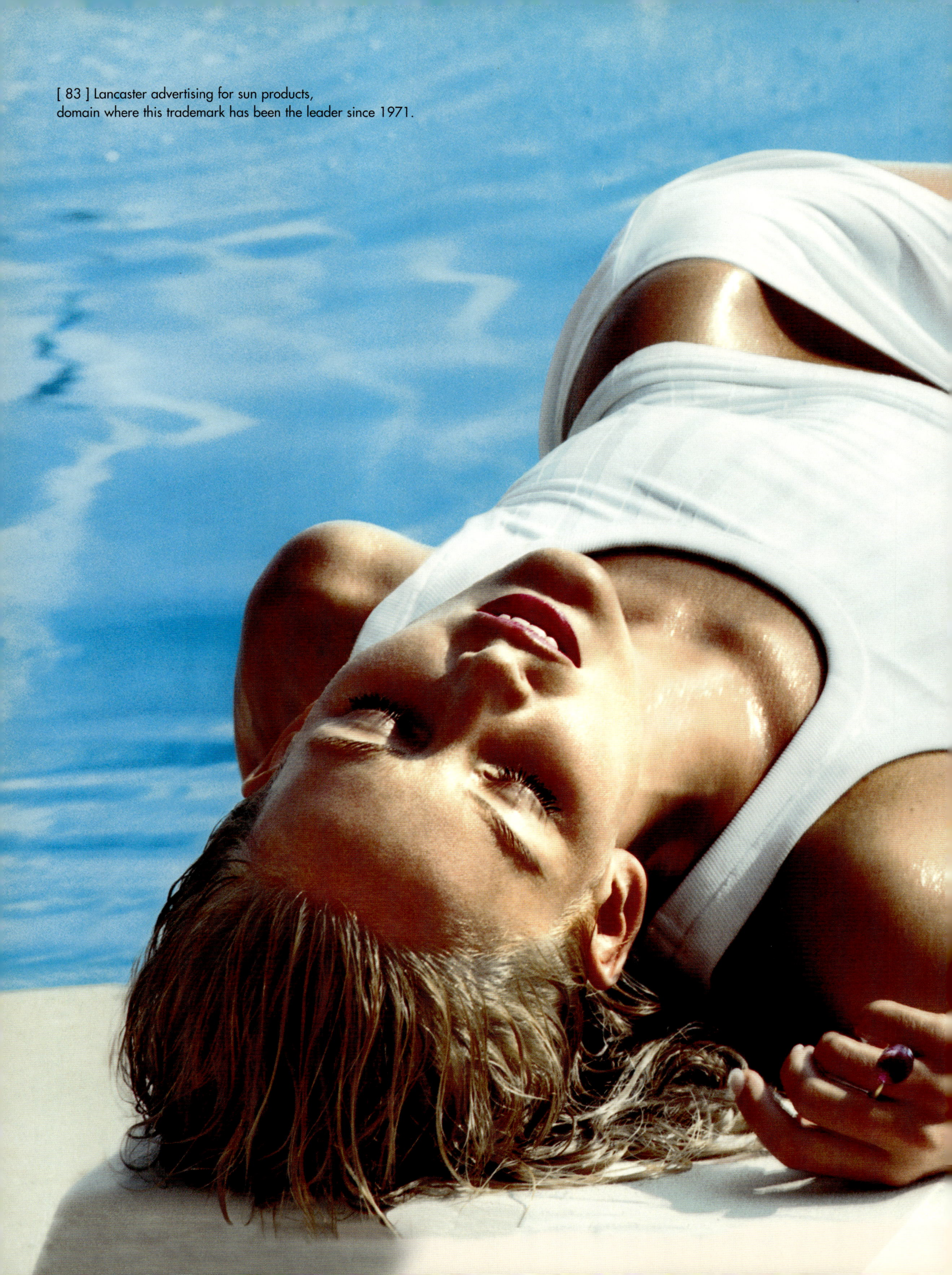

[83] Lancaster advertising for sun products,
domain where this trademark has been the leader since 1971.

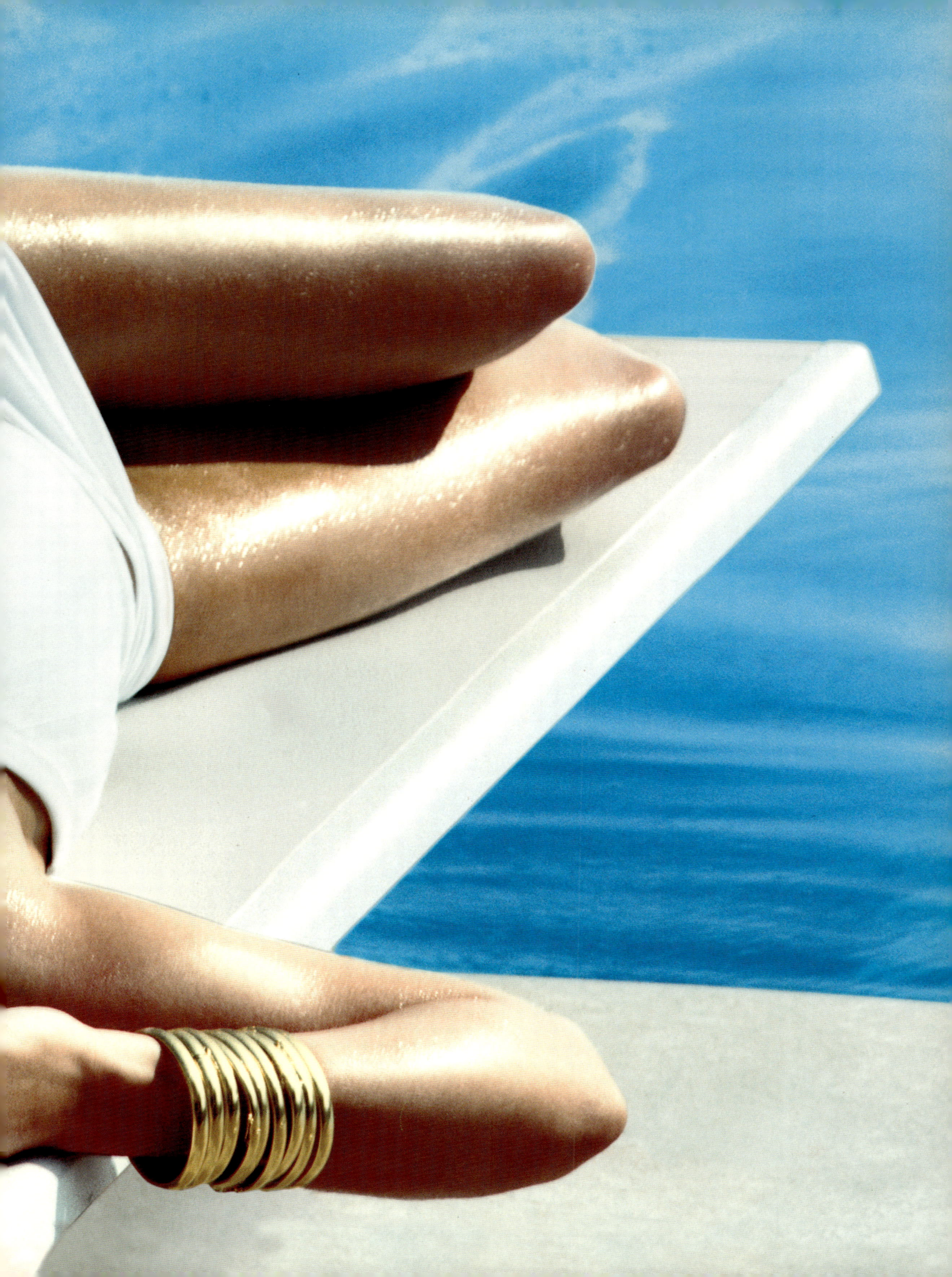

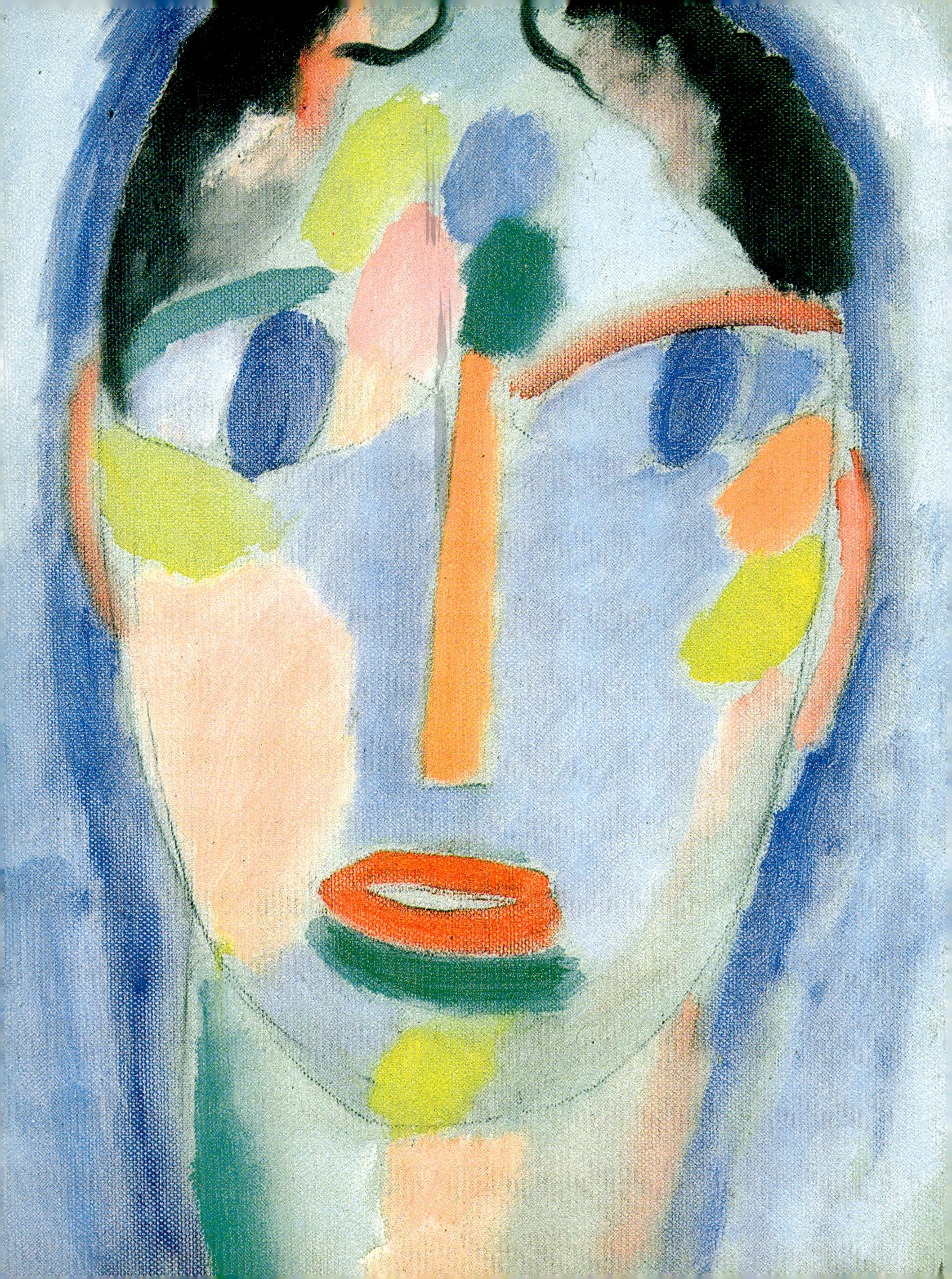

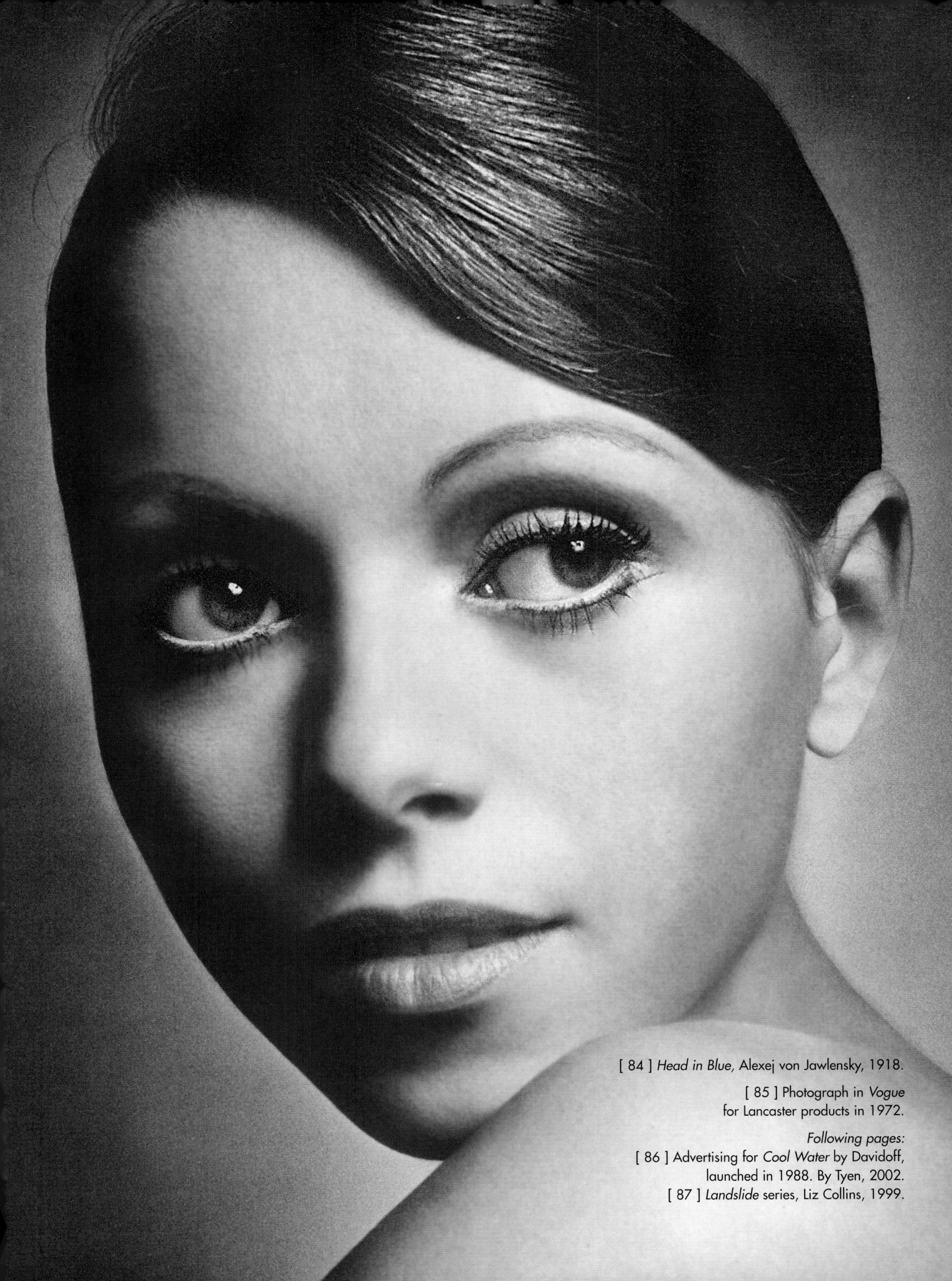

[84] *Head in Blue,* Alexej von Jawlensky, 1918.

[85] Photograph in *Vogue* for Lancaster products in 1972.

Following pages:
[86] Advertising for *Cool Water* by Davidoff, launched in 1988. By Tyen, 2002.
[87] *Landslide* series, Liz Collins, 1999.

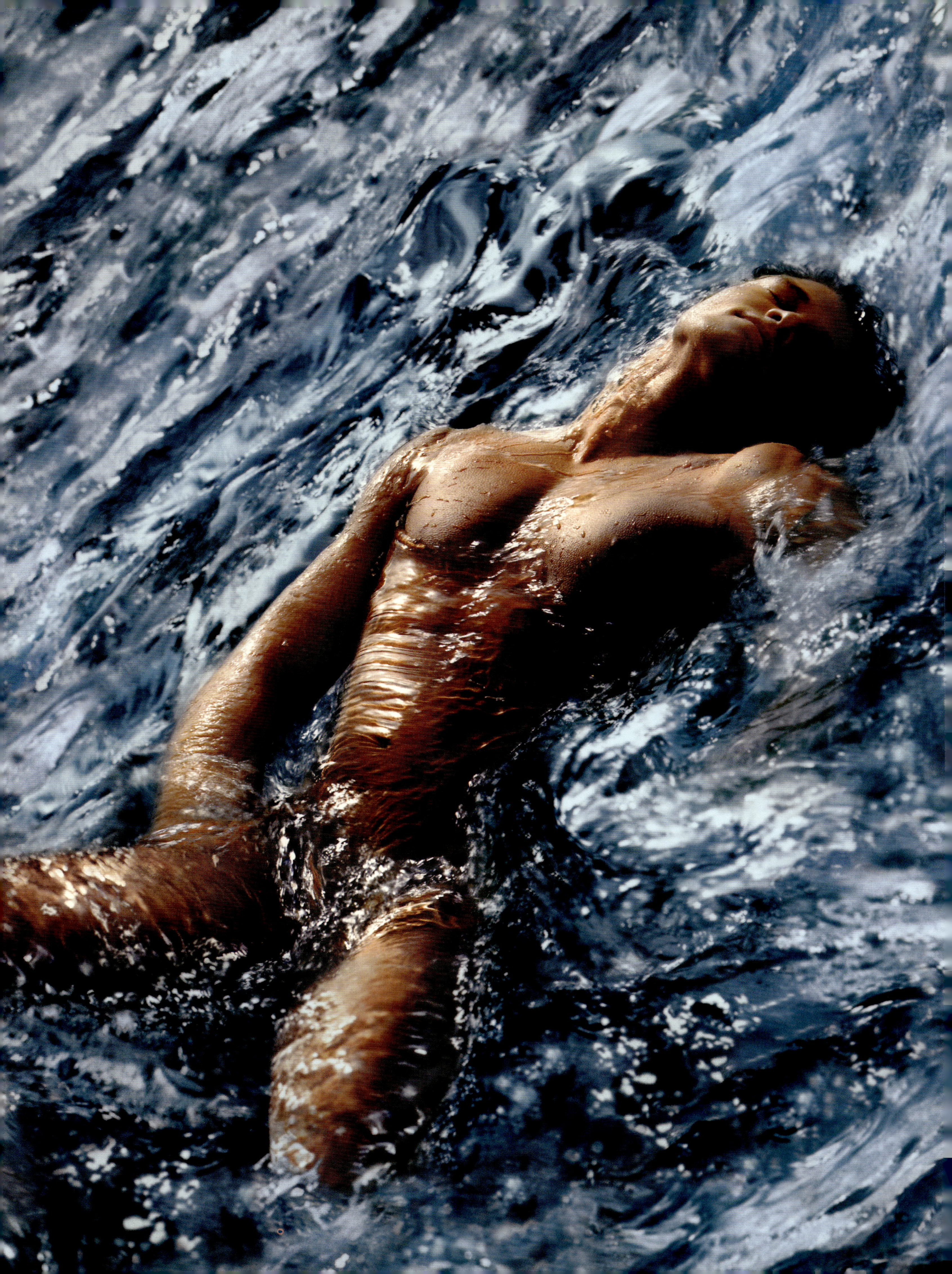

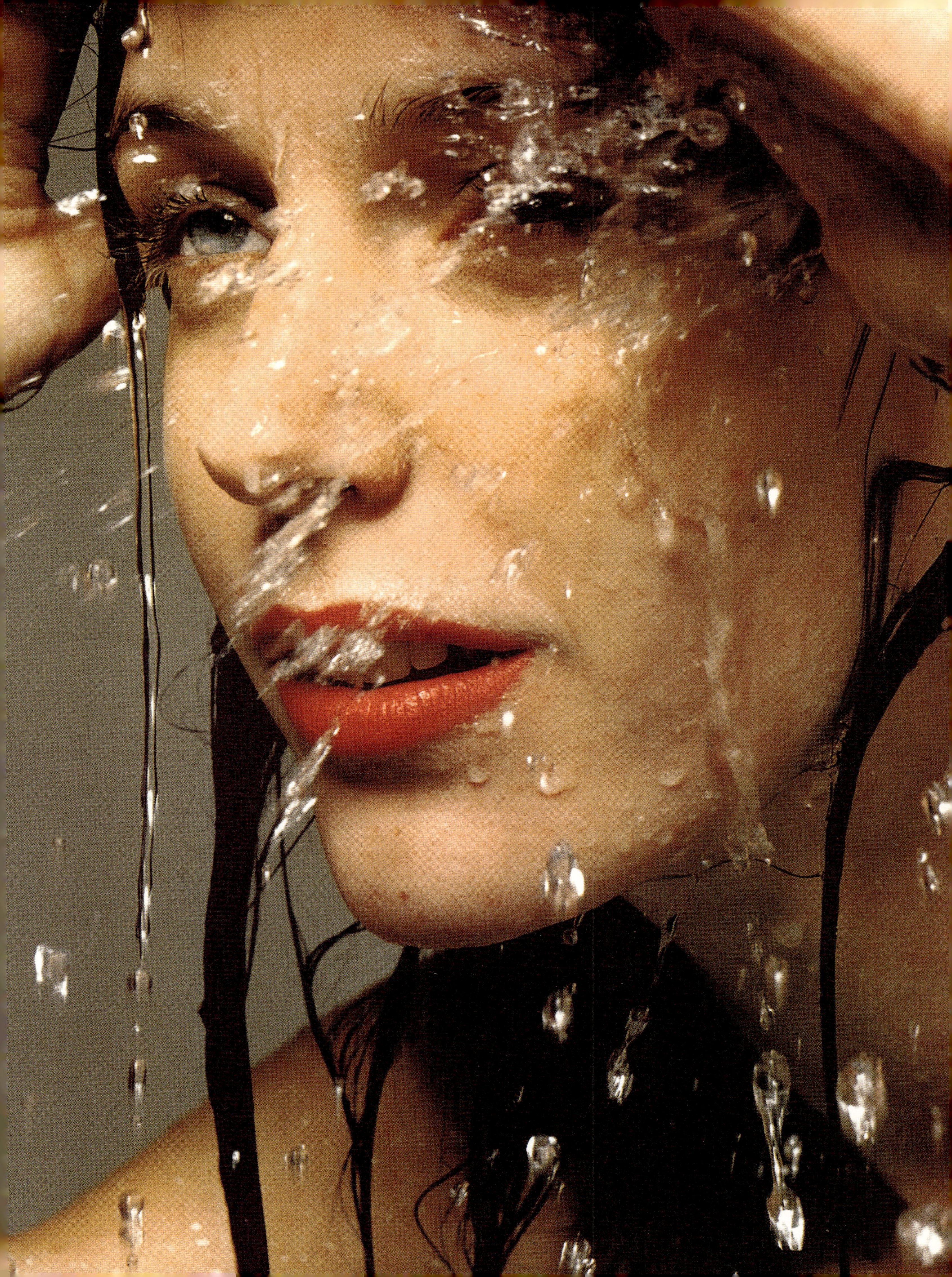

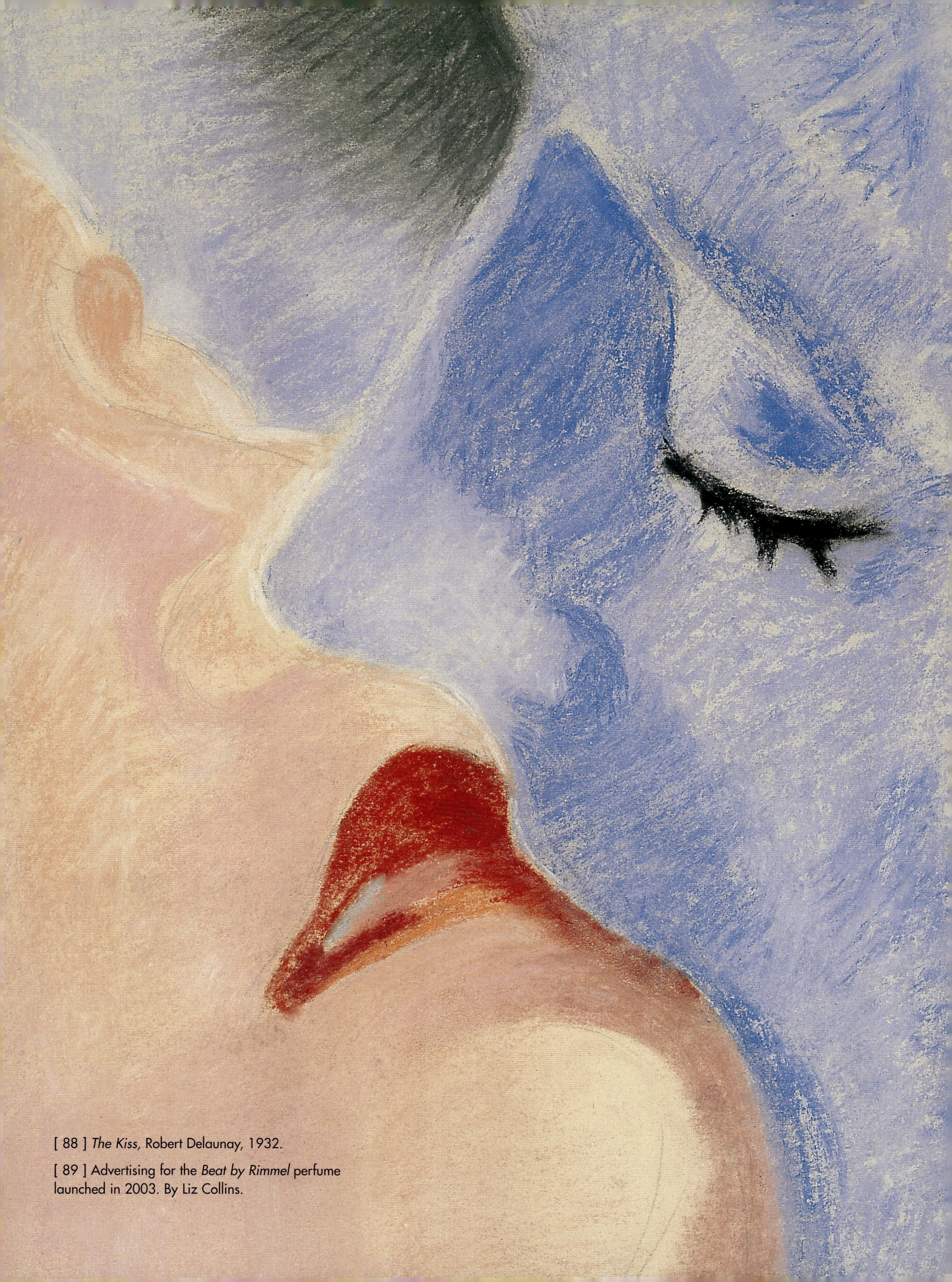

[88] *The Kiss,* Robert Delaunay, 1932.

[89] Advertising for the *Beat by Rimmel* perfume launched in 2003. By Liz Collins.

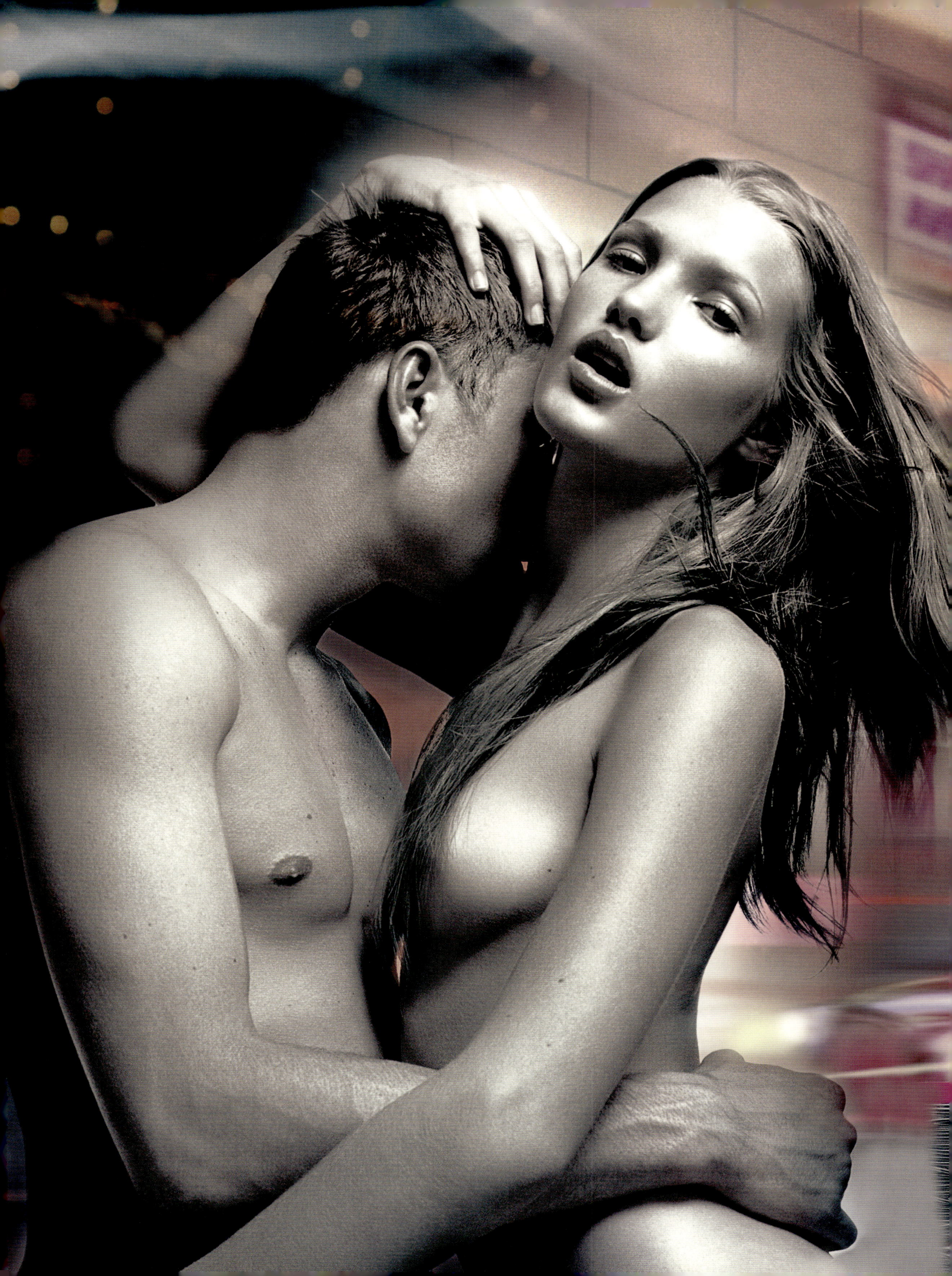

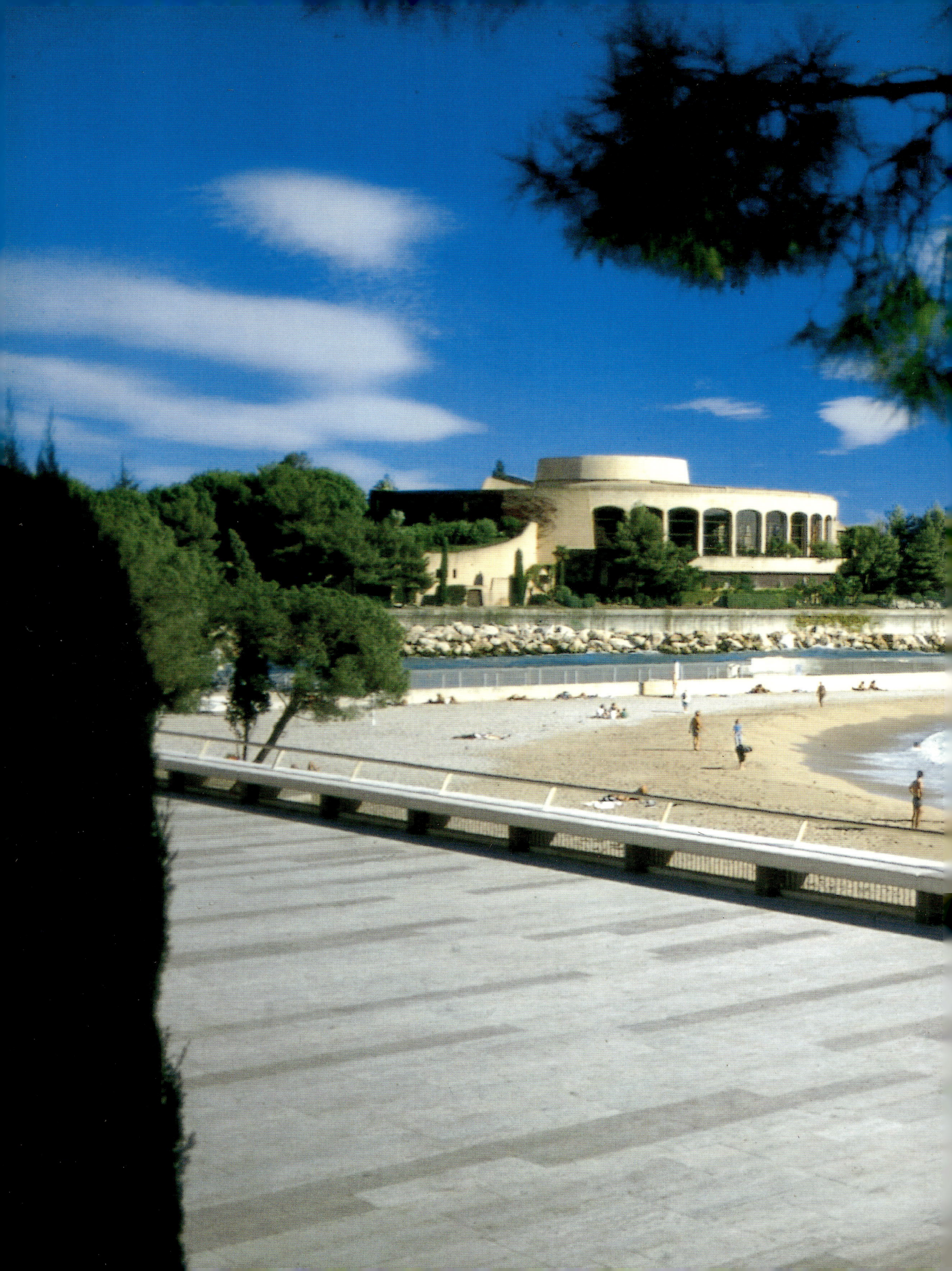

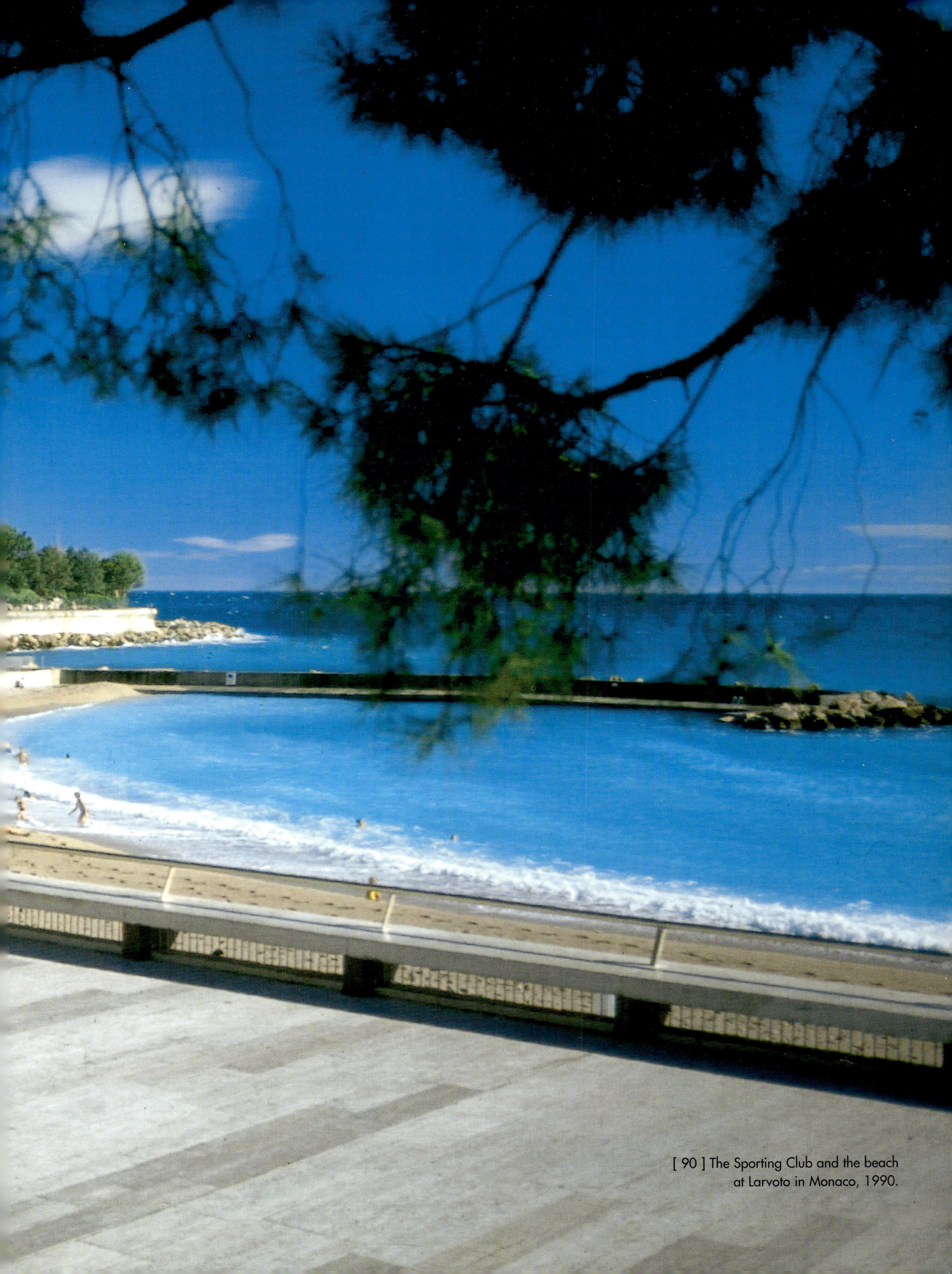

[90] The Sporting Club and the beach
at Larvoto in Monaco, 1990.

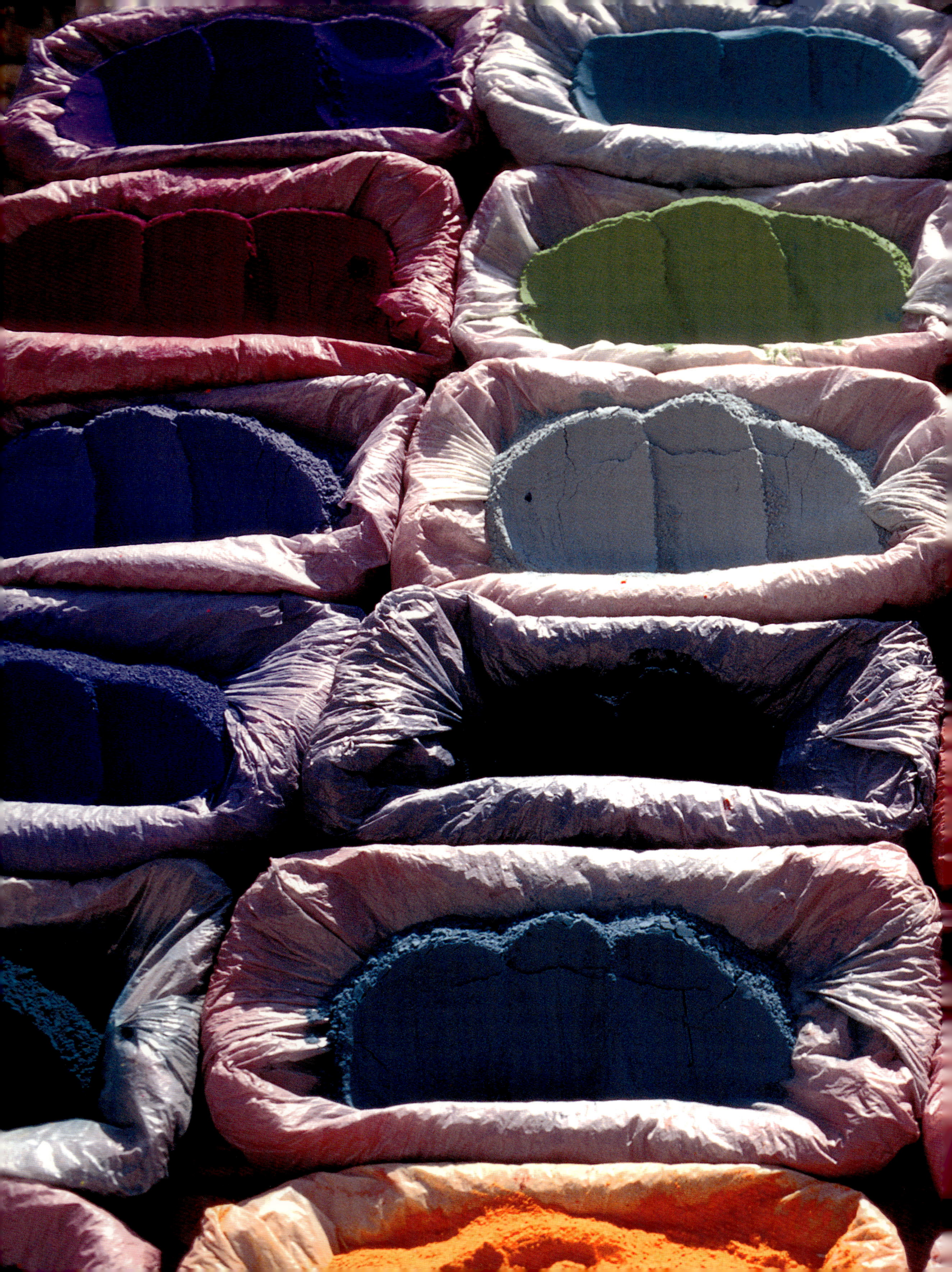

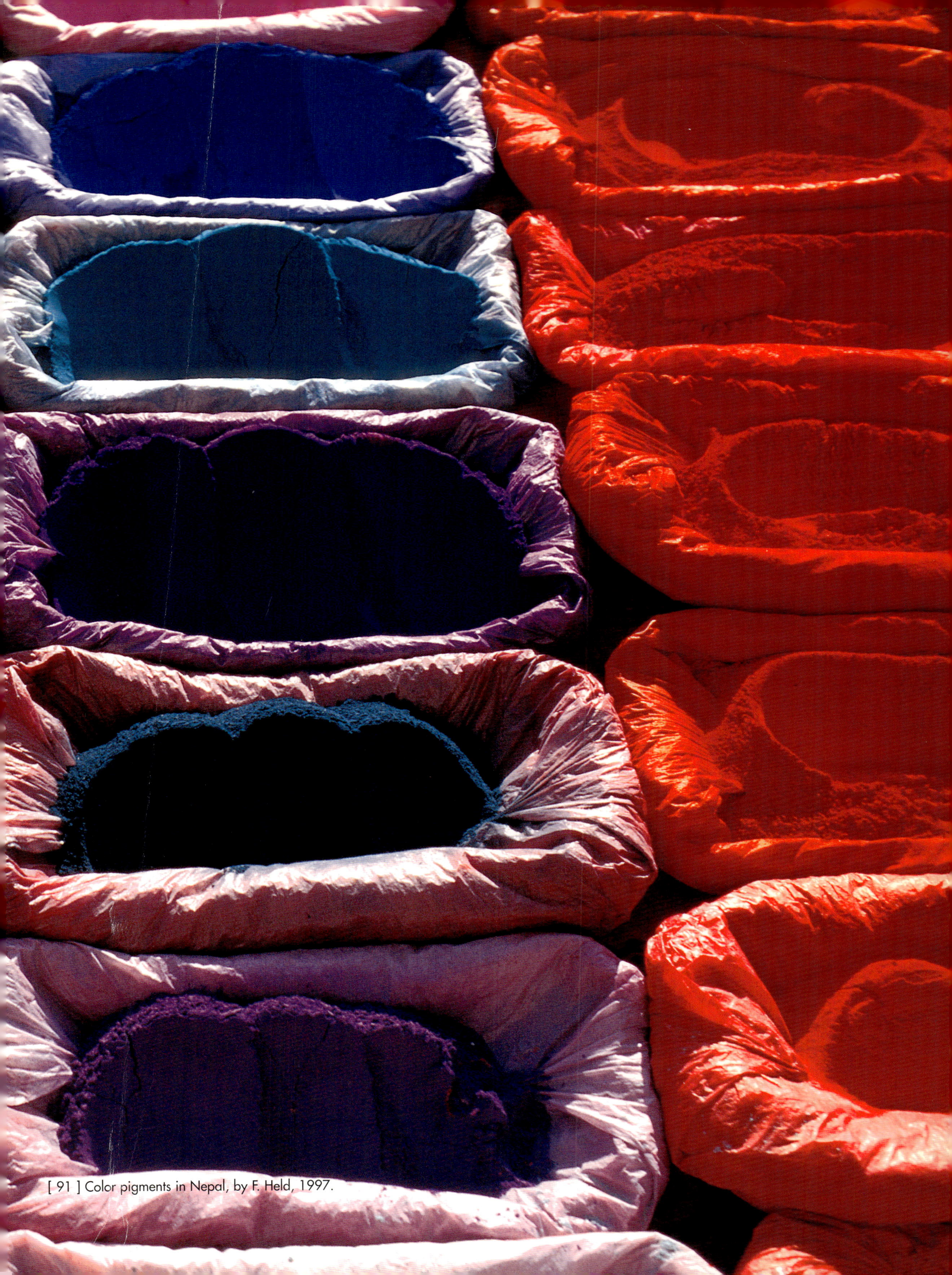
[91] Color pigments in Nepal, by F. Held, 1997.

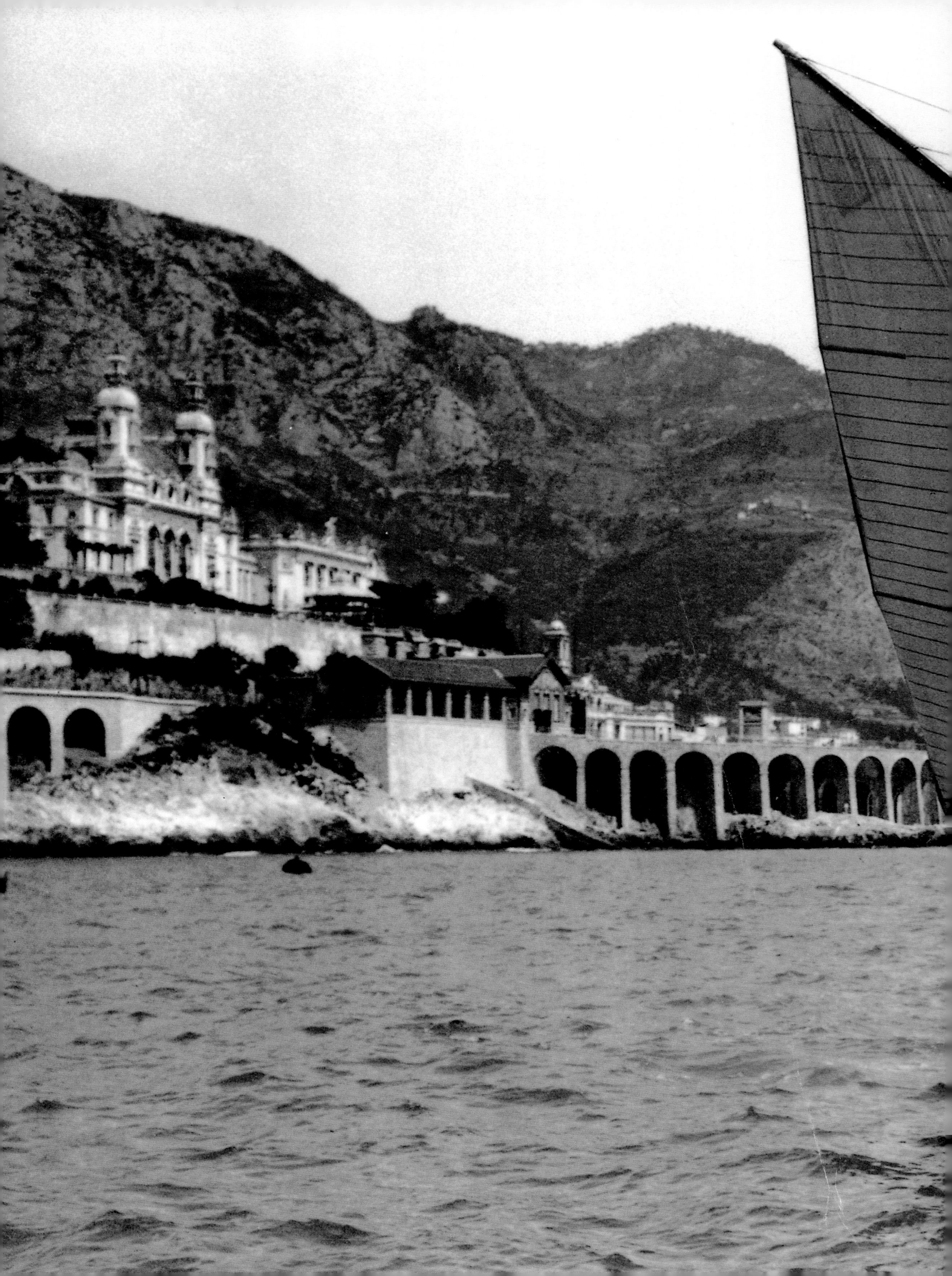

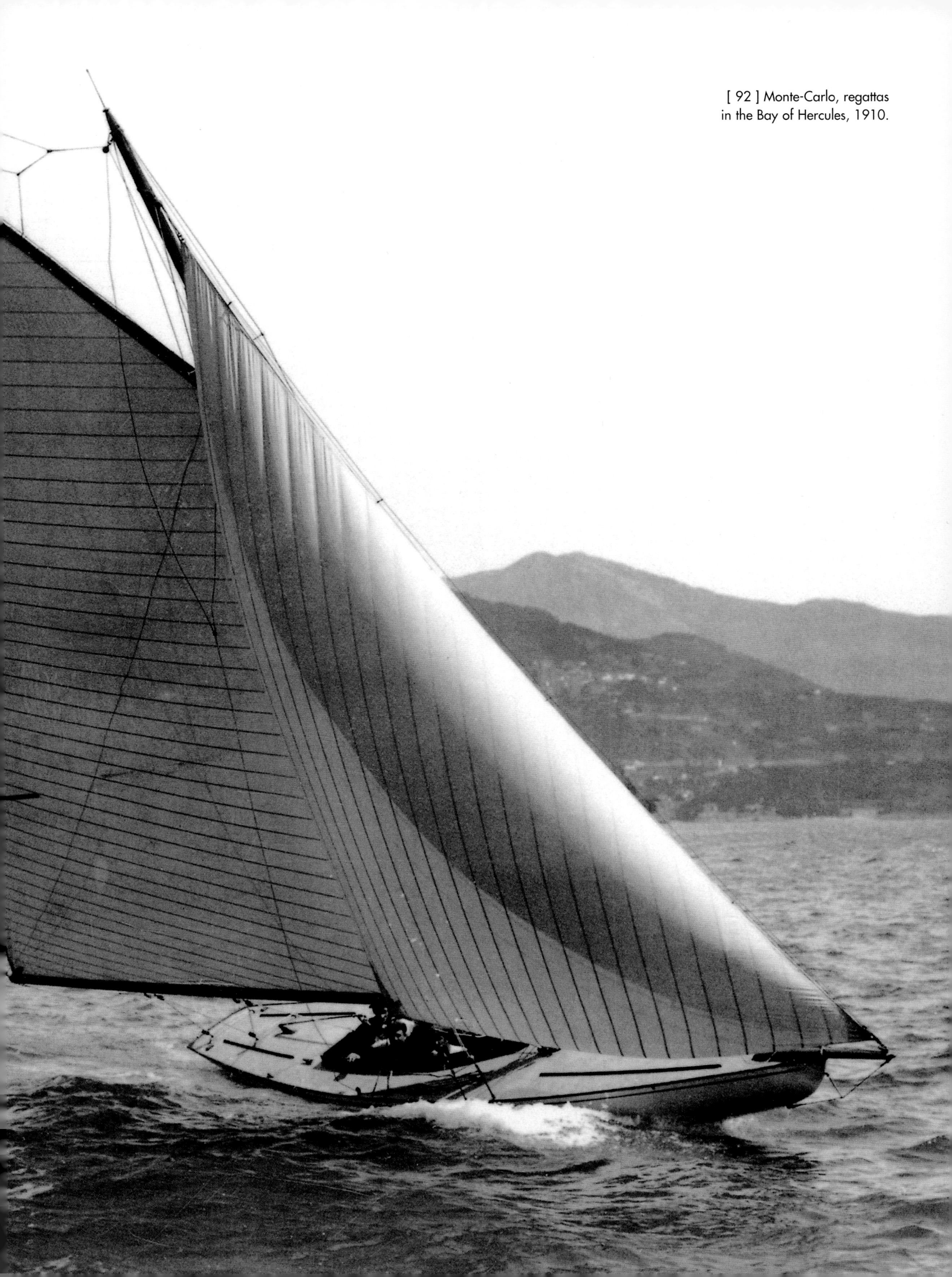

[92] Monte-Carlo, regattas in the Bay of Hercules, 1910.

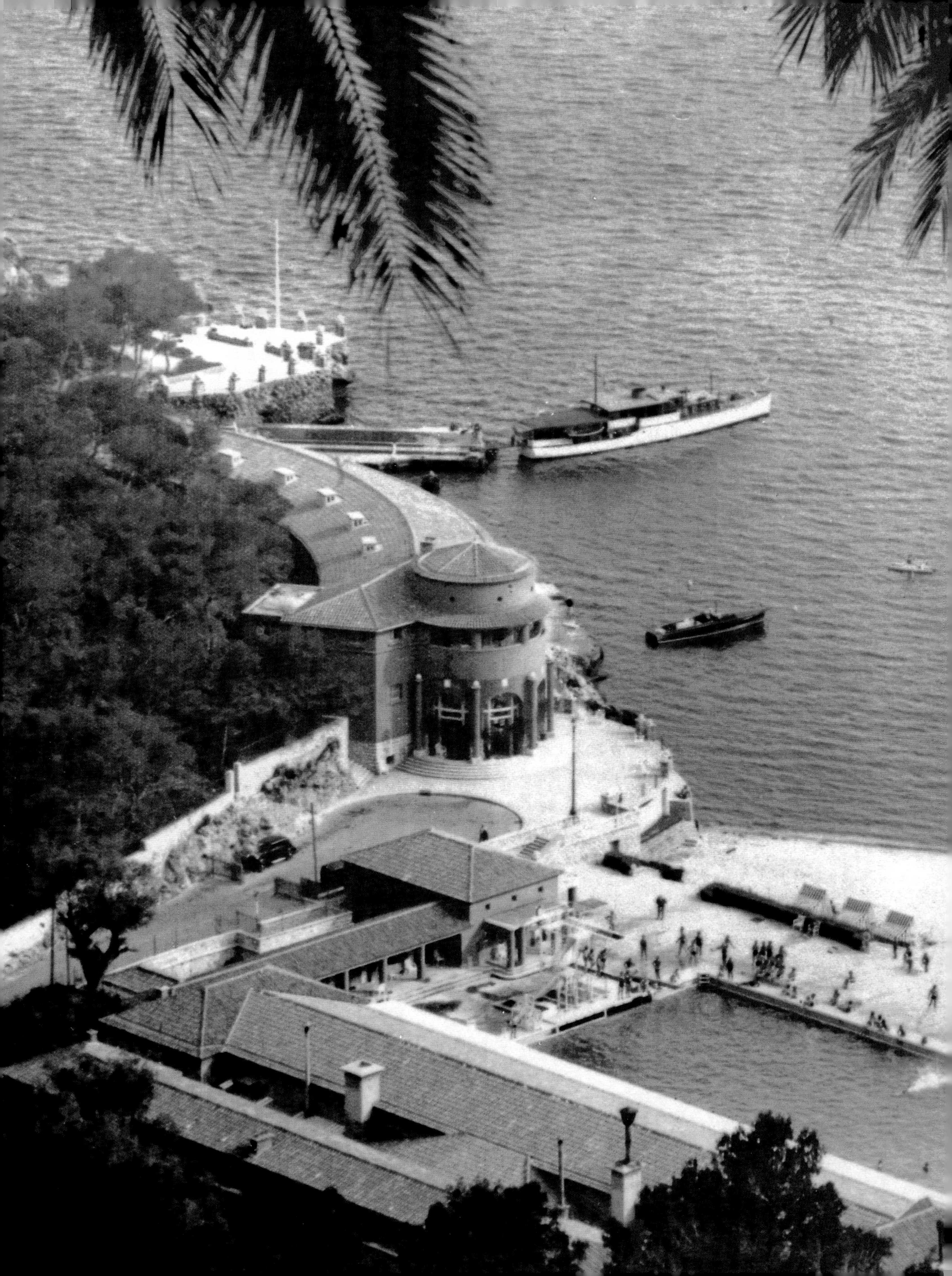

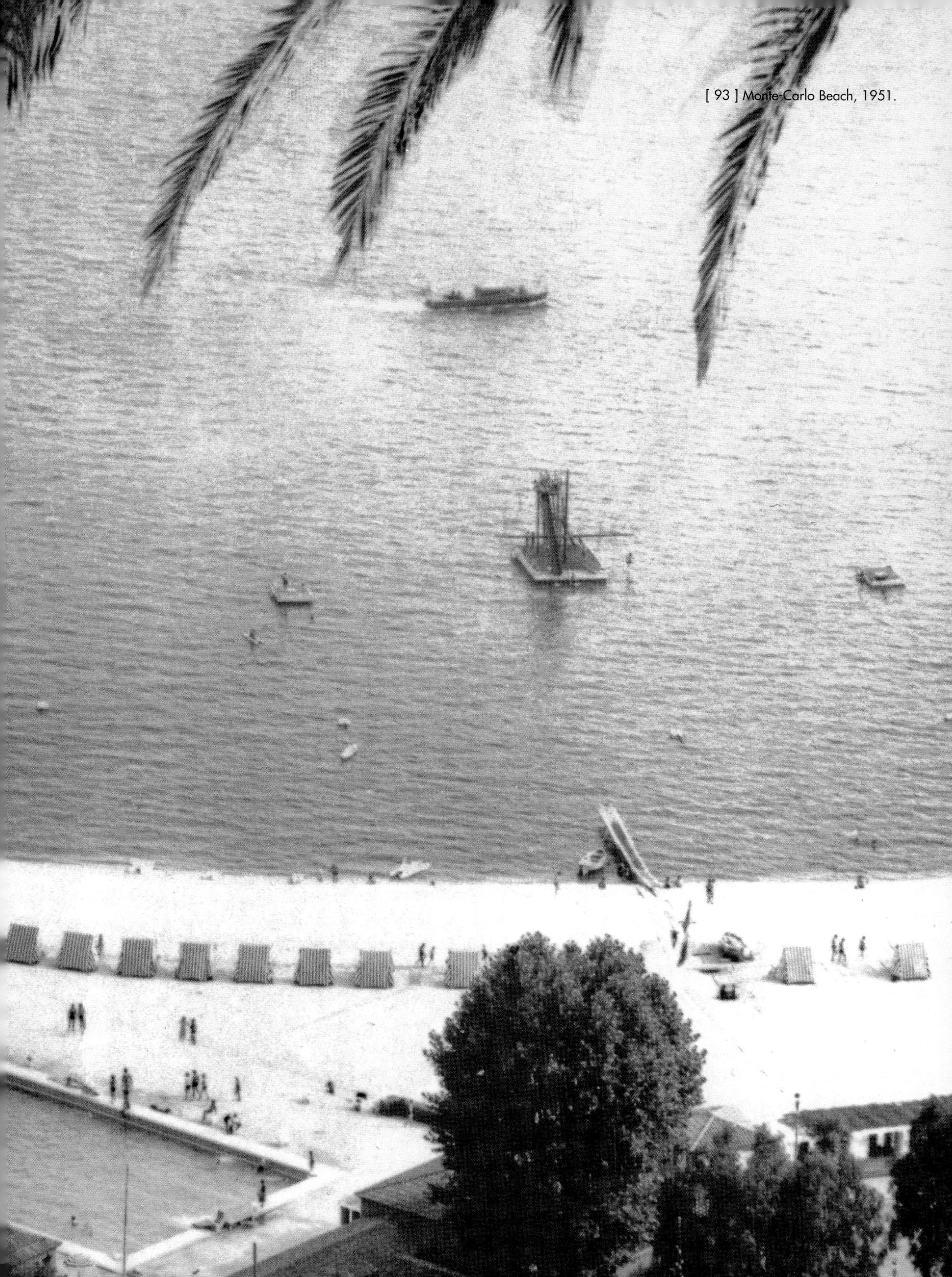

[93] Monte-Carlo Beach, 1951.

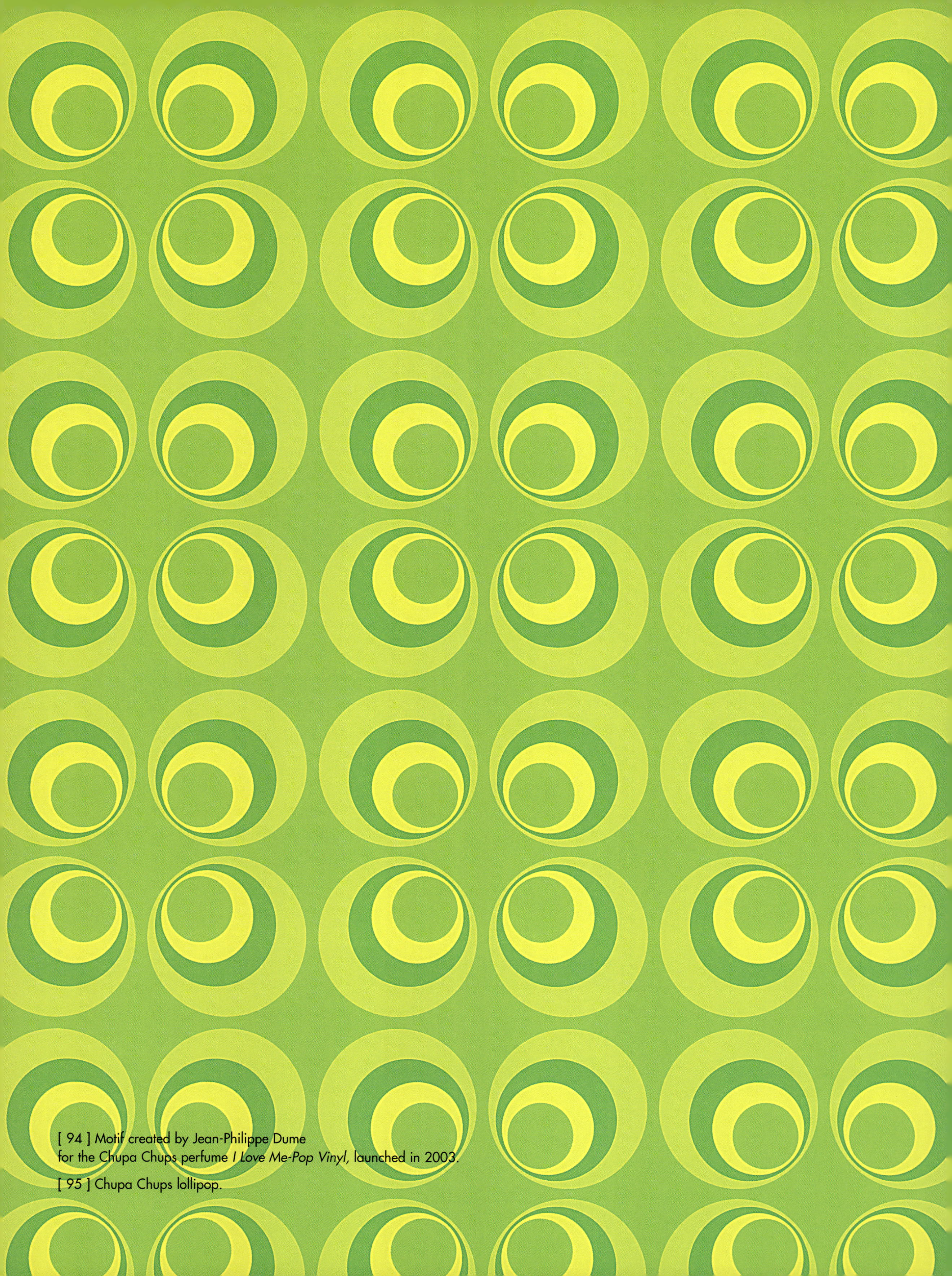

[94] Motif created by Jean-Philippe Dume
for the Chupa Chups perfume *I Love Me-Pop Vinyl,* launched in 2003.

[95] Chupa Chups lollipop.

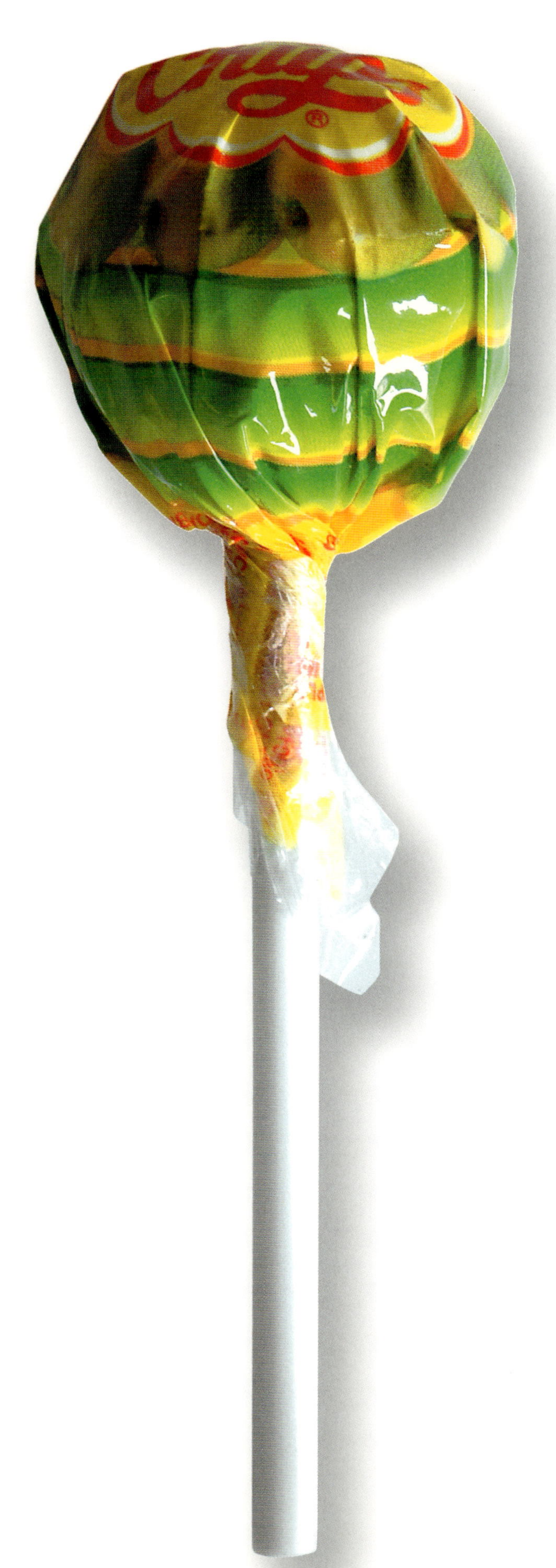

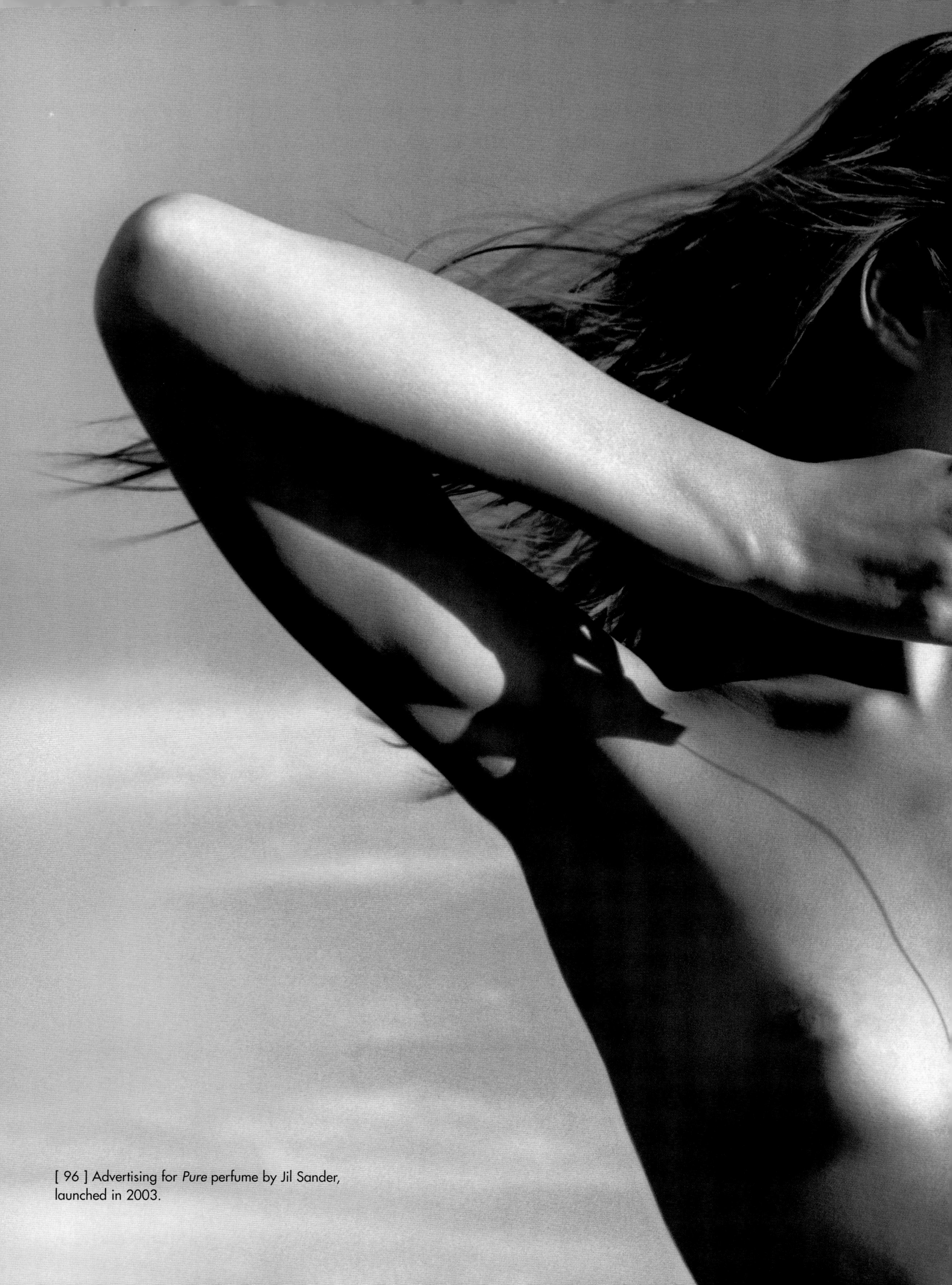

[96] Advertising for *Pure* perfume by Jil Sander, launched in 2003.

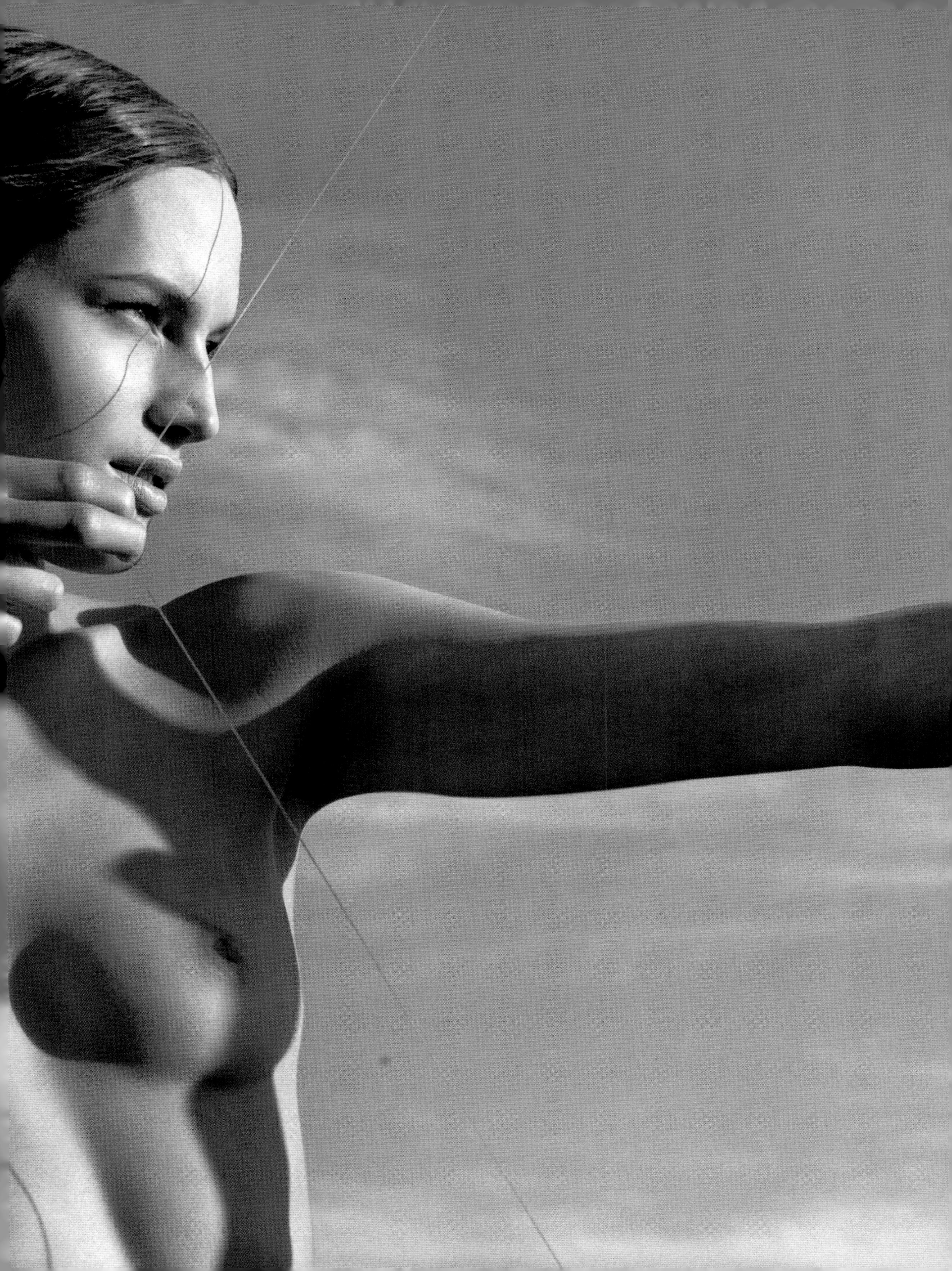

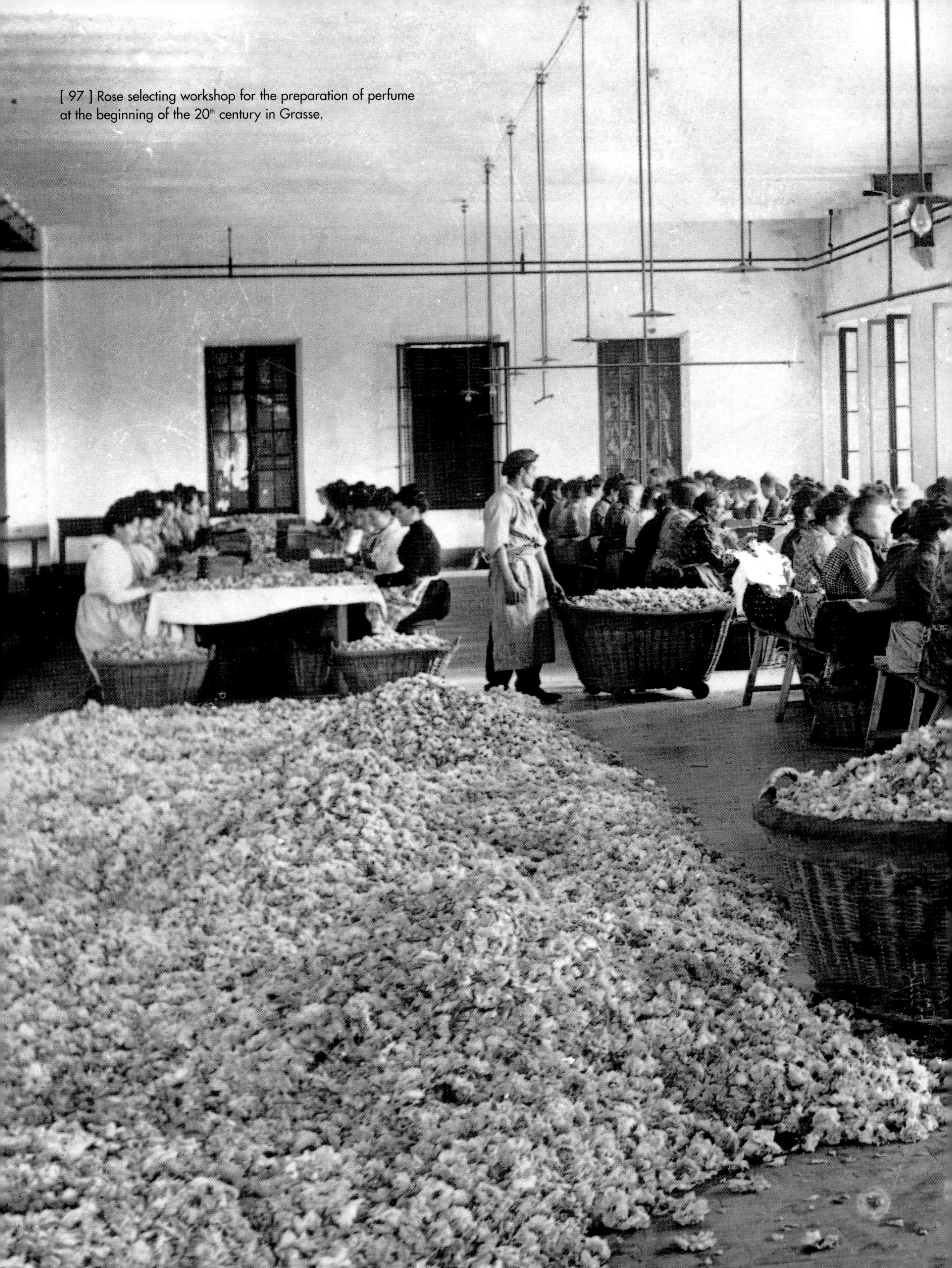

[97] Rose selecting workshop for the preparation of perfume at the beginning of the 20th century in Grasse.

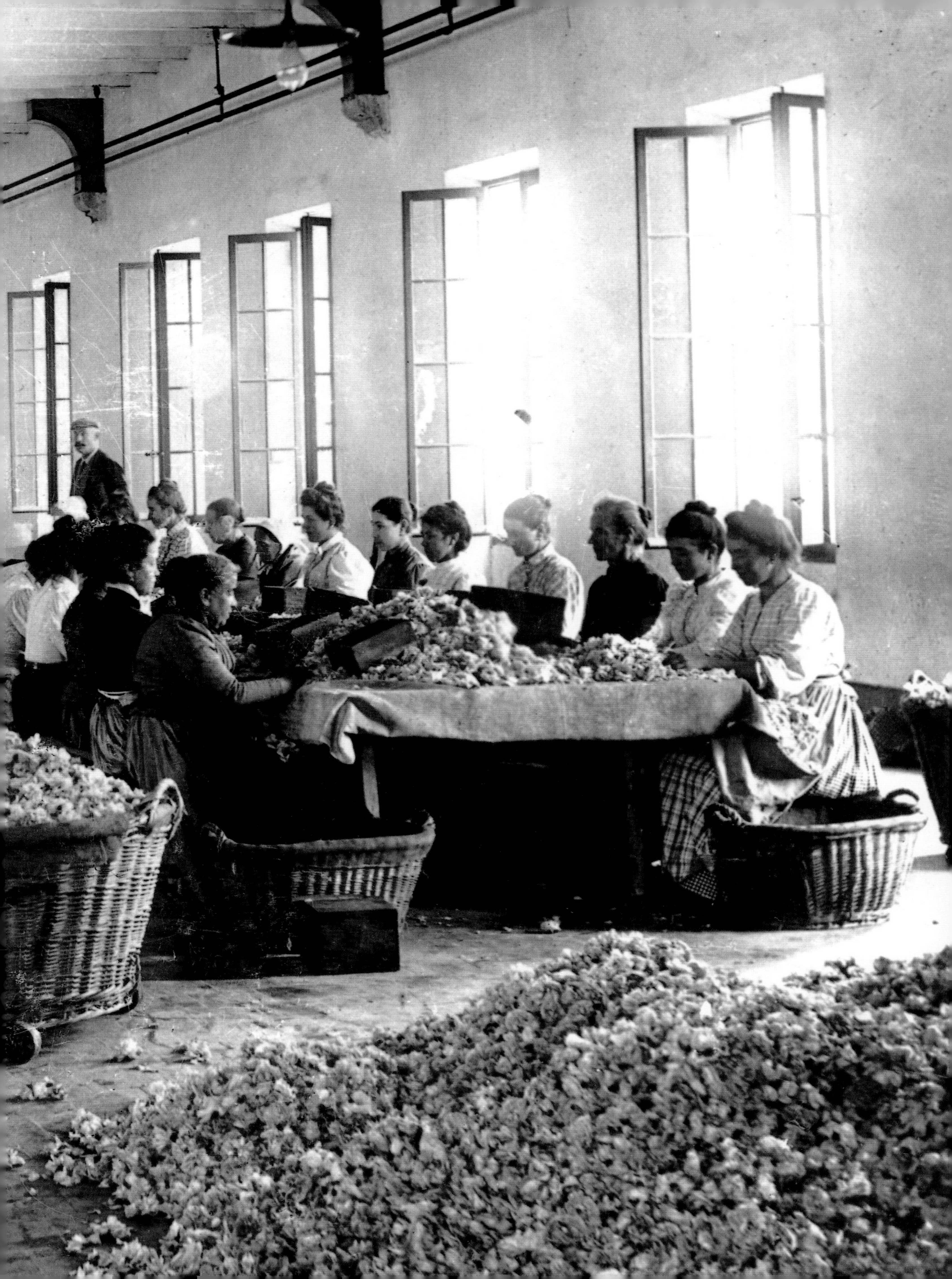

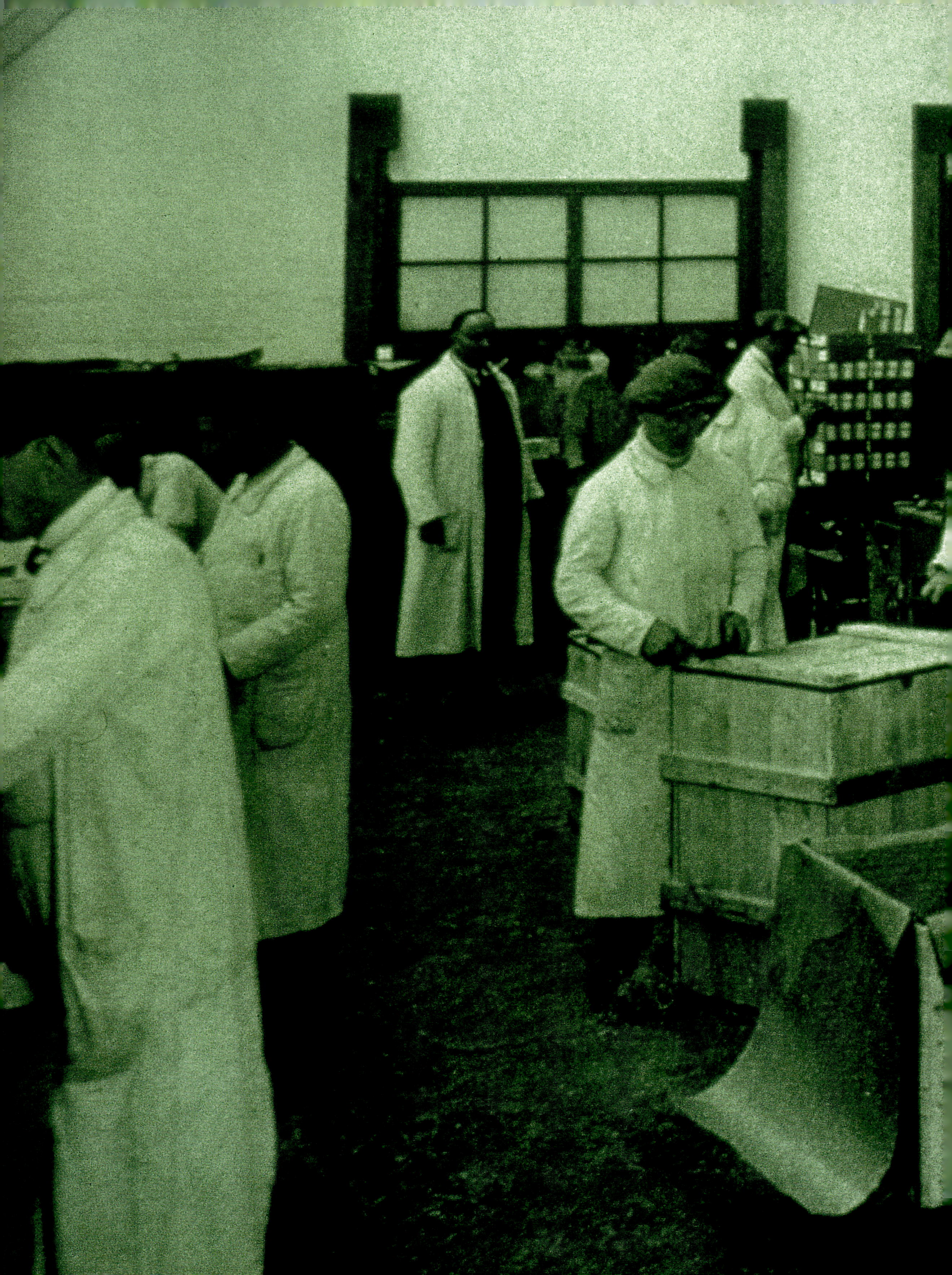

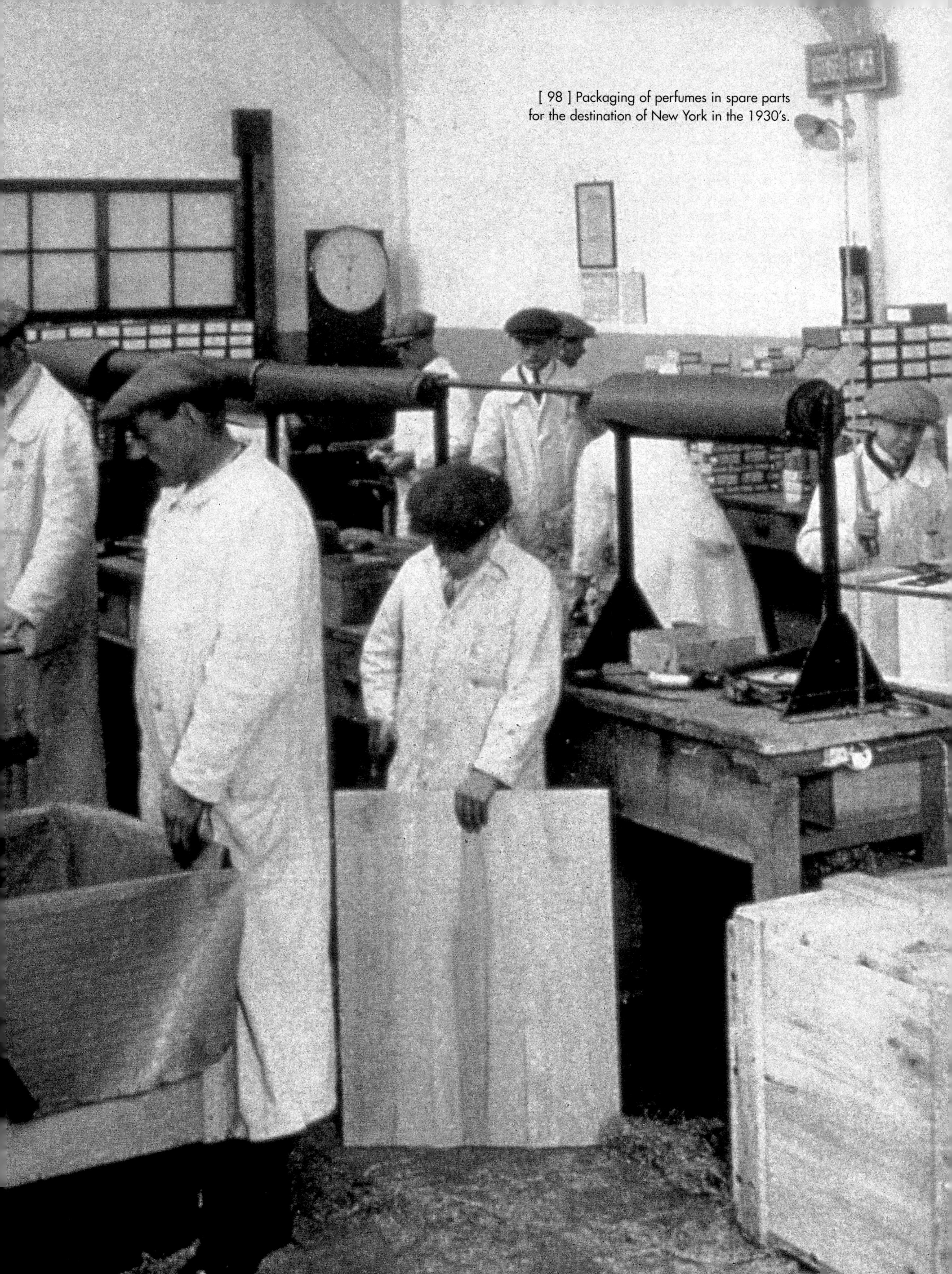

[98] Packaging of perfumes in spare parts for the destination of New York in the 1930's.

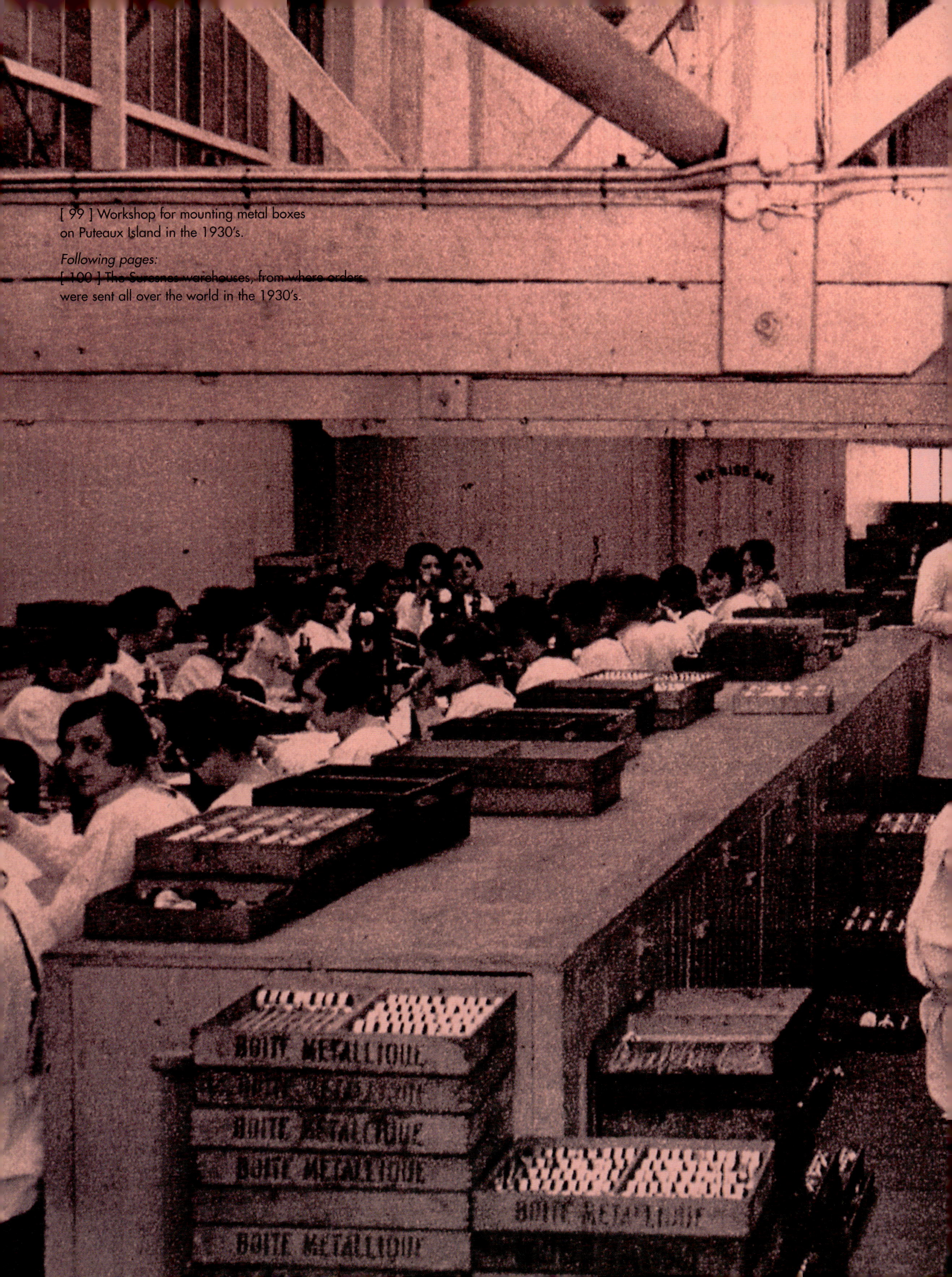

[99] Workshop for mounting metal boxes on Puteaux Island in the 1930's.

Following pages:
[100] The Suresnes warehouses, from where orders were sent all over the world in the 1930's.

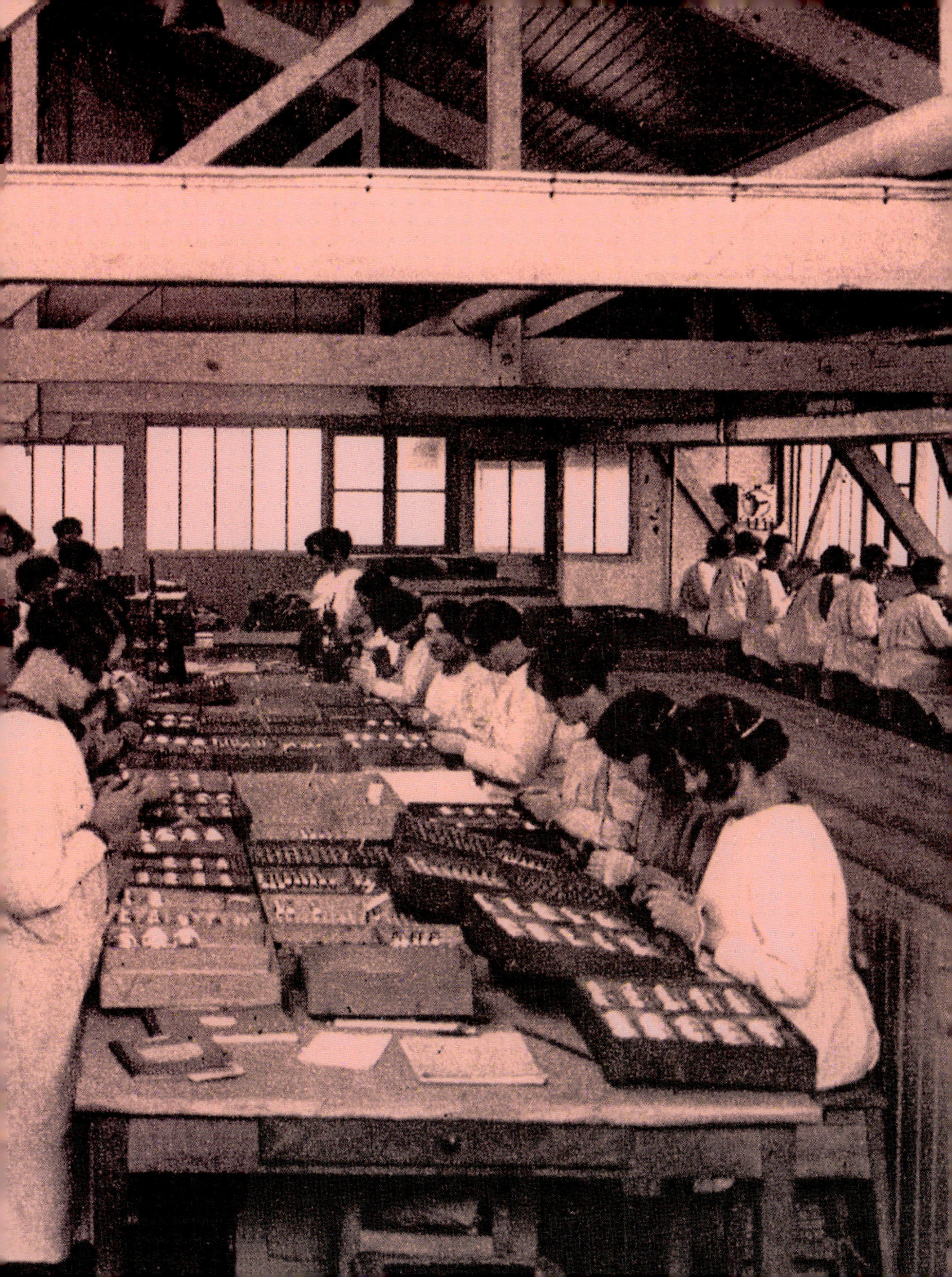

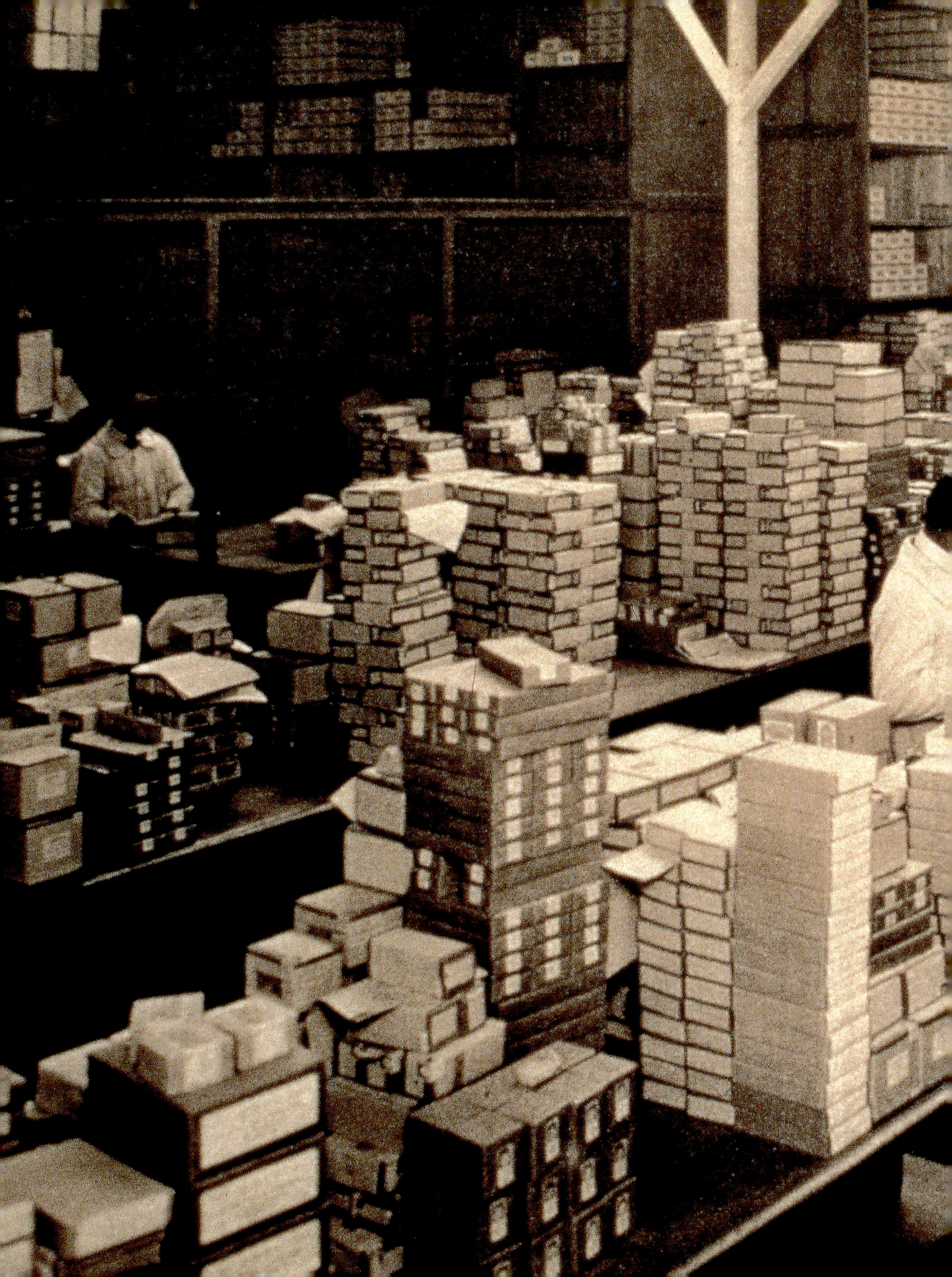

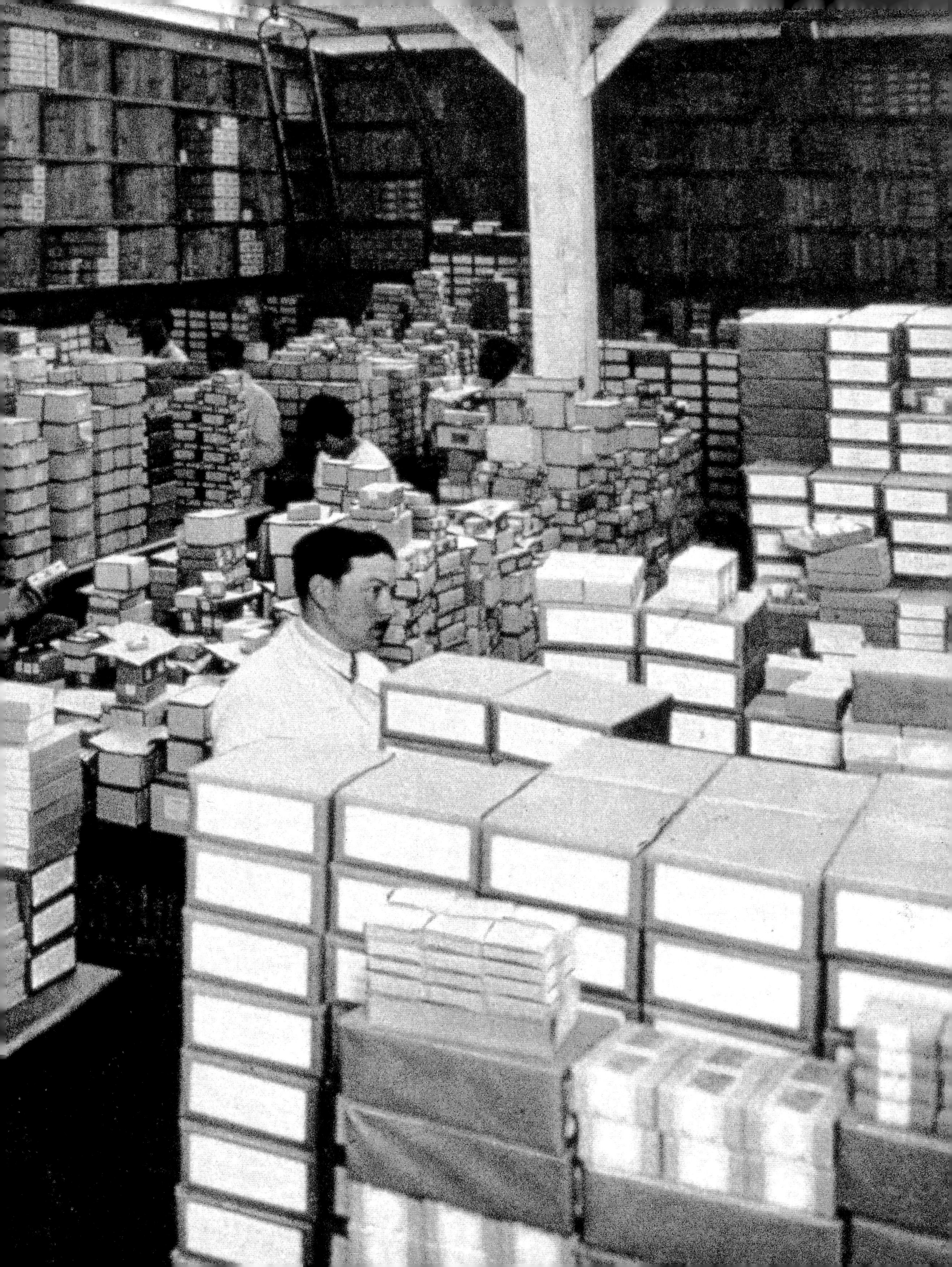

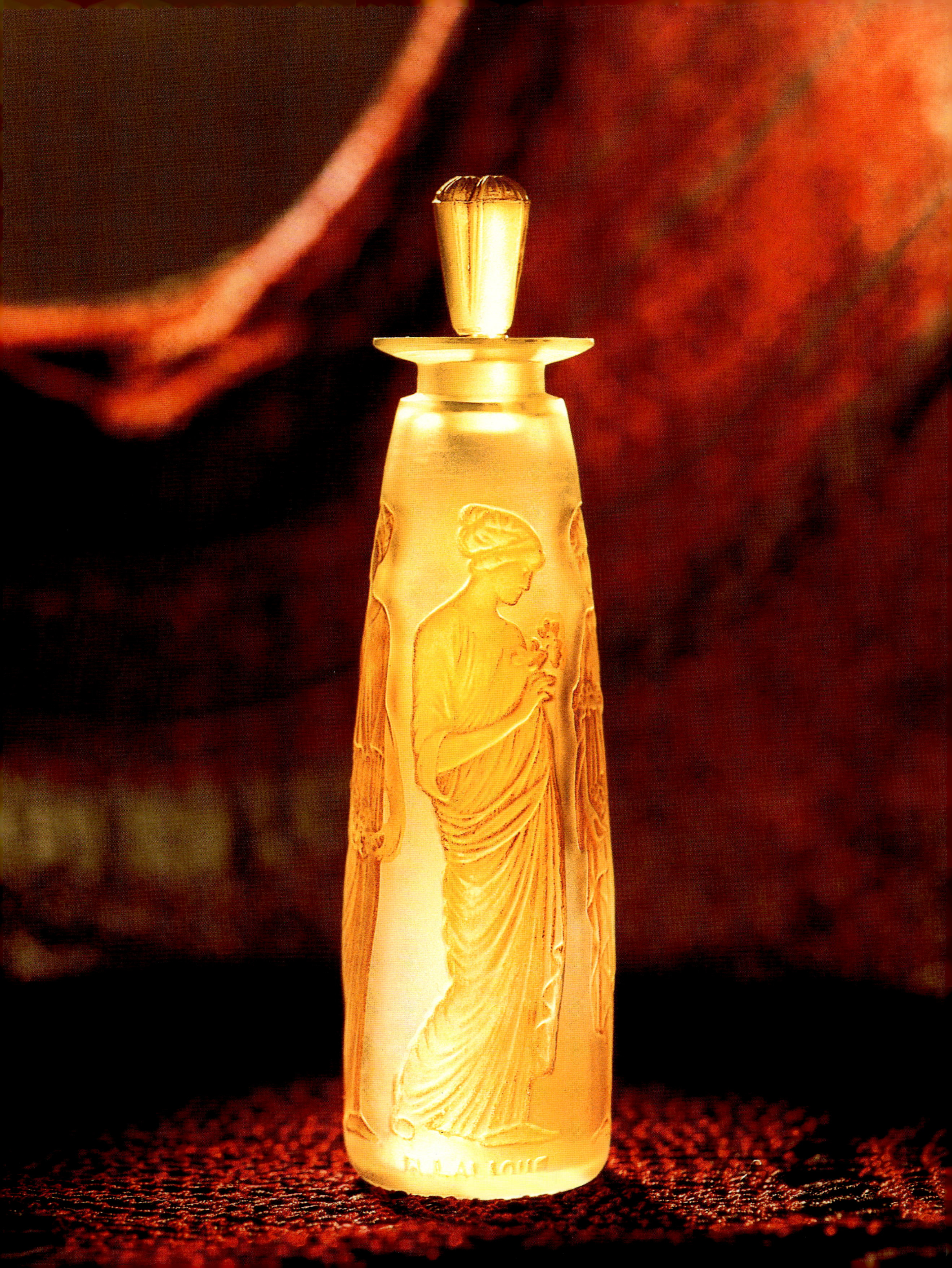

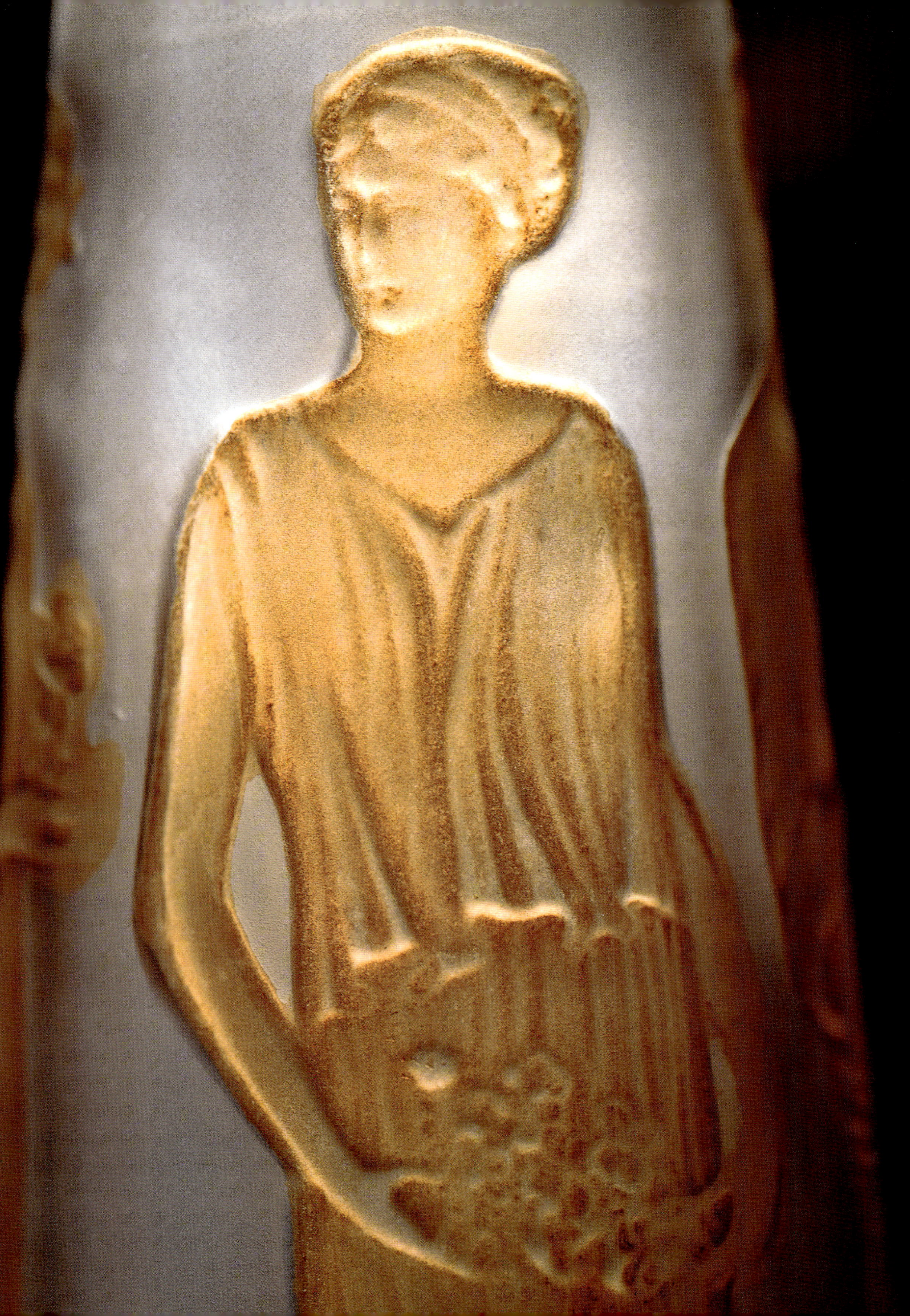

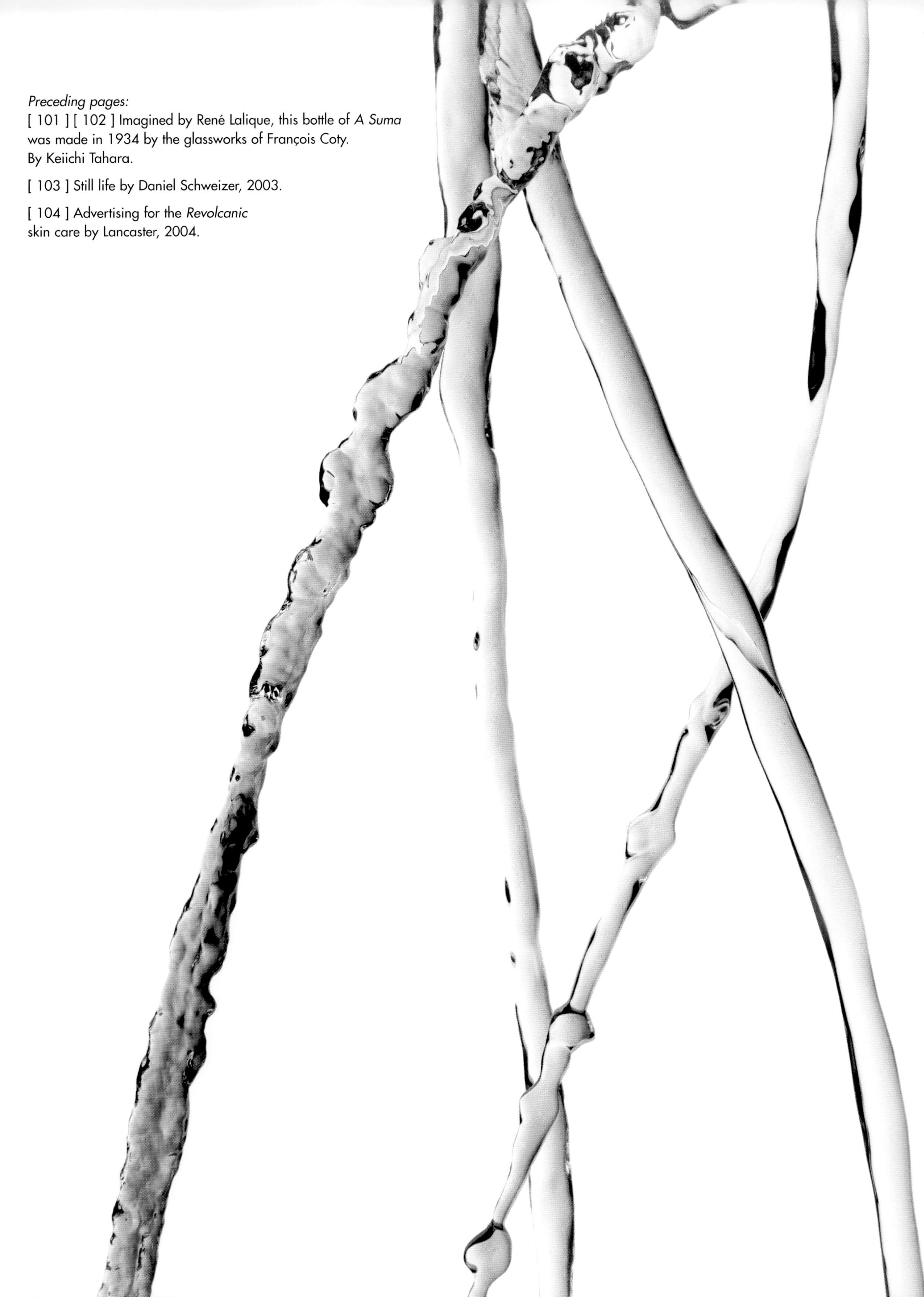

Preceding pages:
[101] [102] Imagined by René Lalique, this bottle of *A Suma* was made in 1934 by the glassworks of François Coty. By Keiichi Tahara.

[103] Still life by Daniel Schweizer, 2003.

[104] Advertising for the *Revolcanic* skin care by Lancaster, 2004.

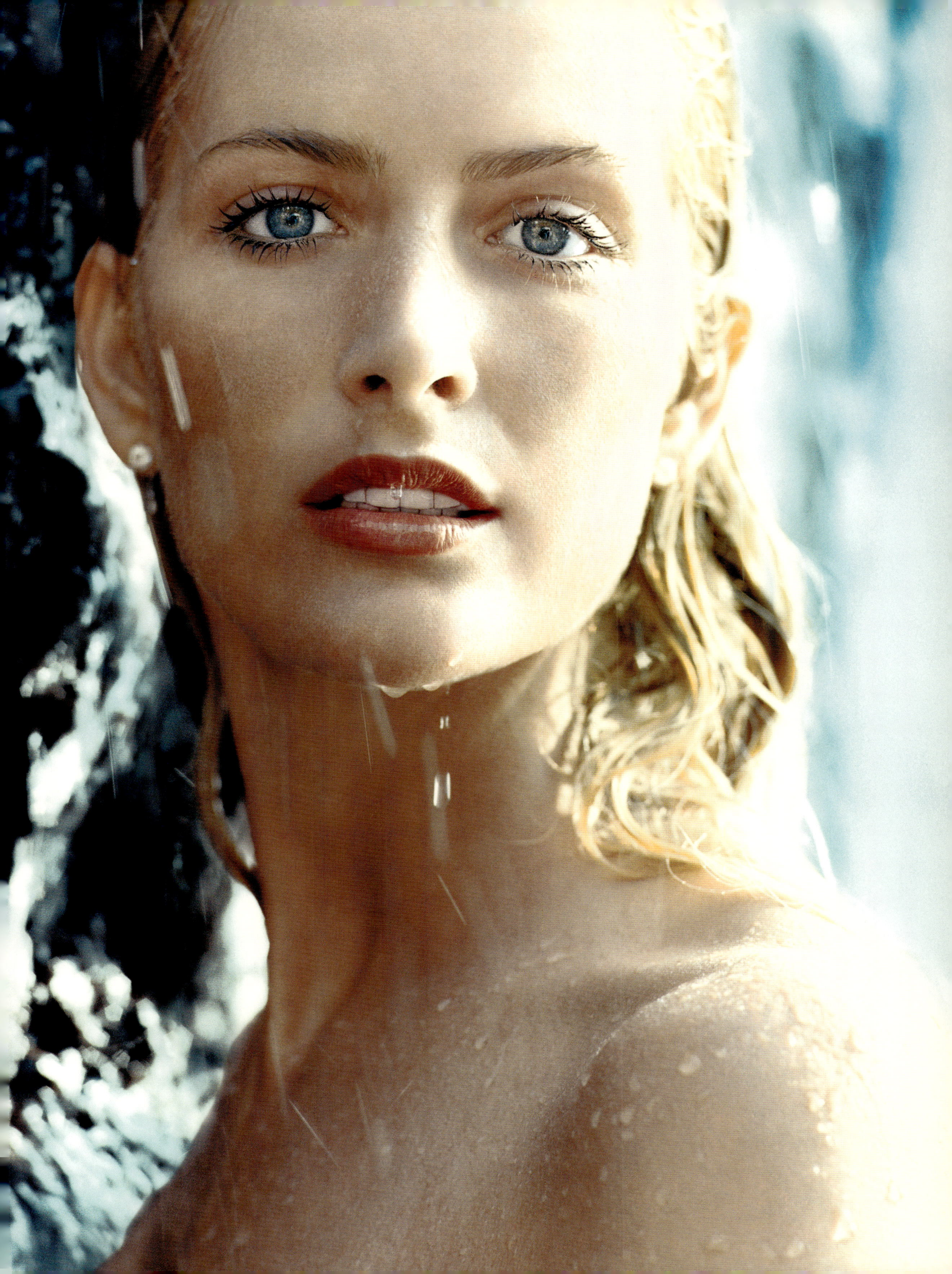

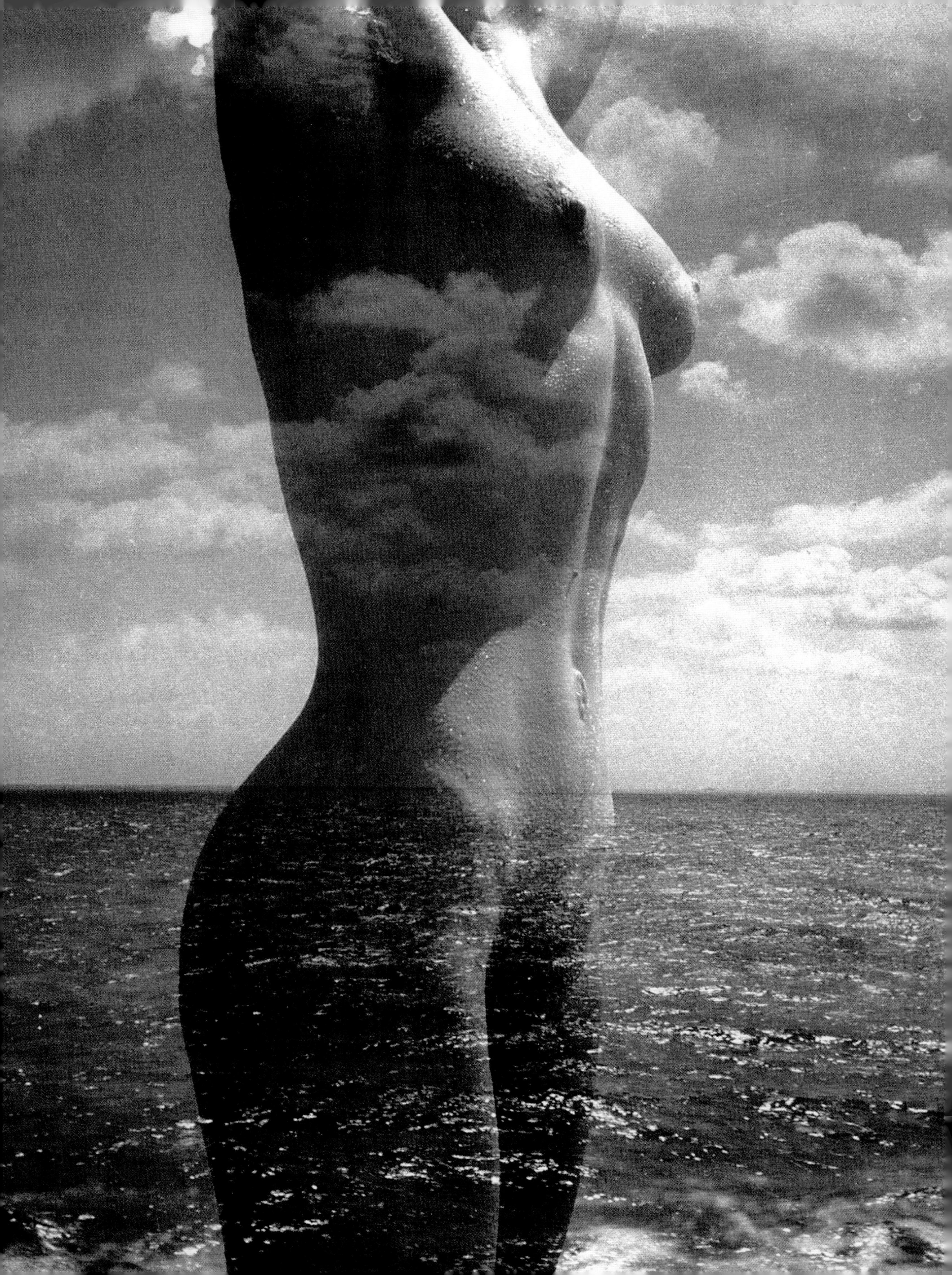

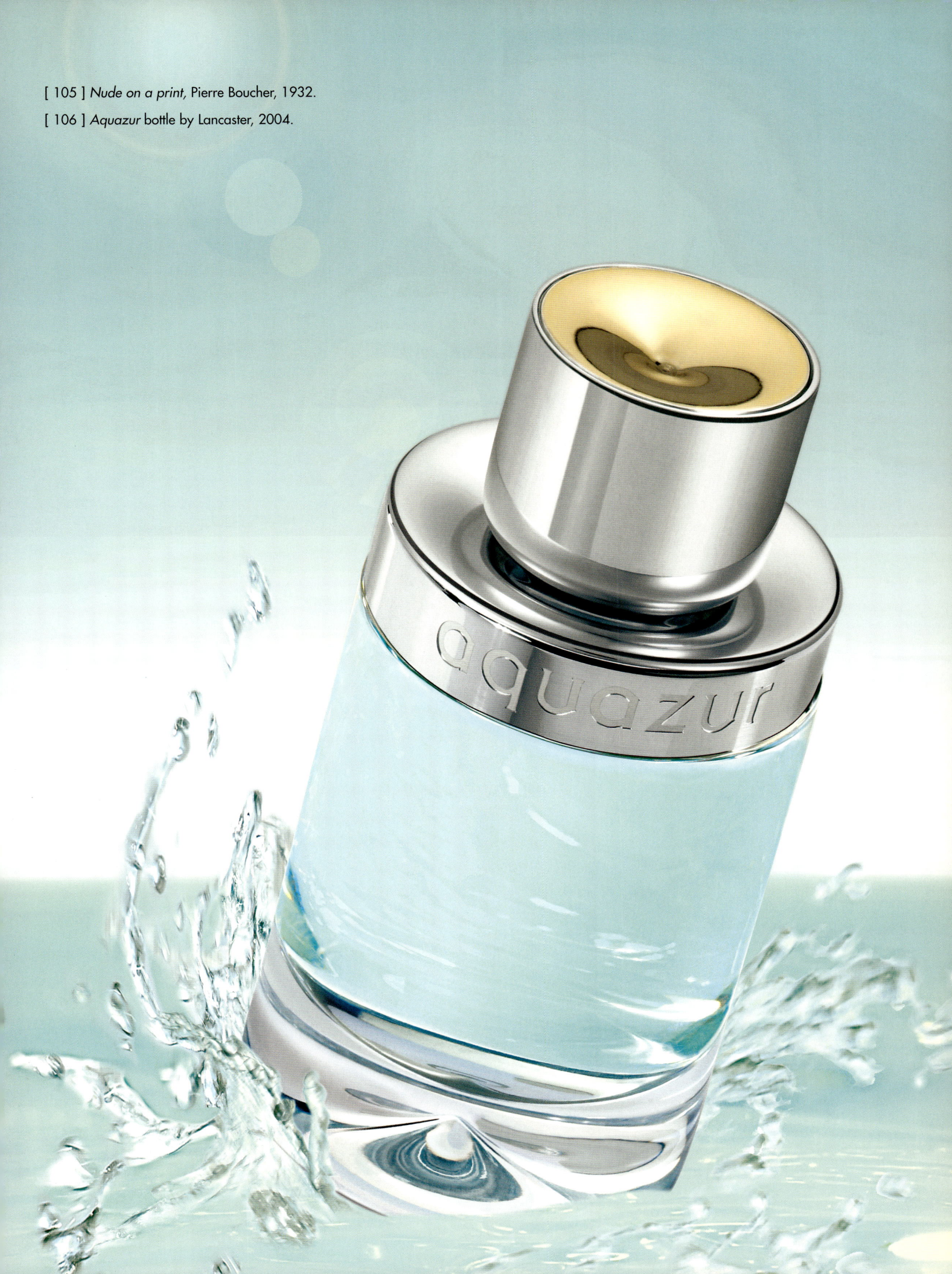

[105] *Nude on a print,* Pierre Boucher, 1932.

[106] *Aquazur* bottle by Lancaster, 2004.

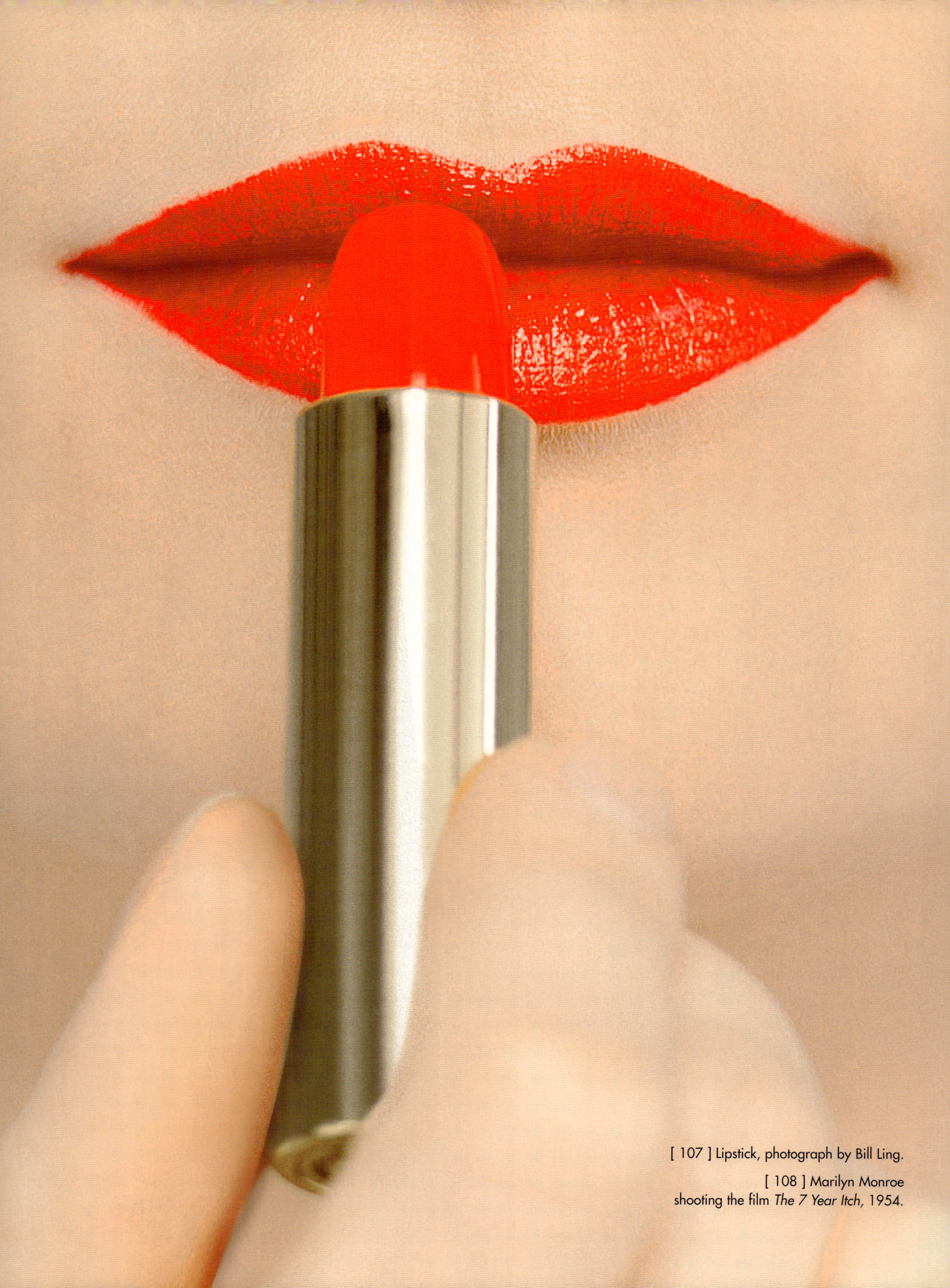

[107] Lipstick, photograph by Bill Ling.

[108] Marilyn Monroe
shooting the film *The 7 Year Itch*, 1954.

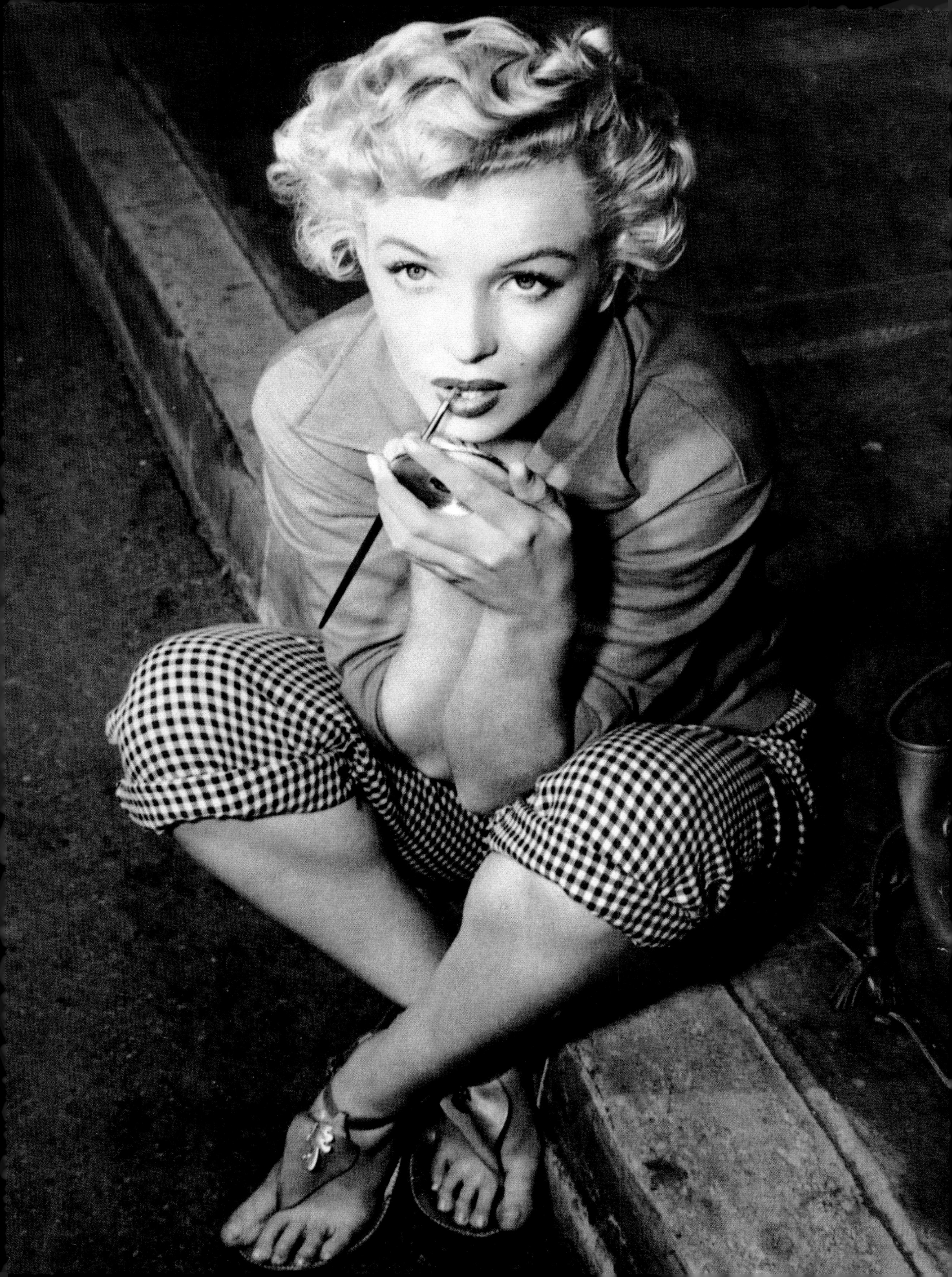

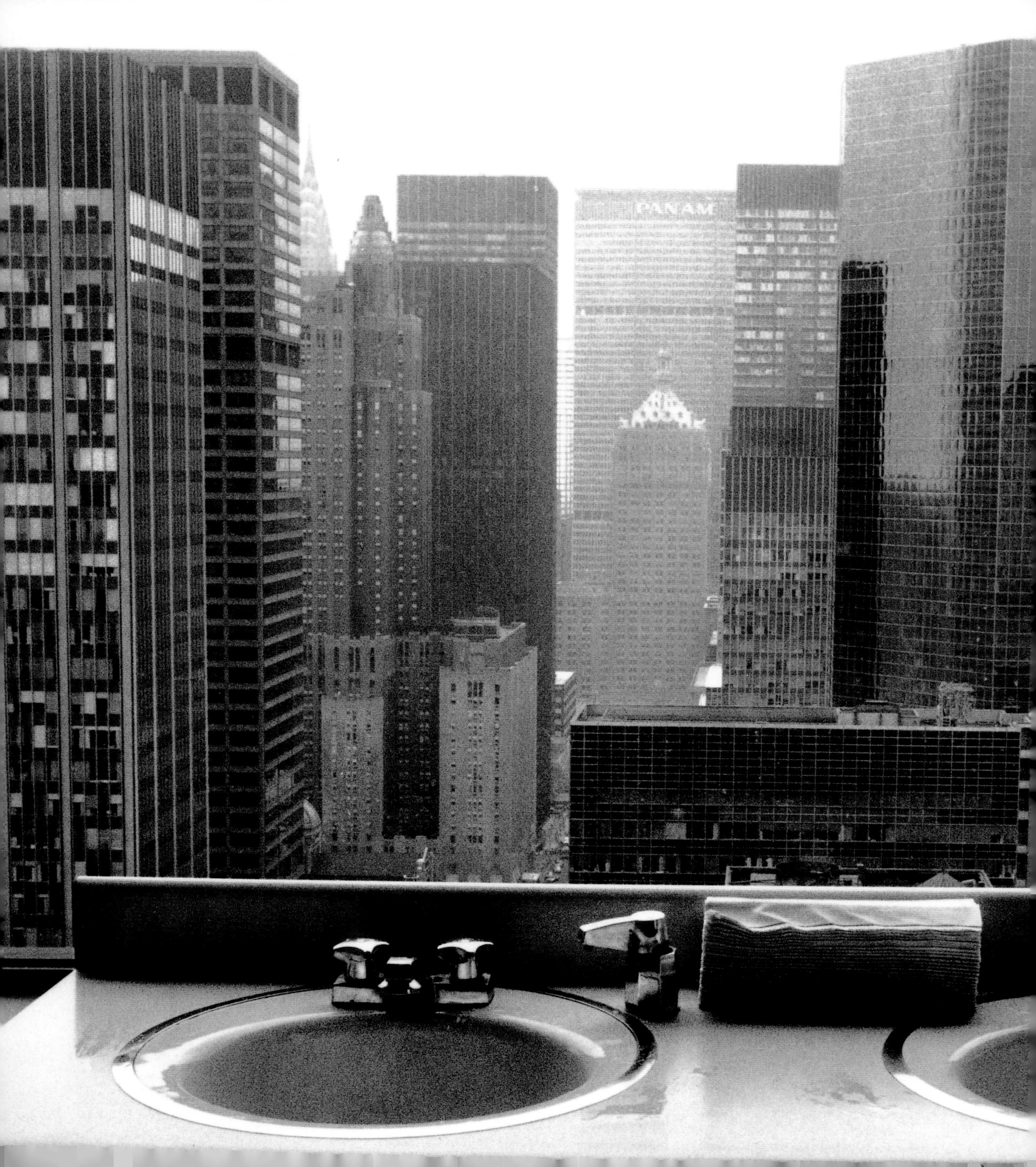
PAN AM

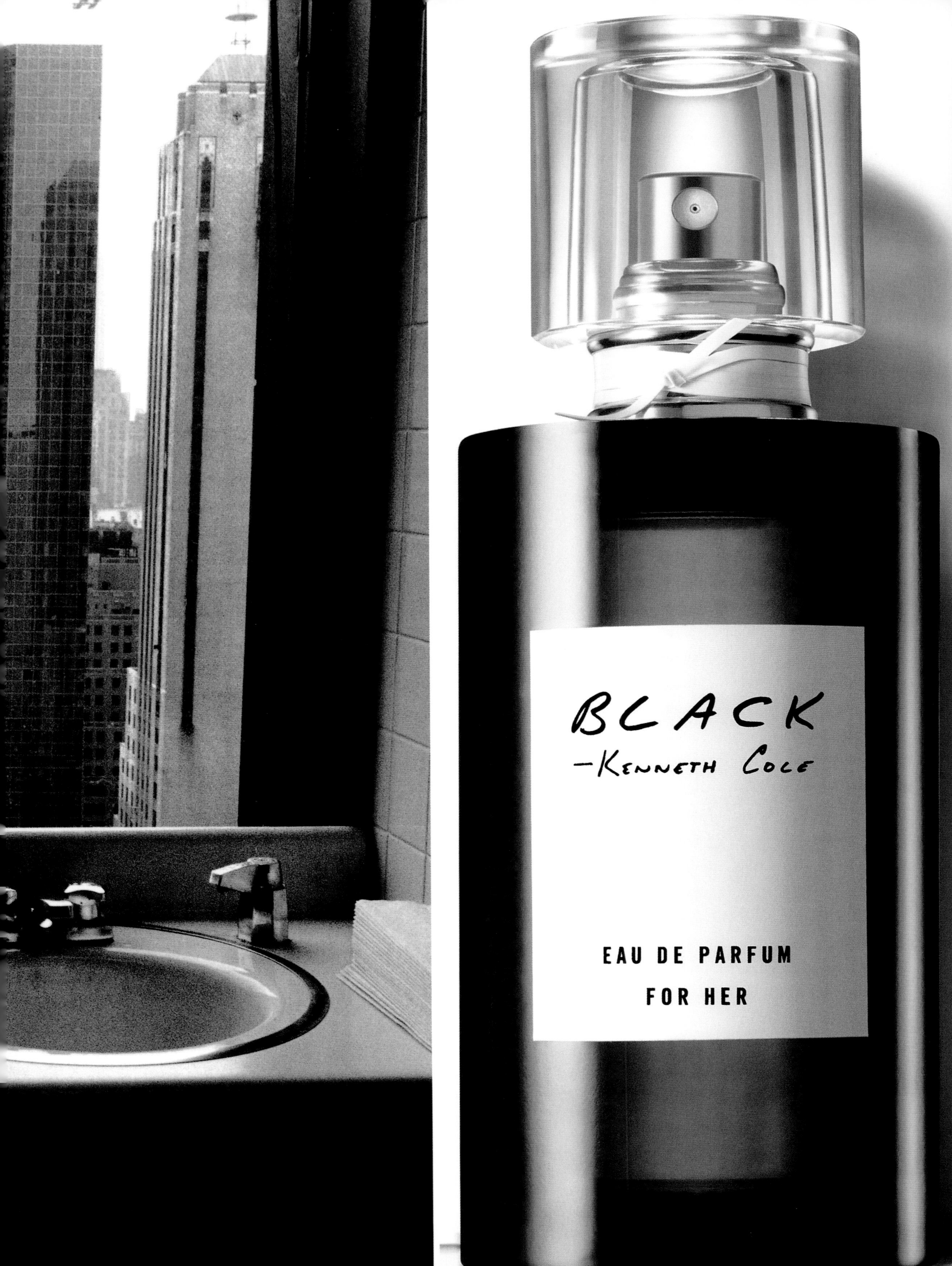
BLACK
–KENNETH COLE
EAU DE PARFUM
FOR HER

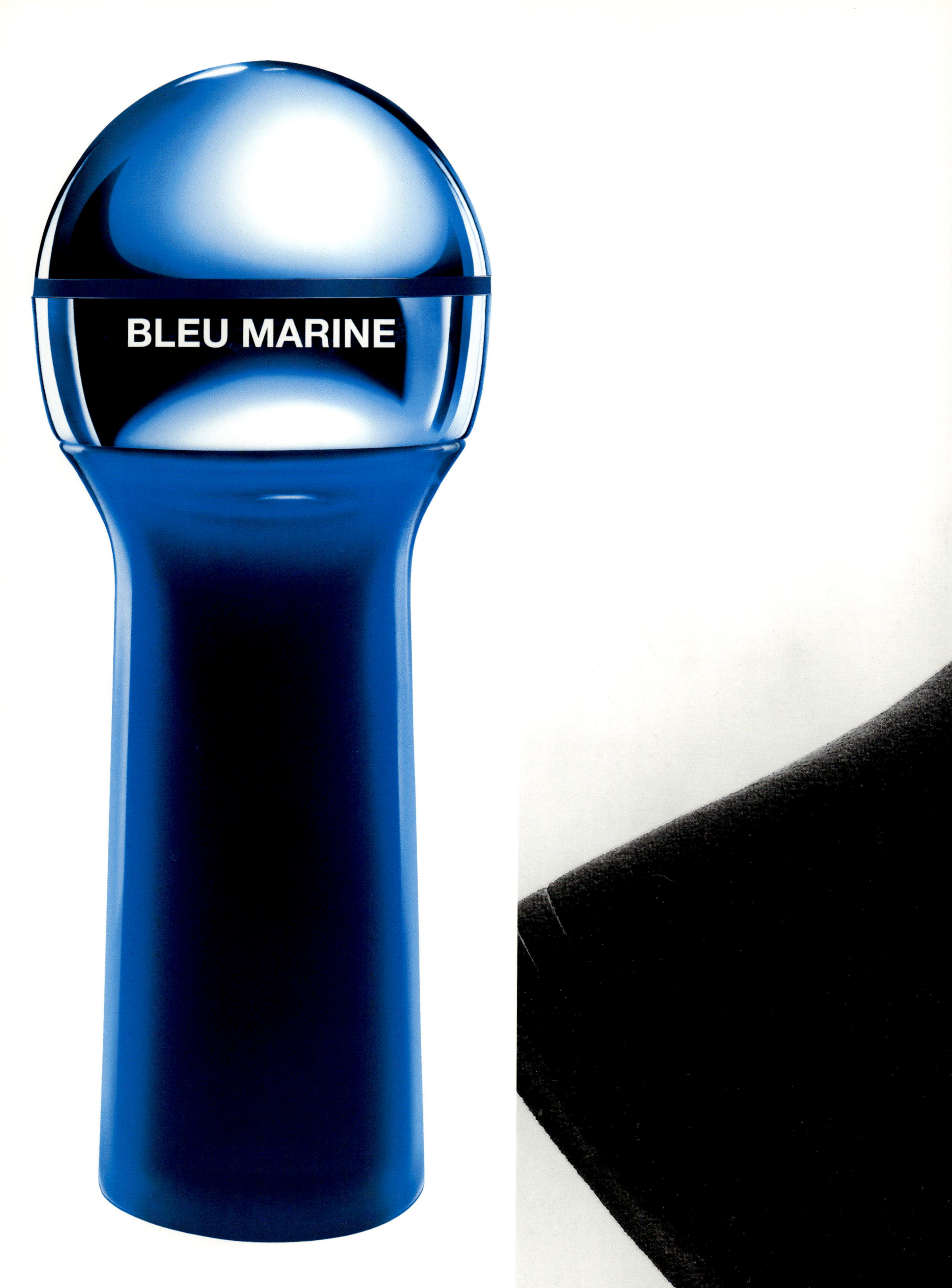
BLEU MARINE

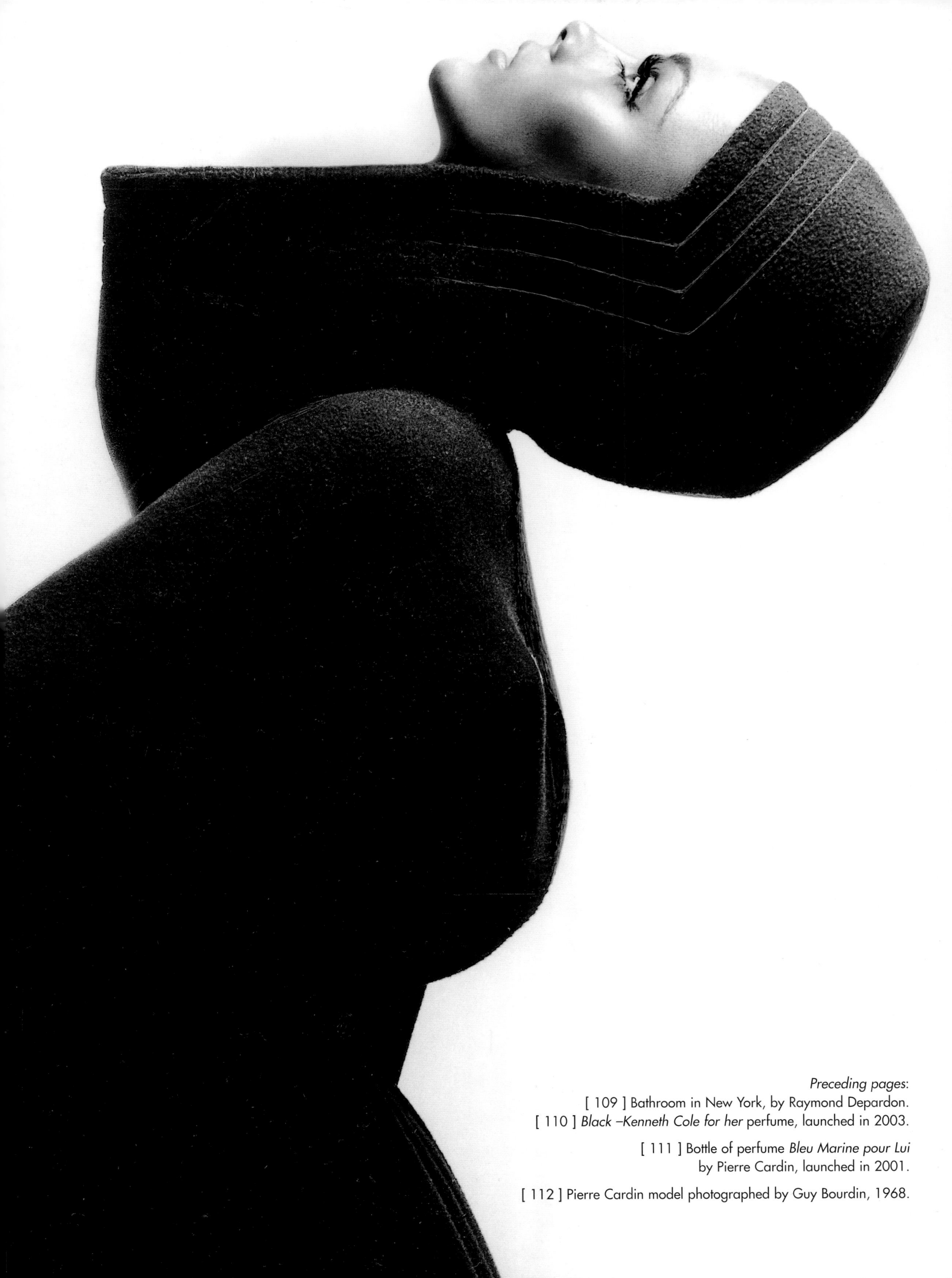

Preceding pages:
[109] Bathroom in New York, by Raymond Depardon.
[110] *Black –Kenneth Cole for her* perfume, launched in 2003.

[111] Bottle of perfume *Bleu Marine pour Lui* by Pierre Cardin, launched in 2001.

[112] Pierre Cardin model photographed by Guy Bourdin, 1968.

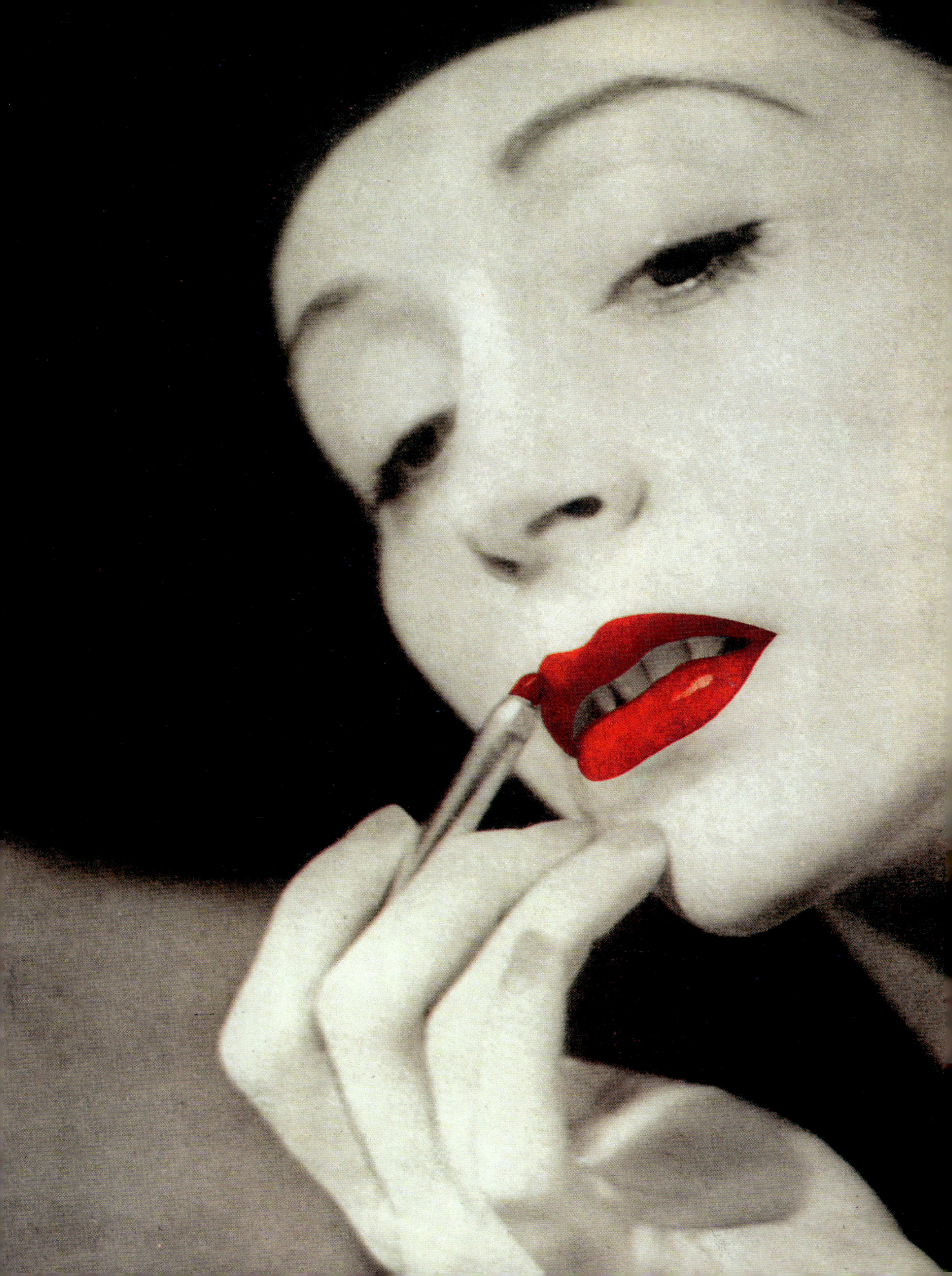

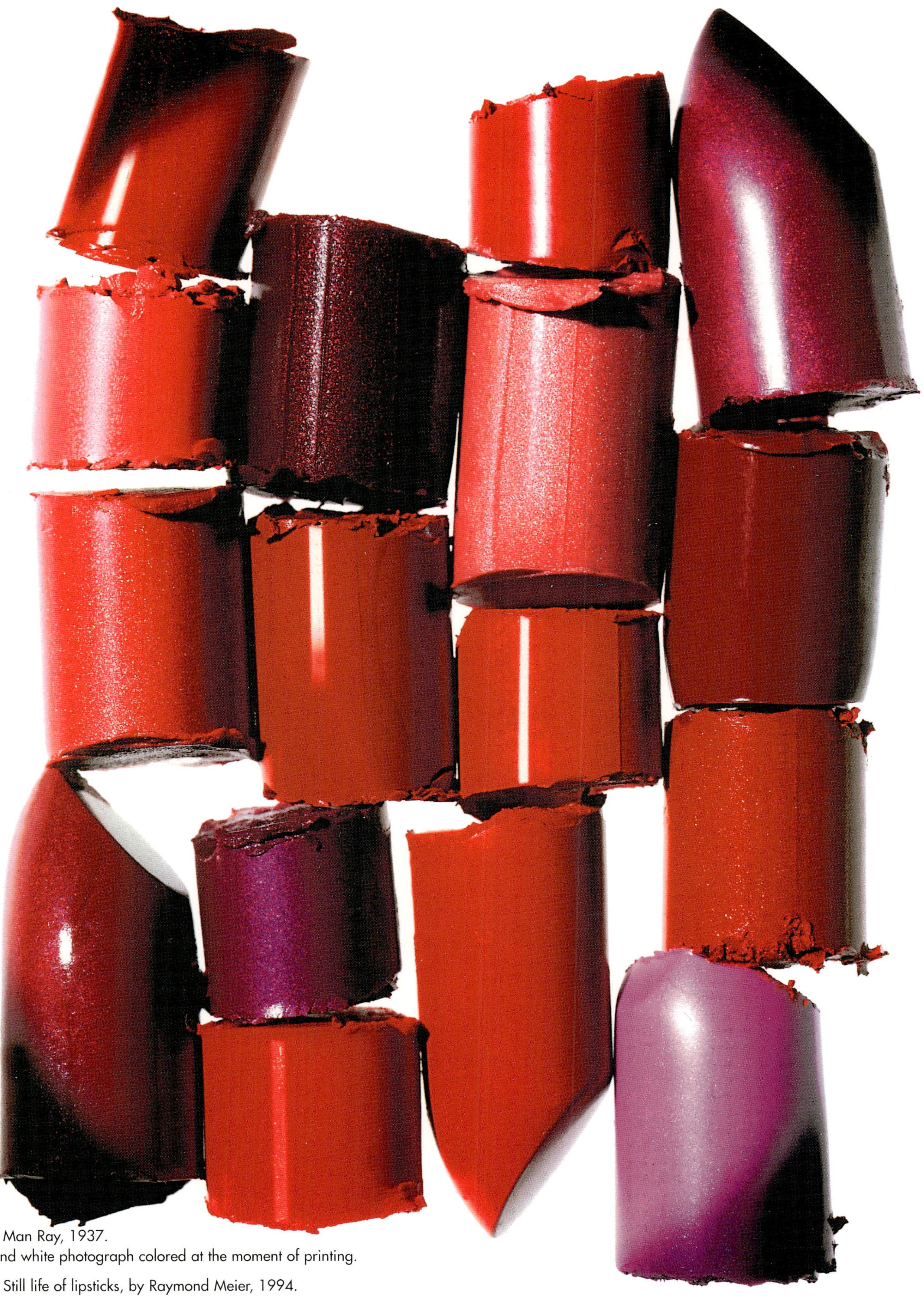

[113] Man Ray, 1937.
Black and white photograph colored at the moment of printing.

[114] Still life of lipsticks, by Raymond Meier, 1994.

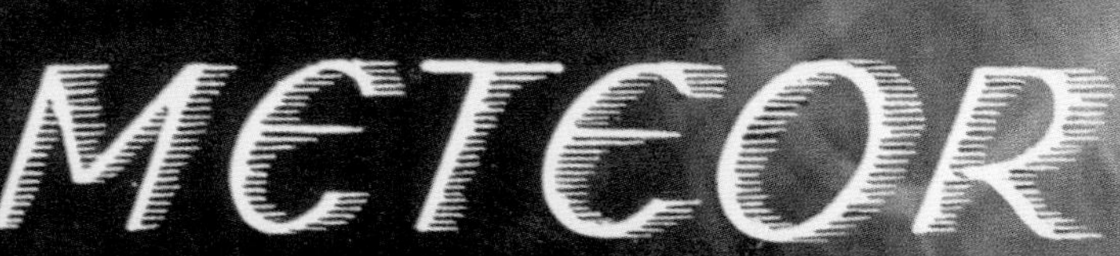

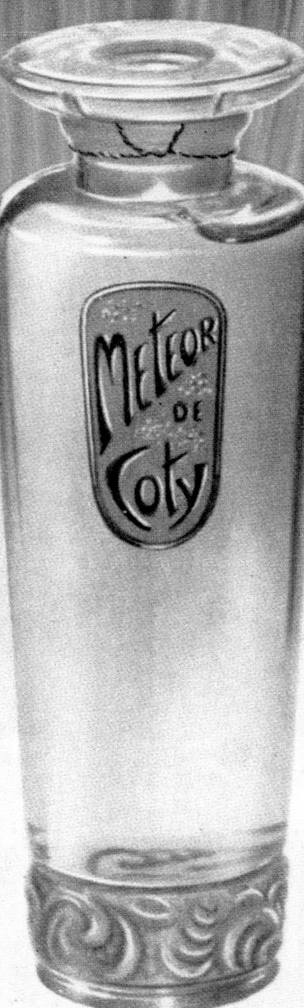

[115] Advertising from 1951 for the *Meteor* perfume by Coty, launched in 1938.

[116] Fireworks.

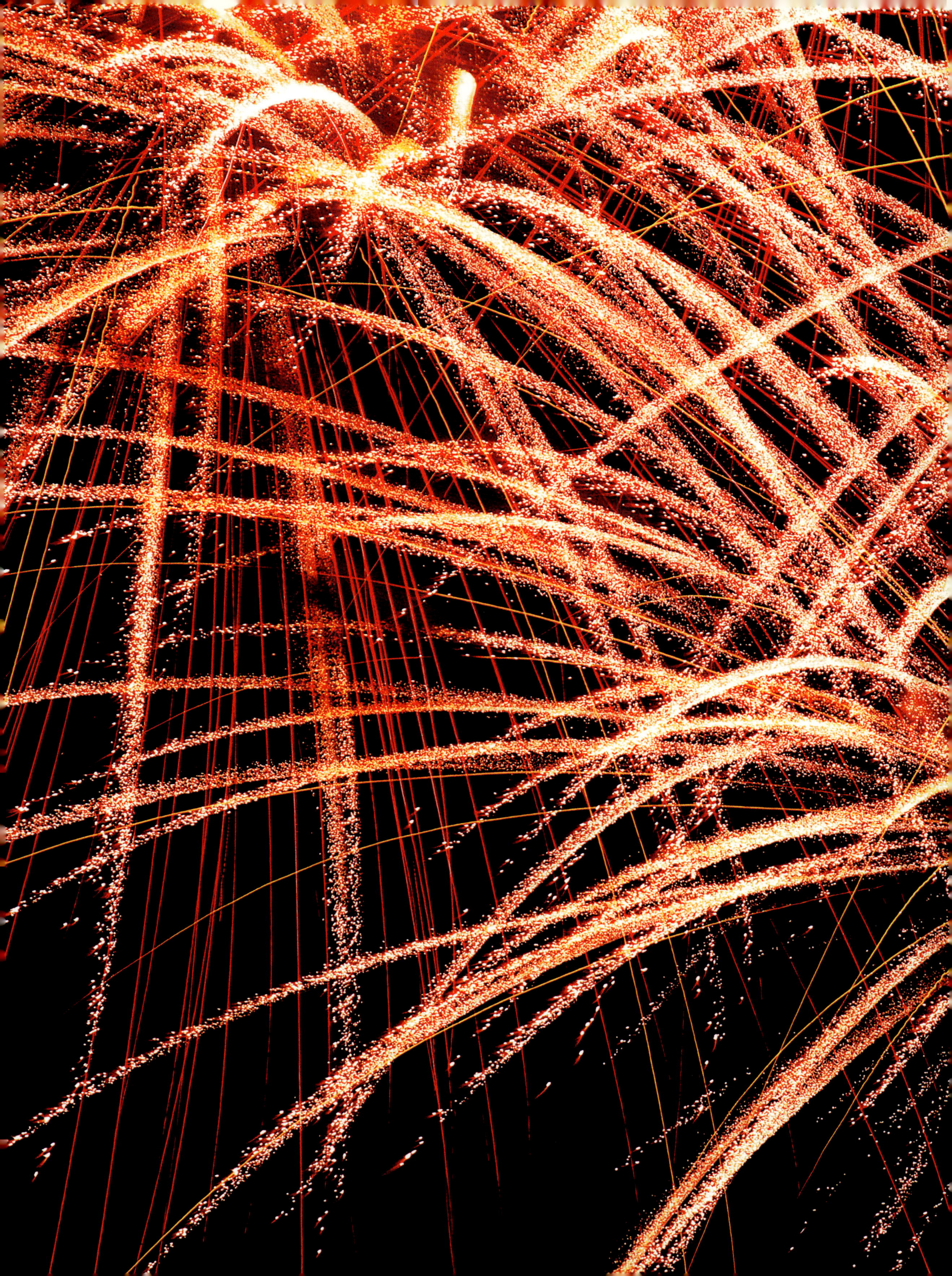

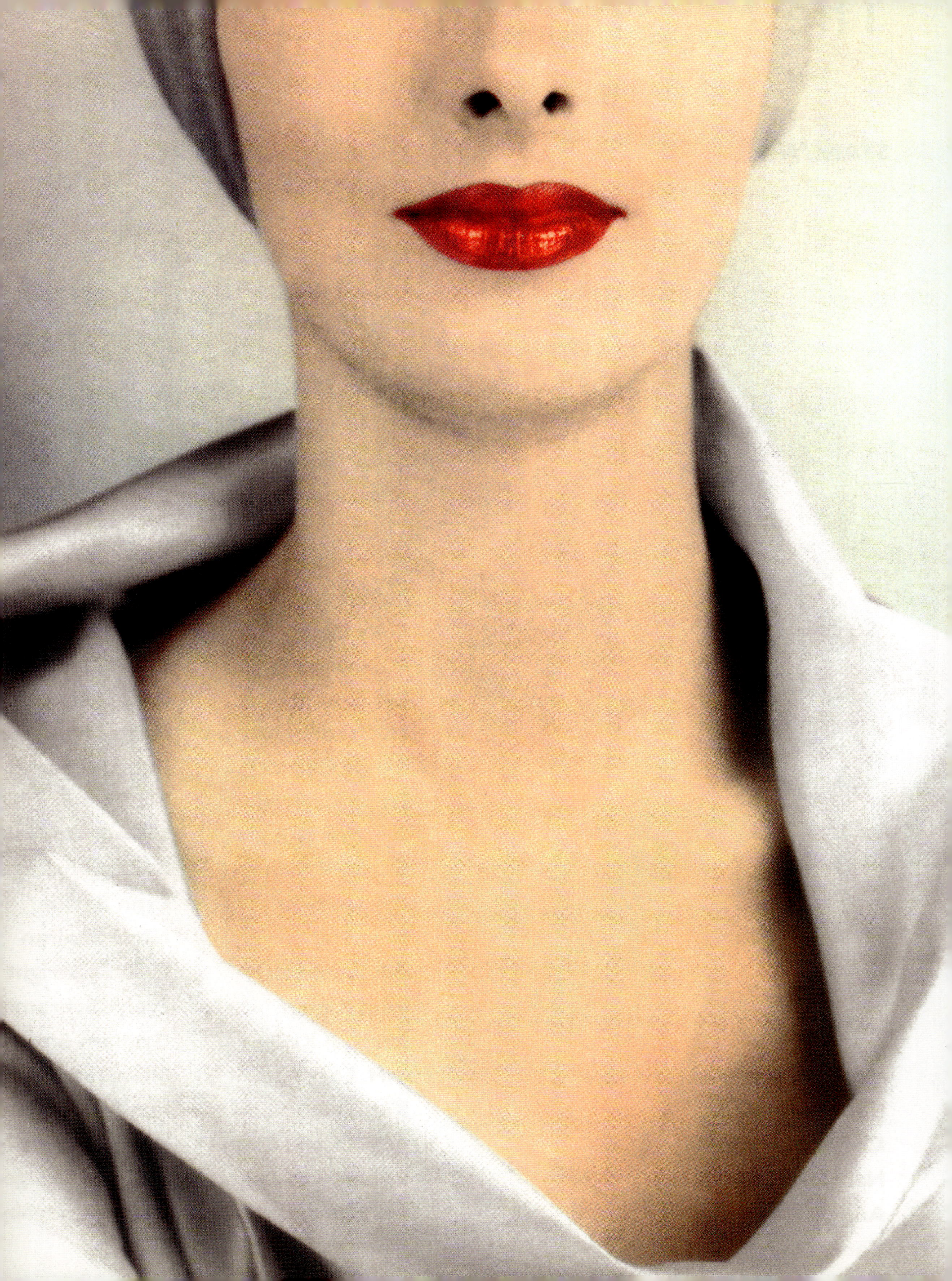

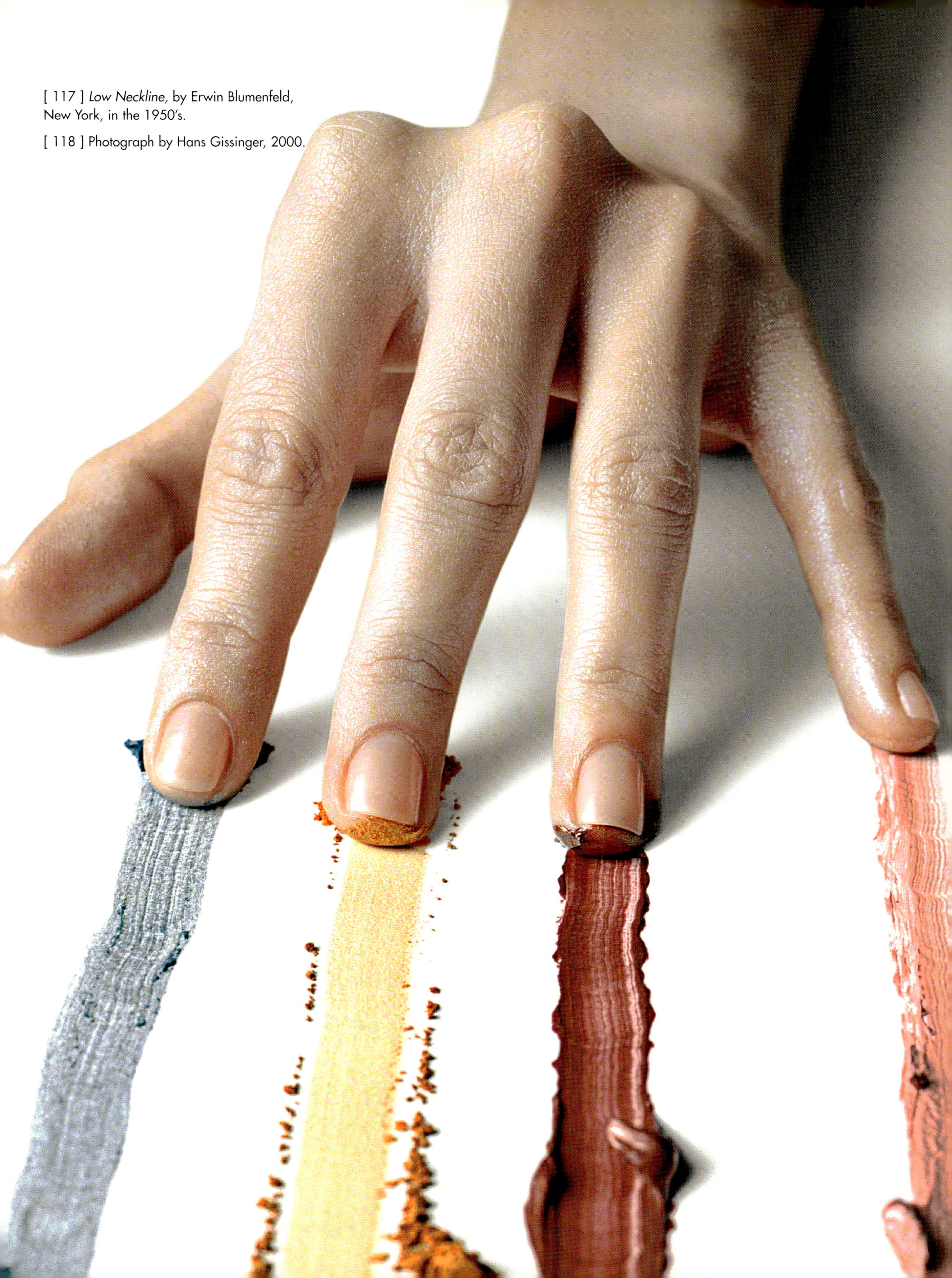

[117] *Low Neckline,* by Erwin Blumenfeld, New York, in the 1950's.

[118] Photograph by Hans Gissinger, 2000.

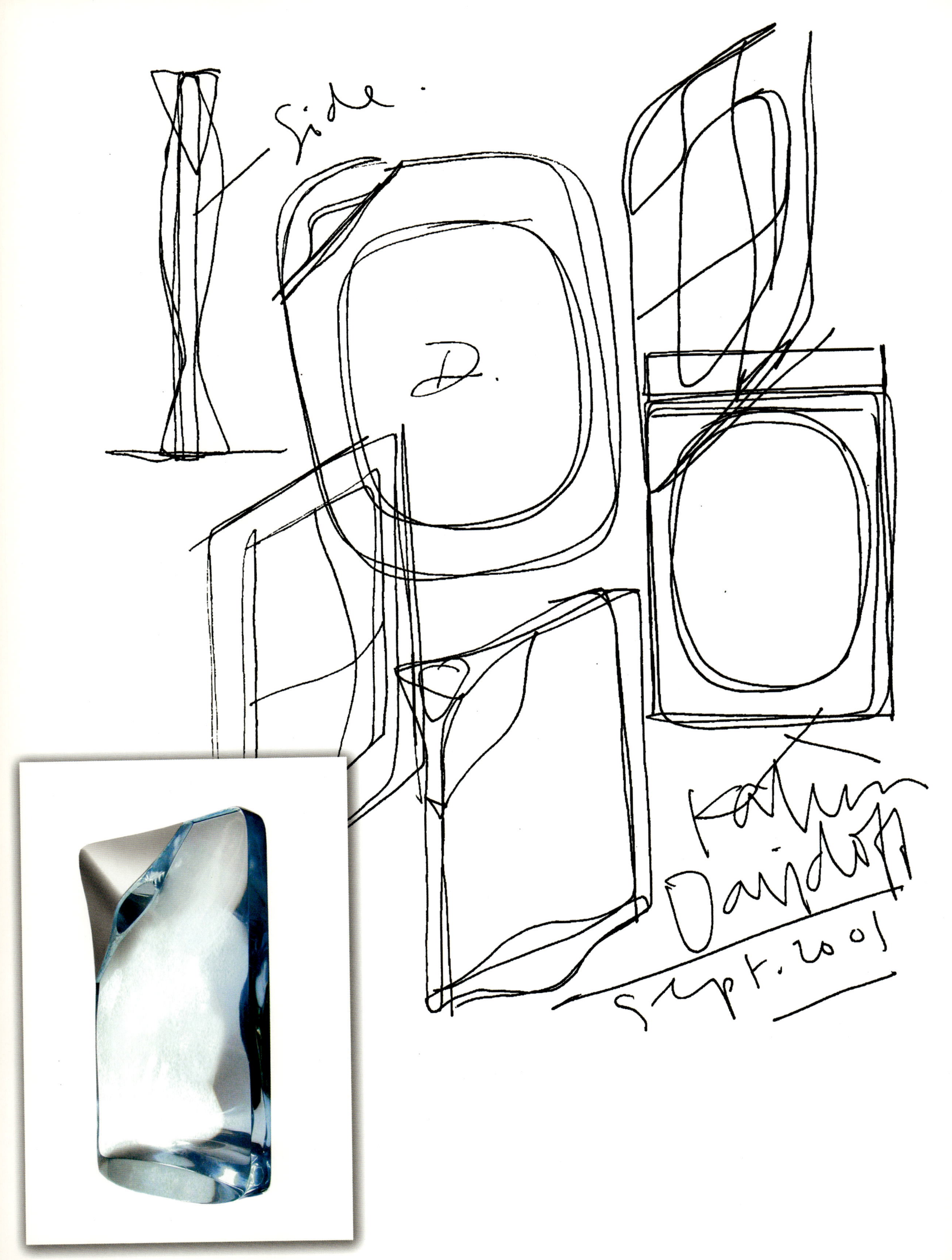
Side.
D.
Karim
Davidoff
Sept. 2001

[119] Karim Rashid, sketches of the Davidoff *Echo* bottle, perfume launched in 2003.

[120] *Echo* bottle by Davidoff, photographed by Henry Dunoyer de Segonzac.

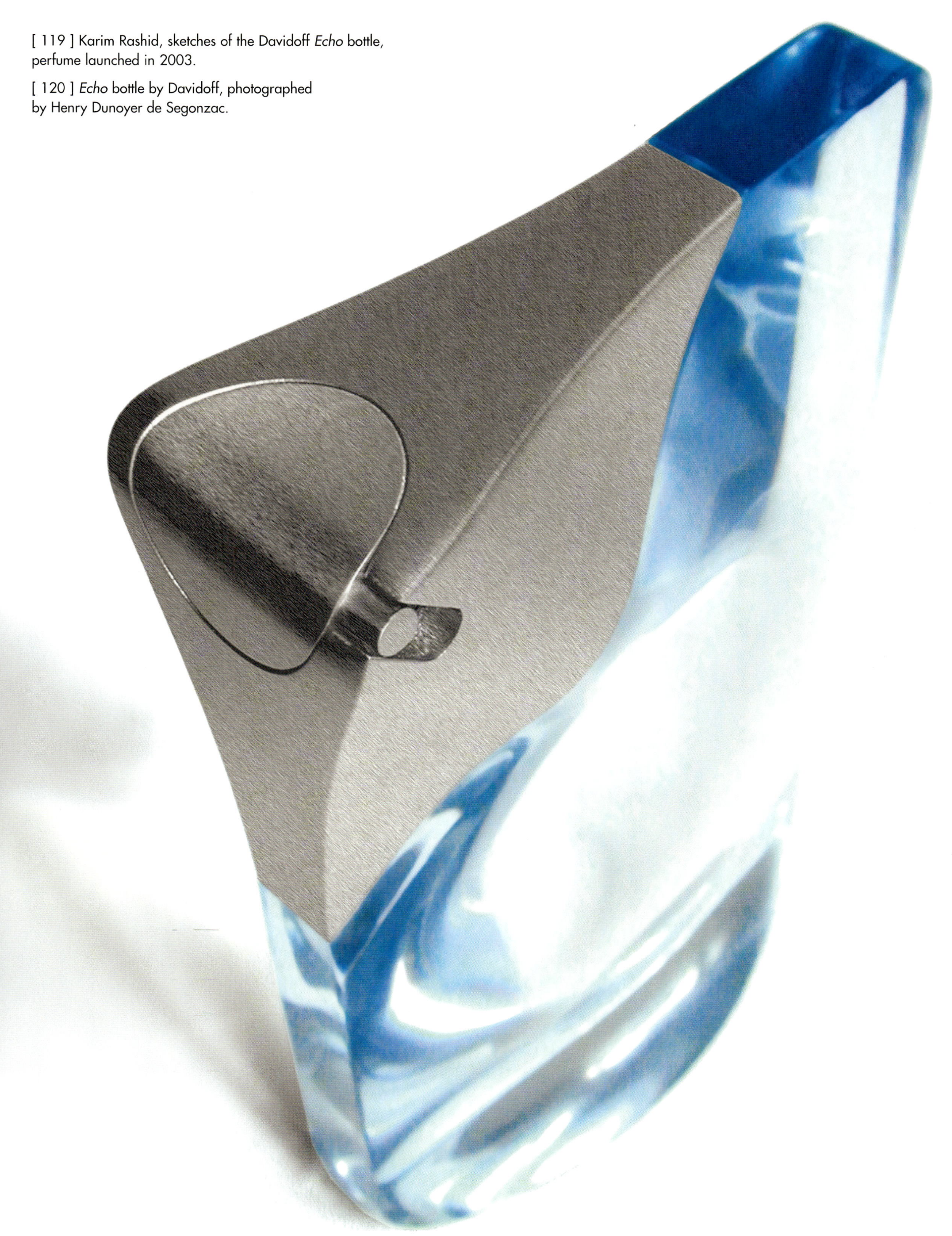

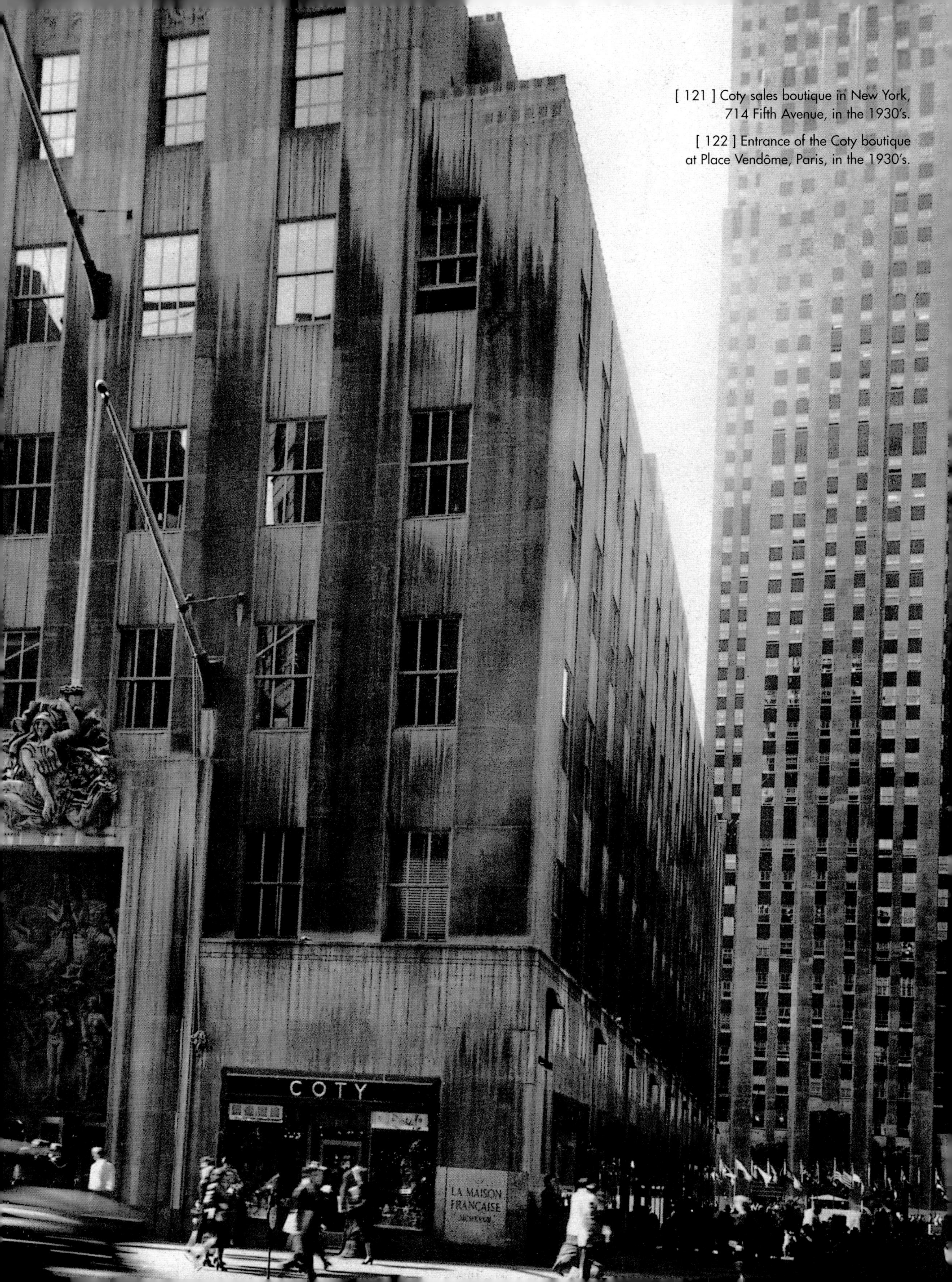

[121] Coty sales boutique in New York, 714 Fifth Avenue, in the 1930's.

[122] Entrance of the Coty boutique at Place Vendôme, Paris, in the 1930's.

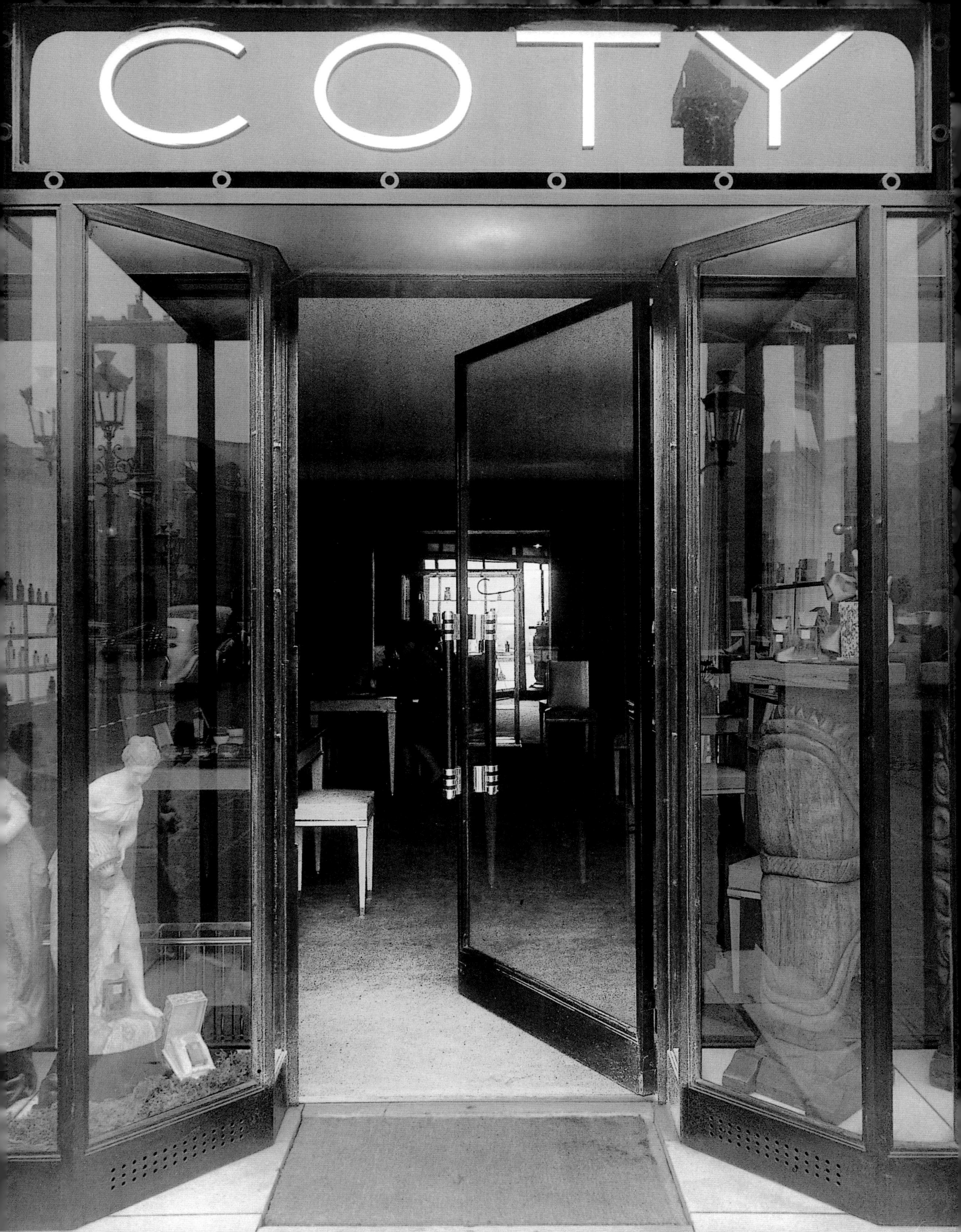
COTY

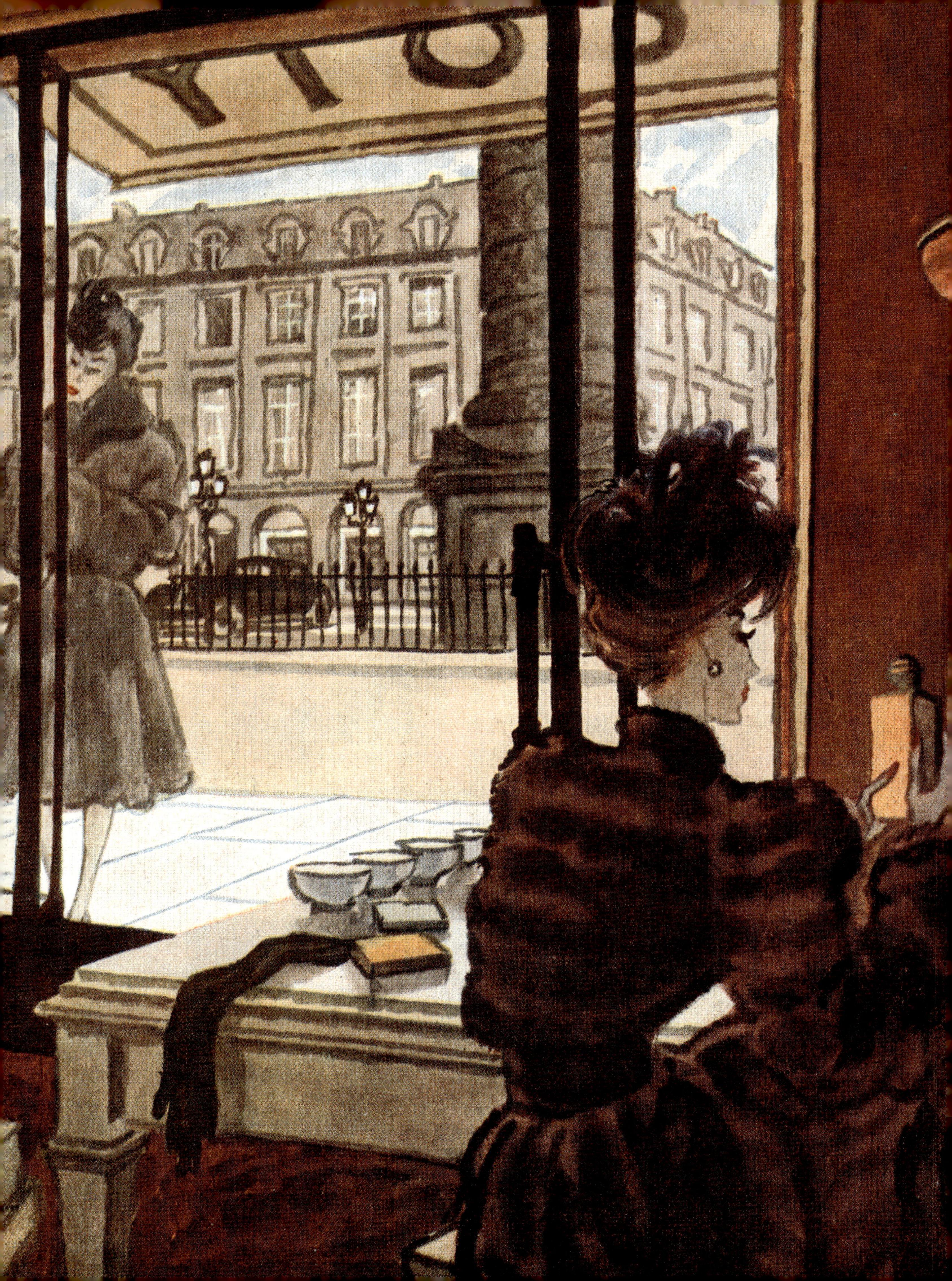

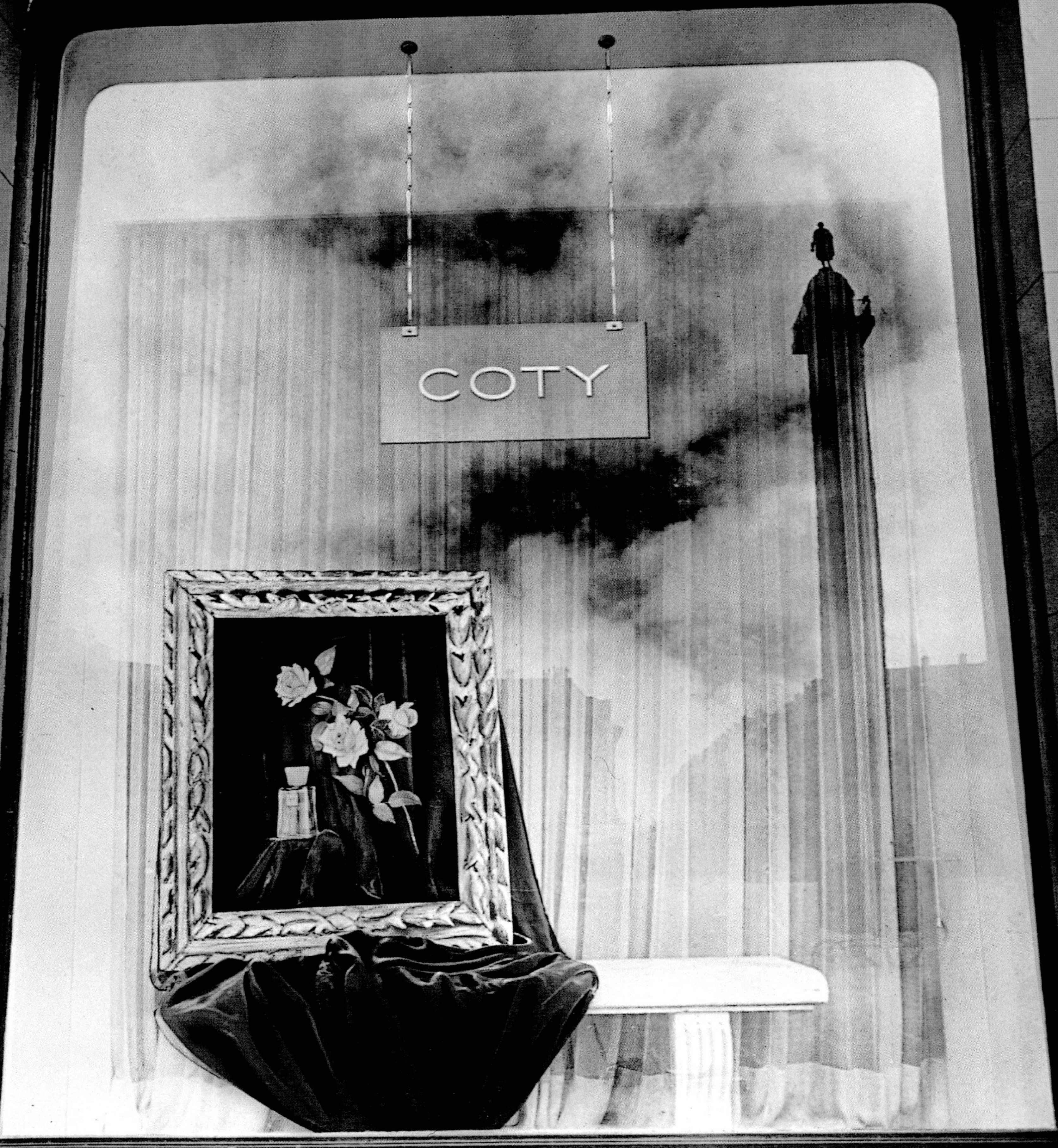

[123] View of the Place Vendôme from the Coty boutique, advertising from 1945.

[124] Shop window of the Coty boutique on the Place Vendôme.

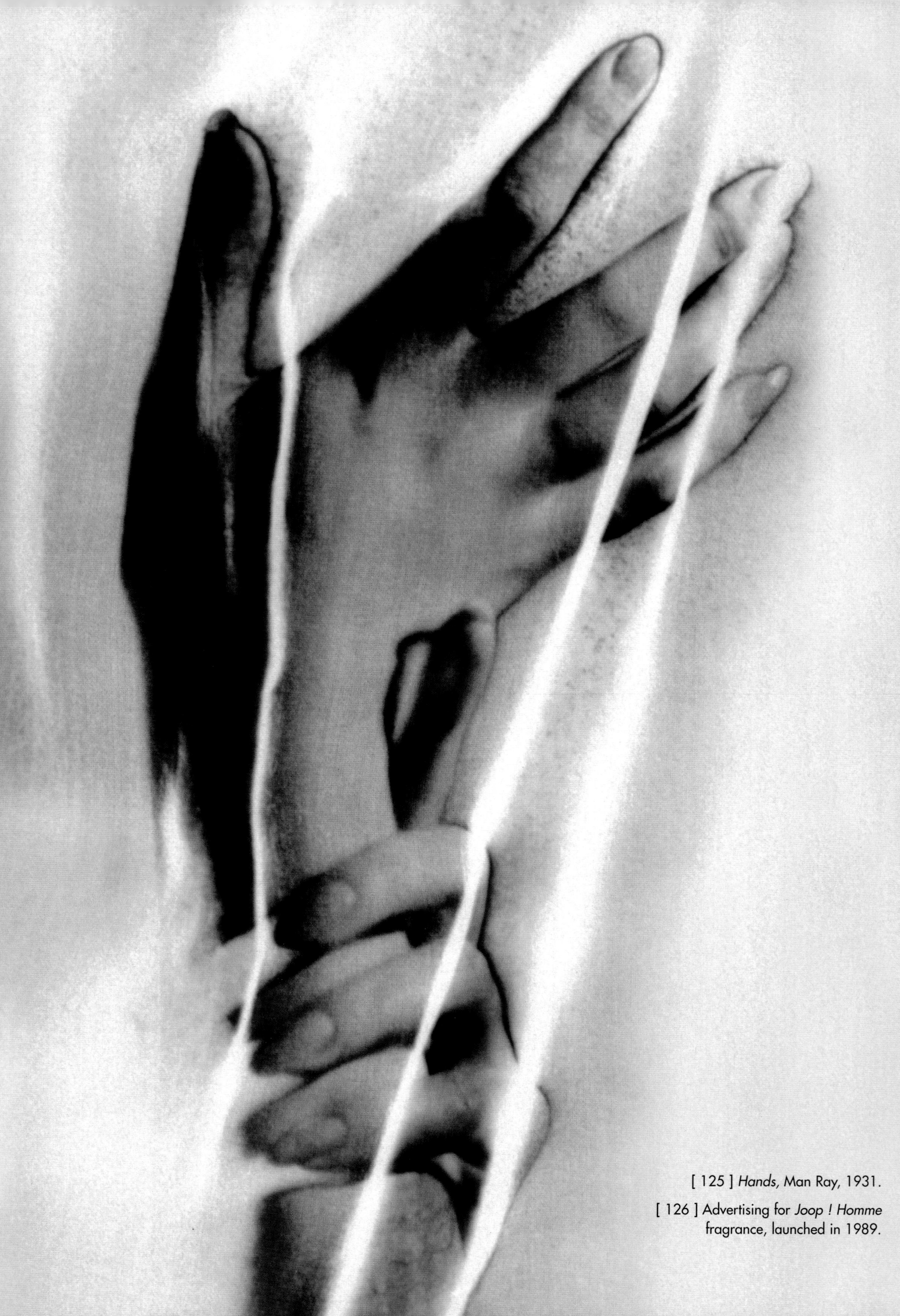

[125] *Hands,* Man Ray, 1931.

[126] Advertising for *Joop ! Homme* fragrance, launched in 1989.

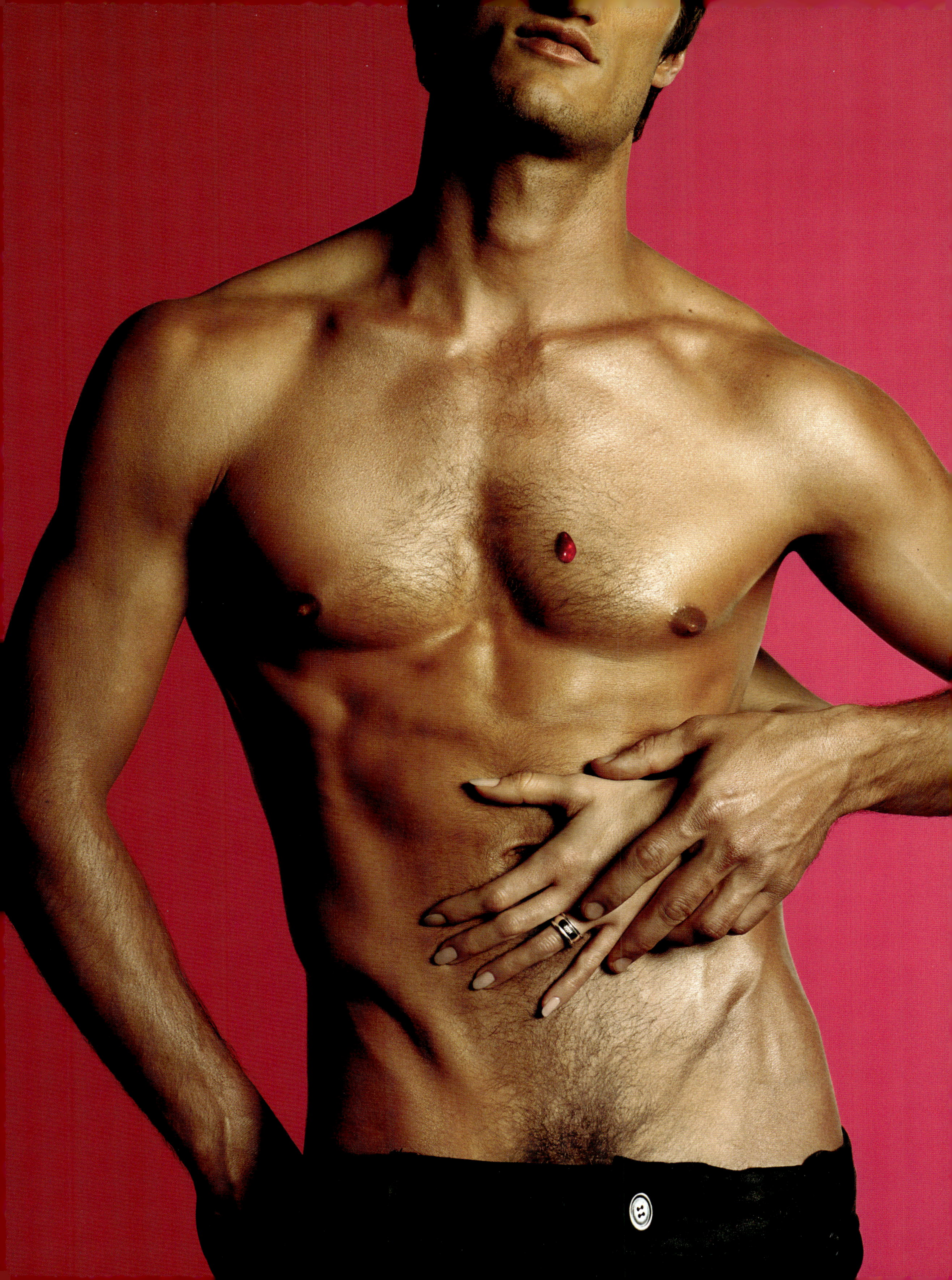

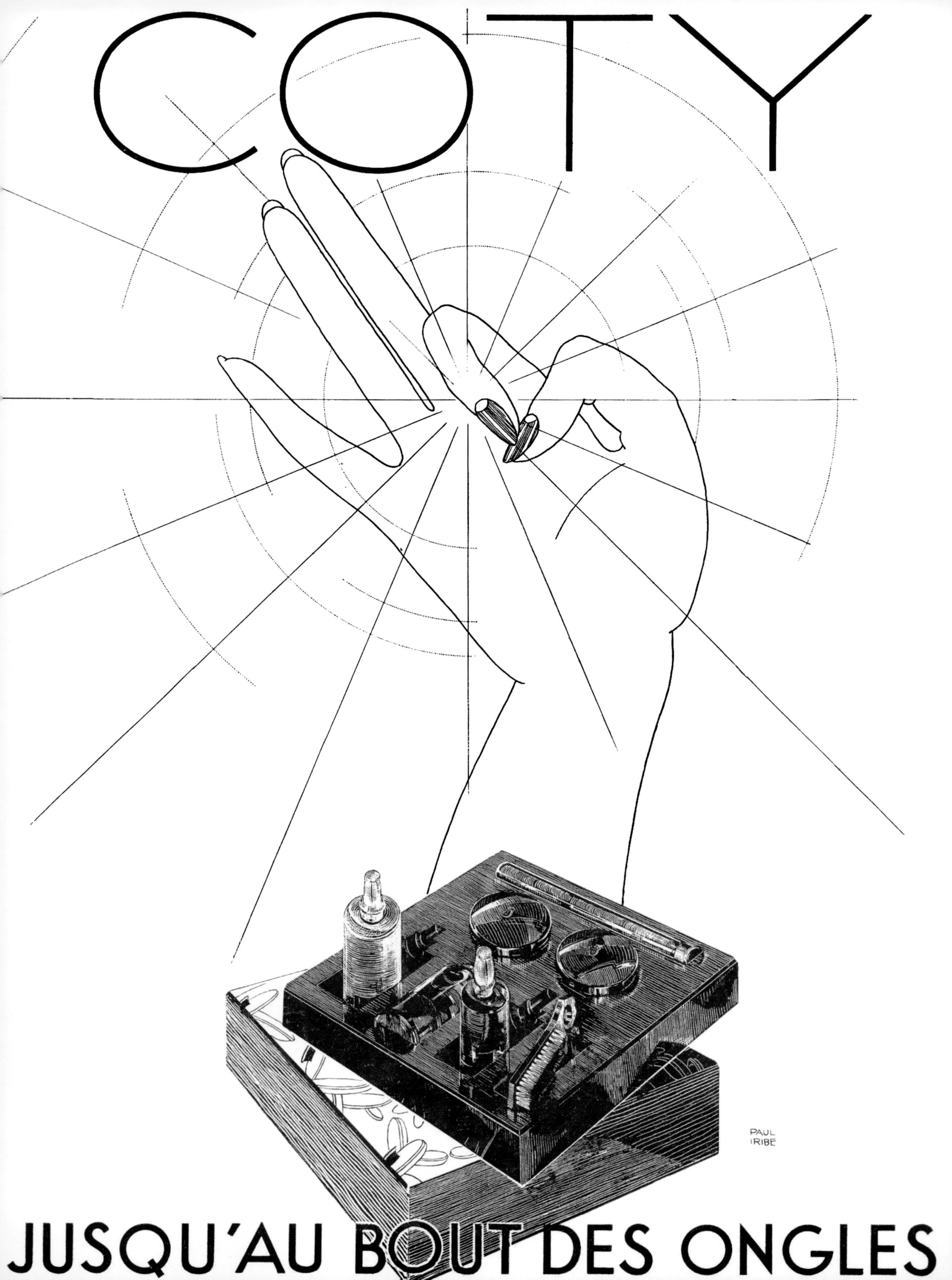
COTY
PAUL
IRIBE
JUSQU'AU BOUT DES ONGLES

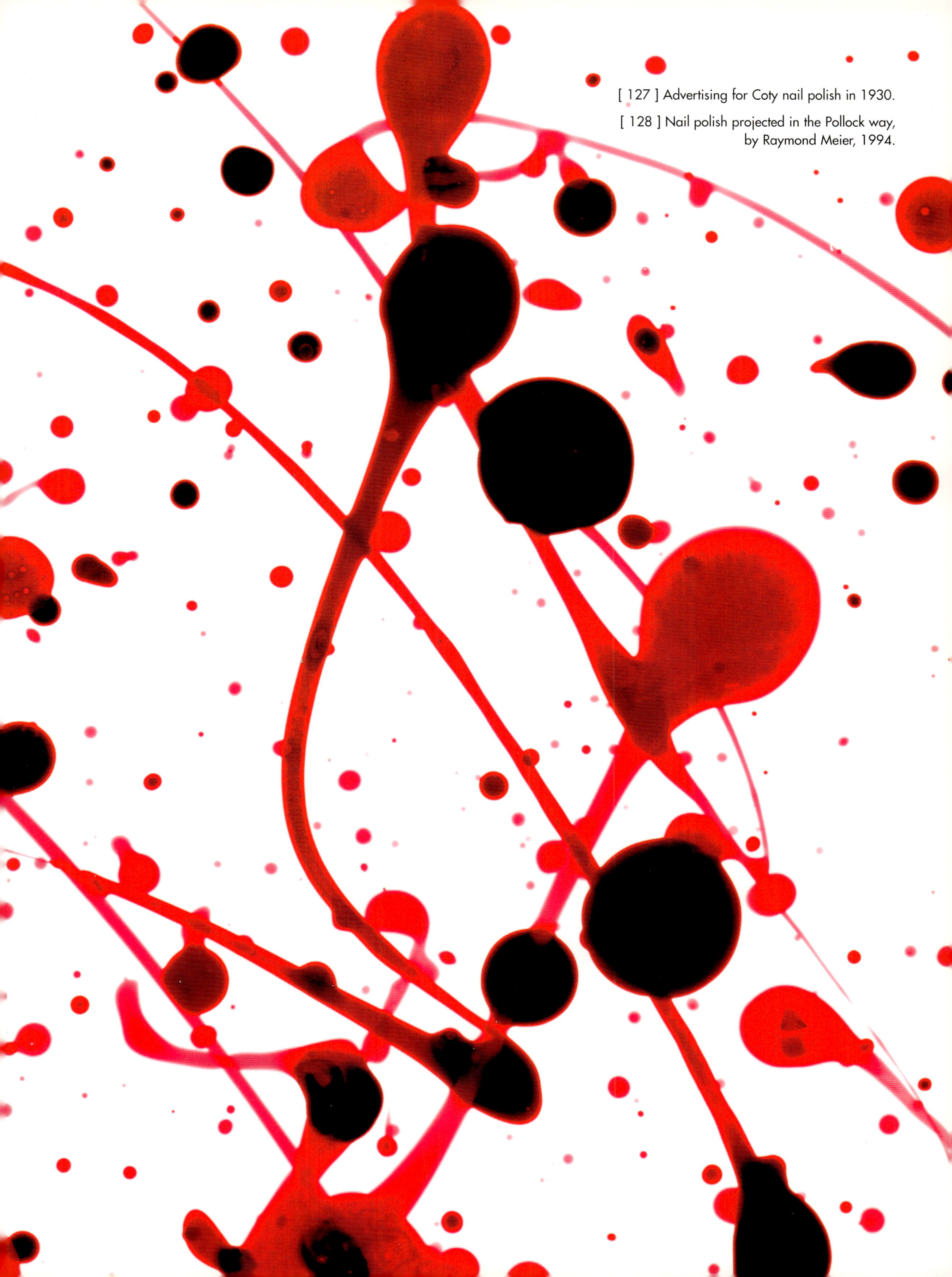

[127] Advertising for Coty nail polish in 1930.

[128] Nail polish projected in the Pollock way, by Raymond Meier, 1994.

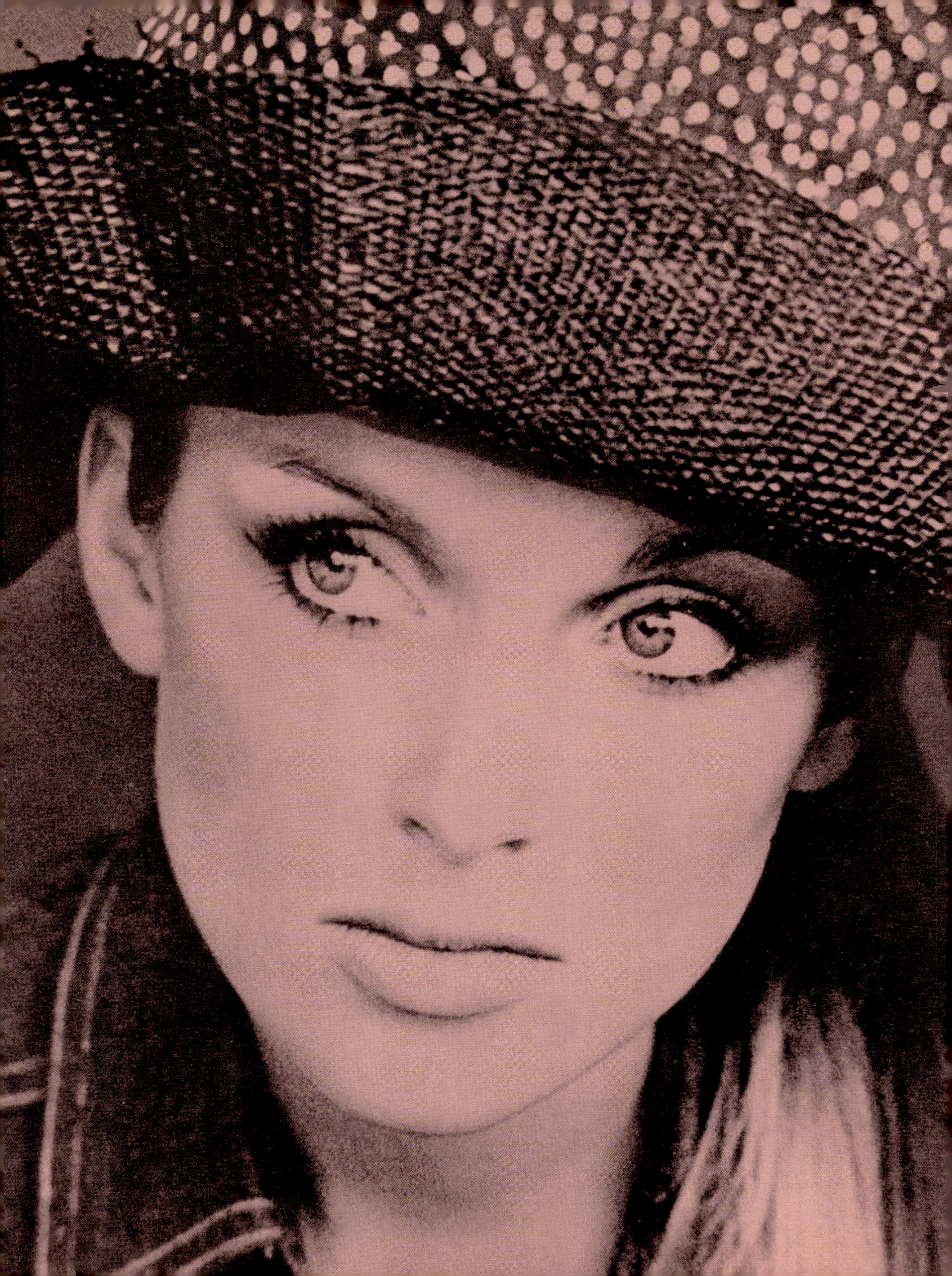

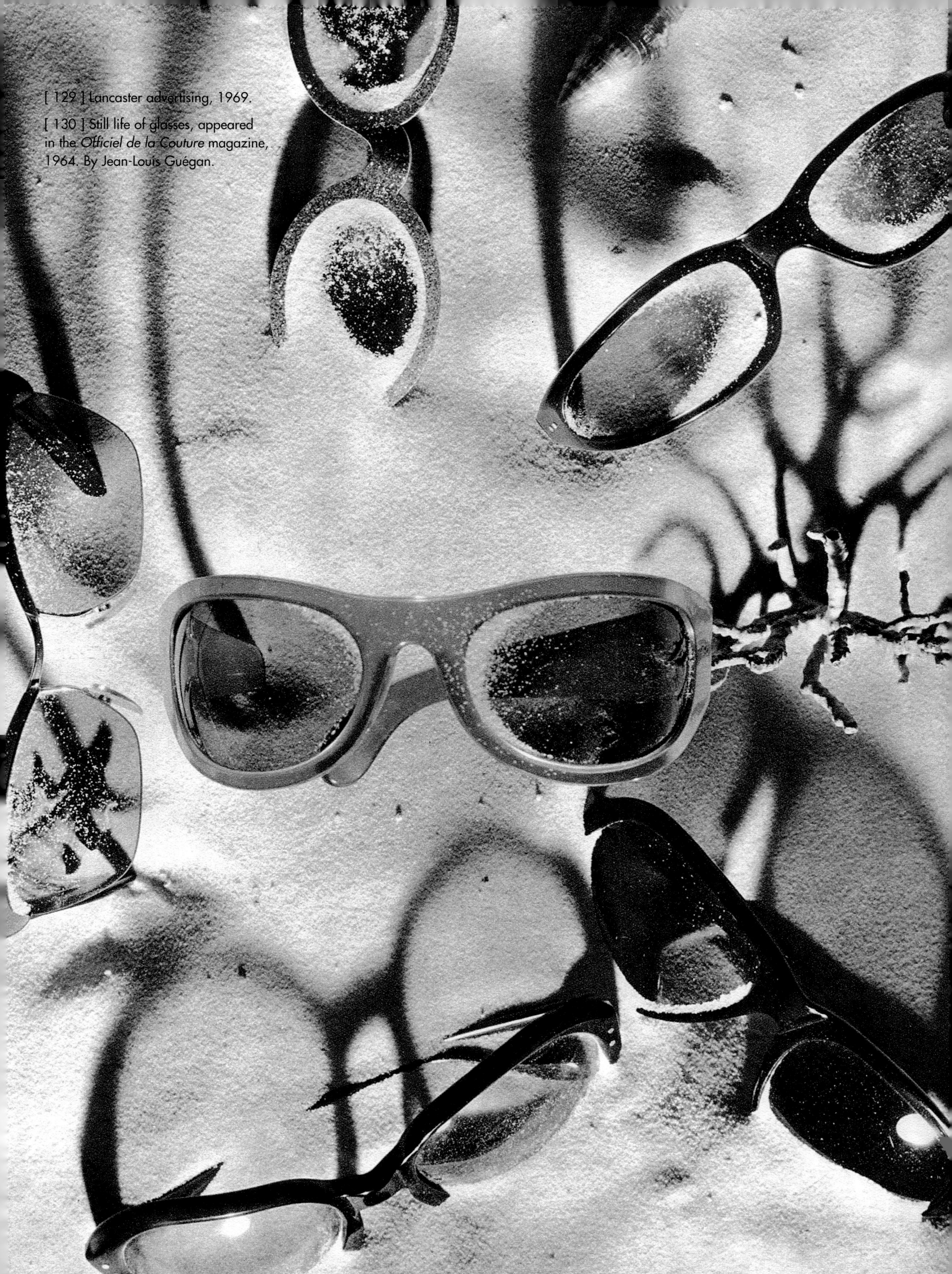

[129] Lancaster advertising, 1969.

[130] Still life of glasses, appeared in the *Officiel de la Couture* magazine, 1964. By Jean-Louis Guégan.

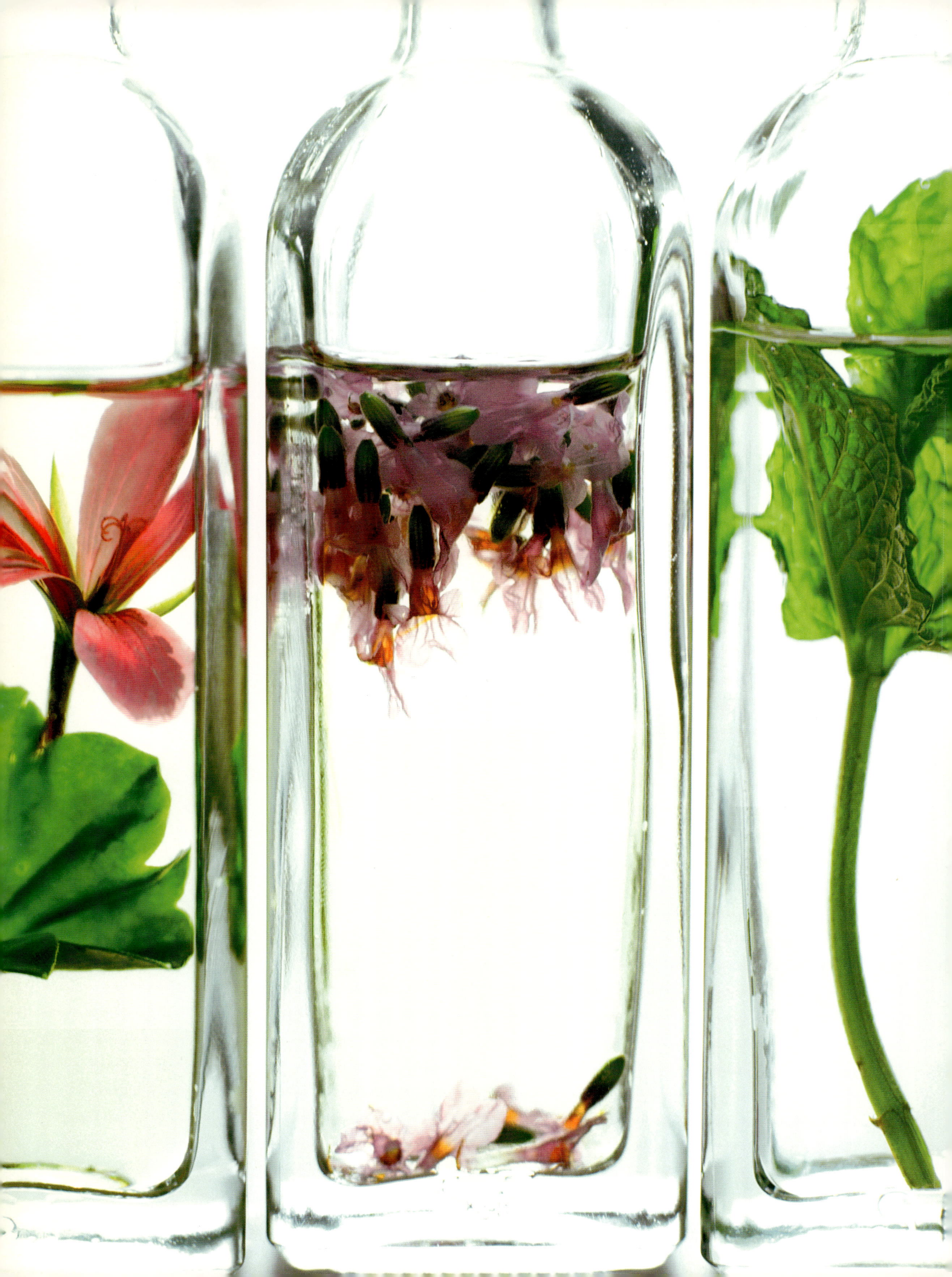

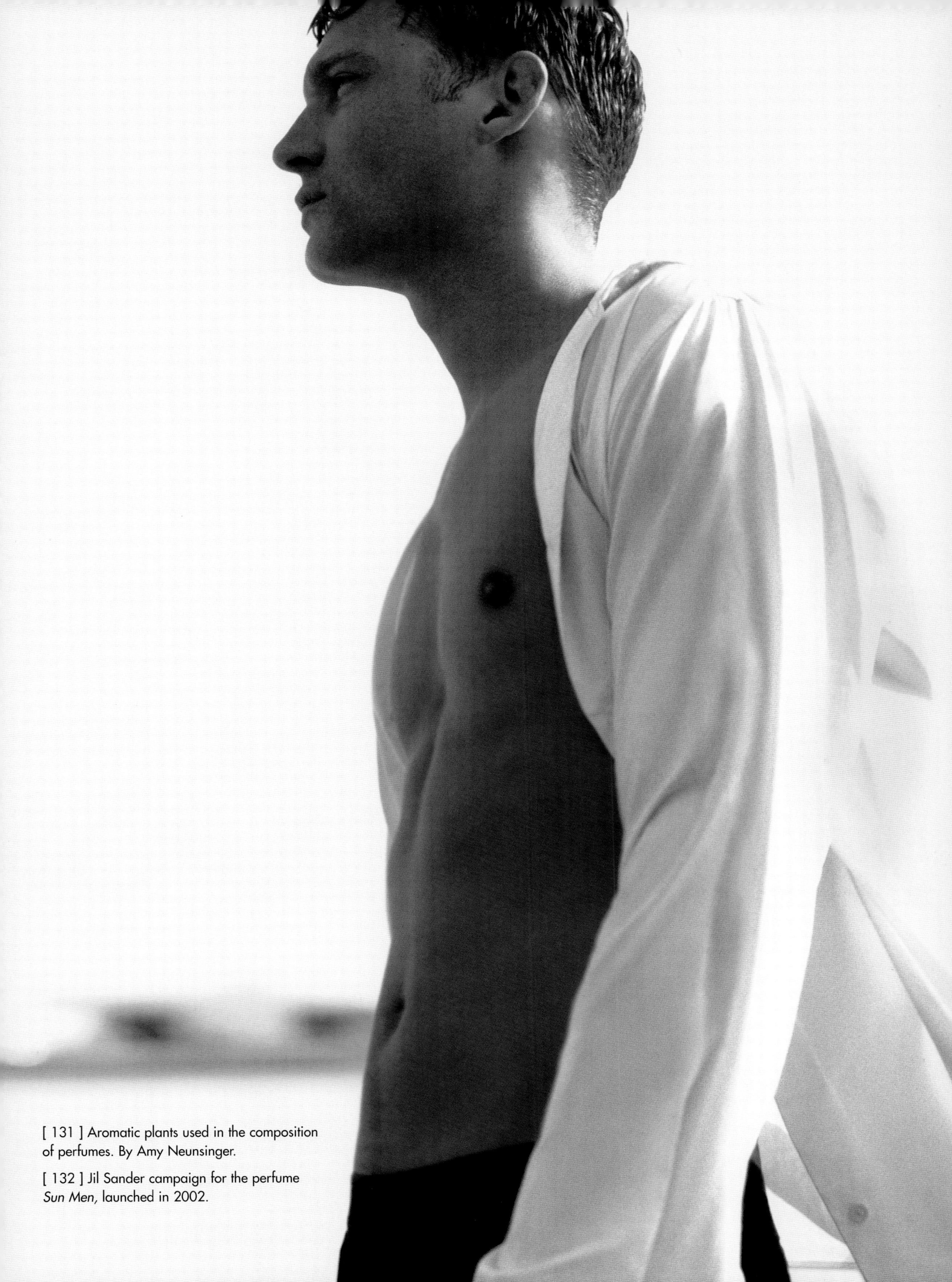

[131] Aromatic plants used in the composition of perfumes. By Amy Neunsinger.

[132] Jil Sander campaign for the perfume *Sun Men,* launched in 2002.

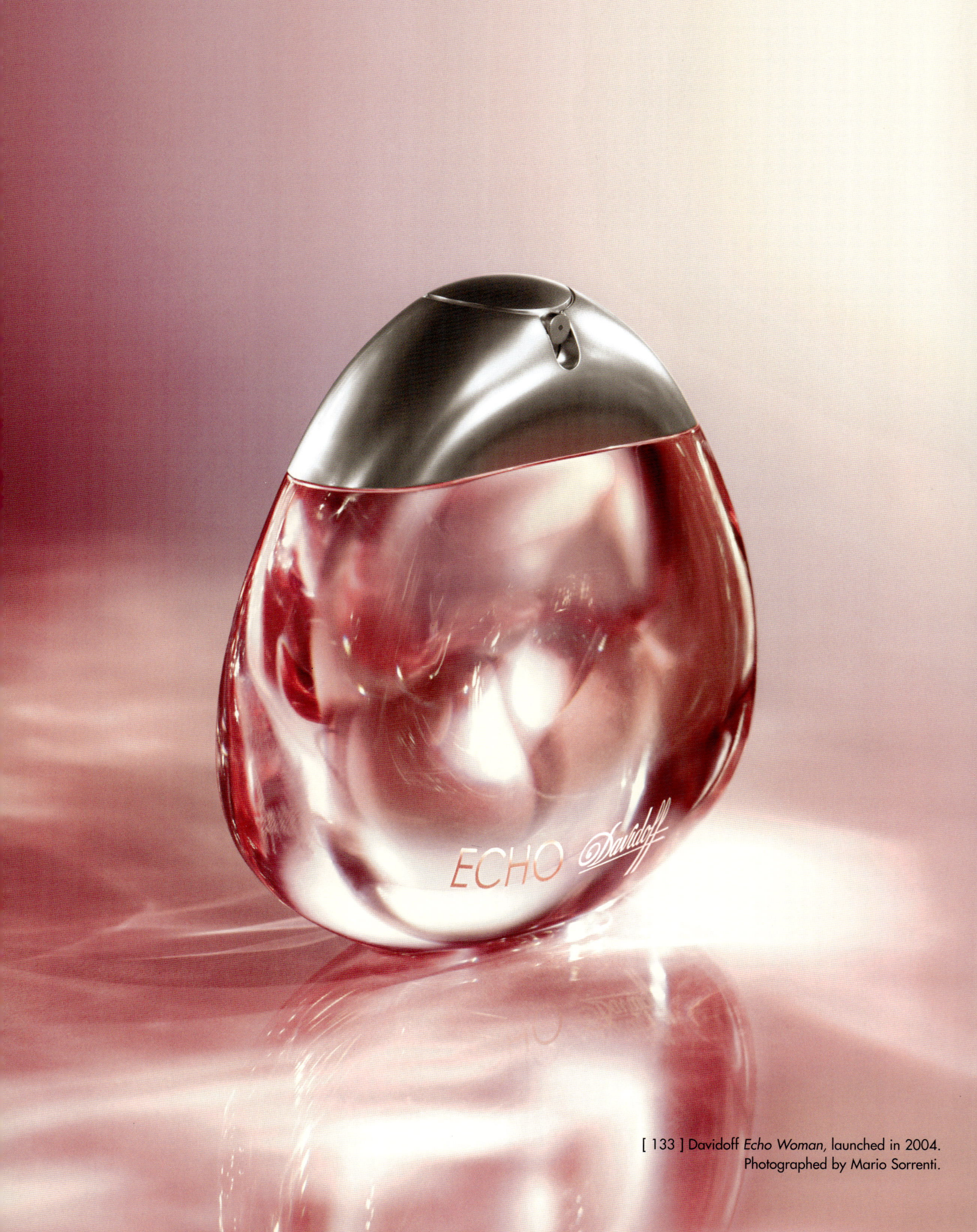

[133] Davidoff *Echo Woman,* launched in 2004.
Photographed by Mario Sorrenti.

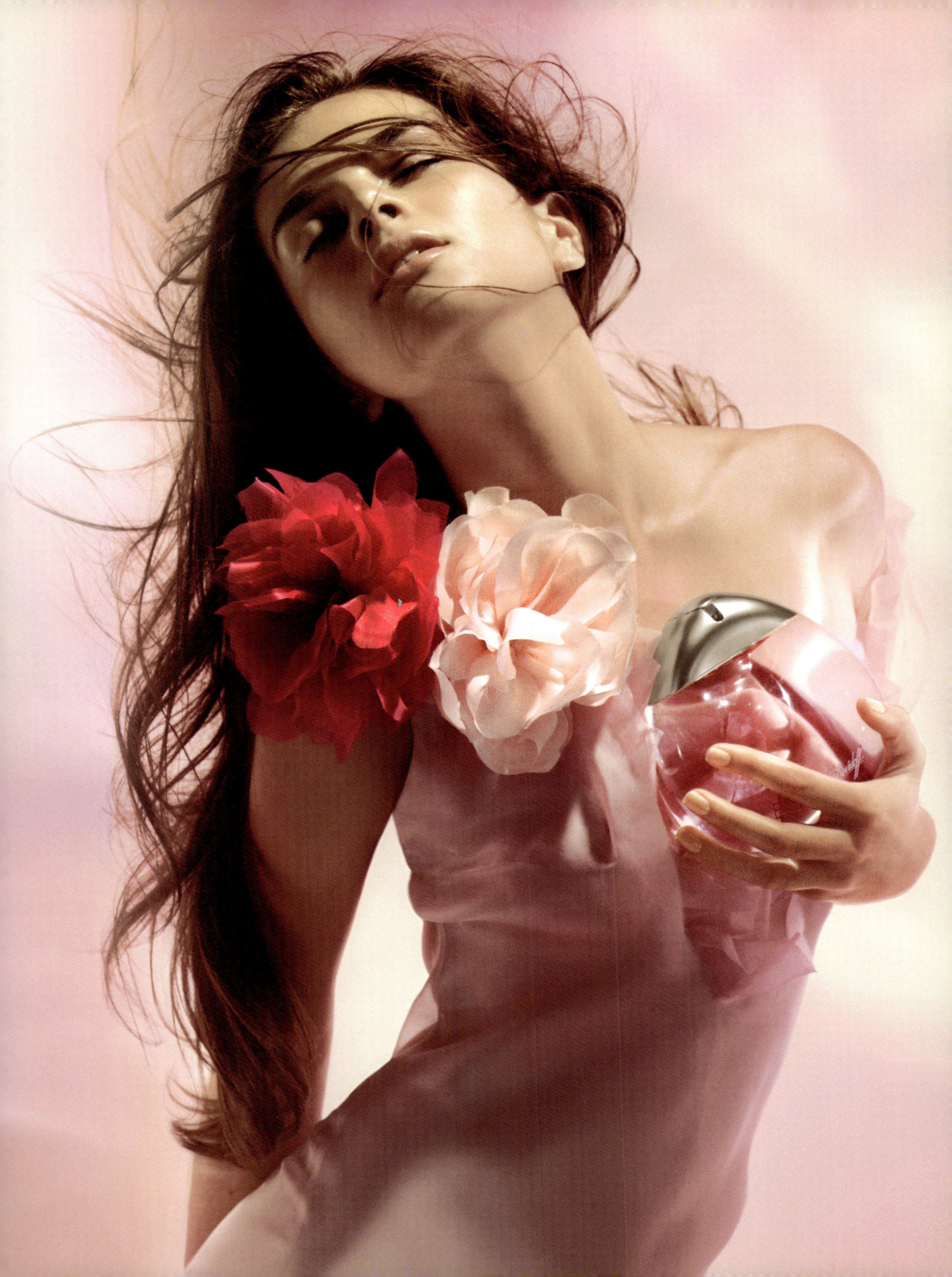

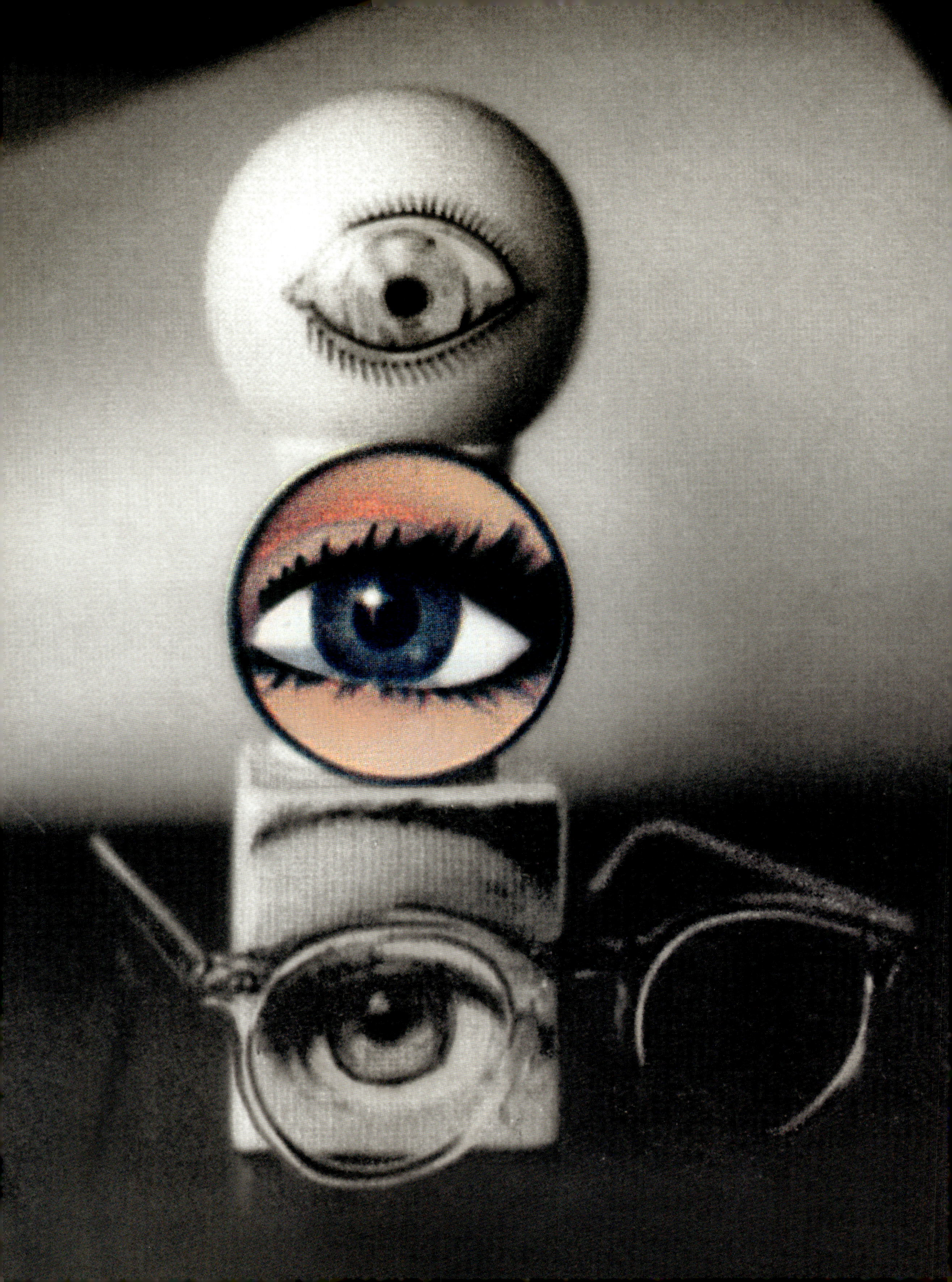

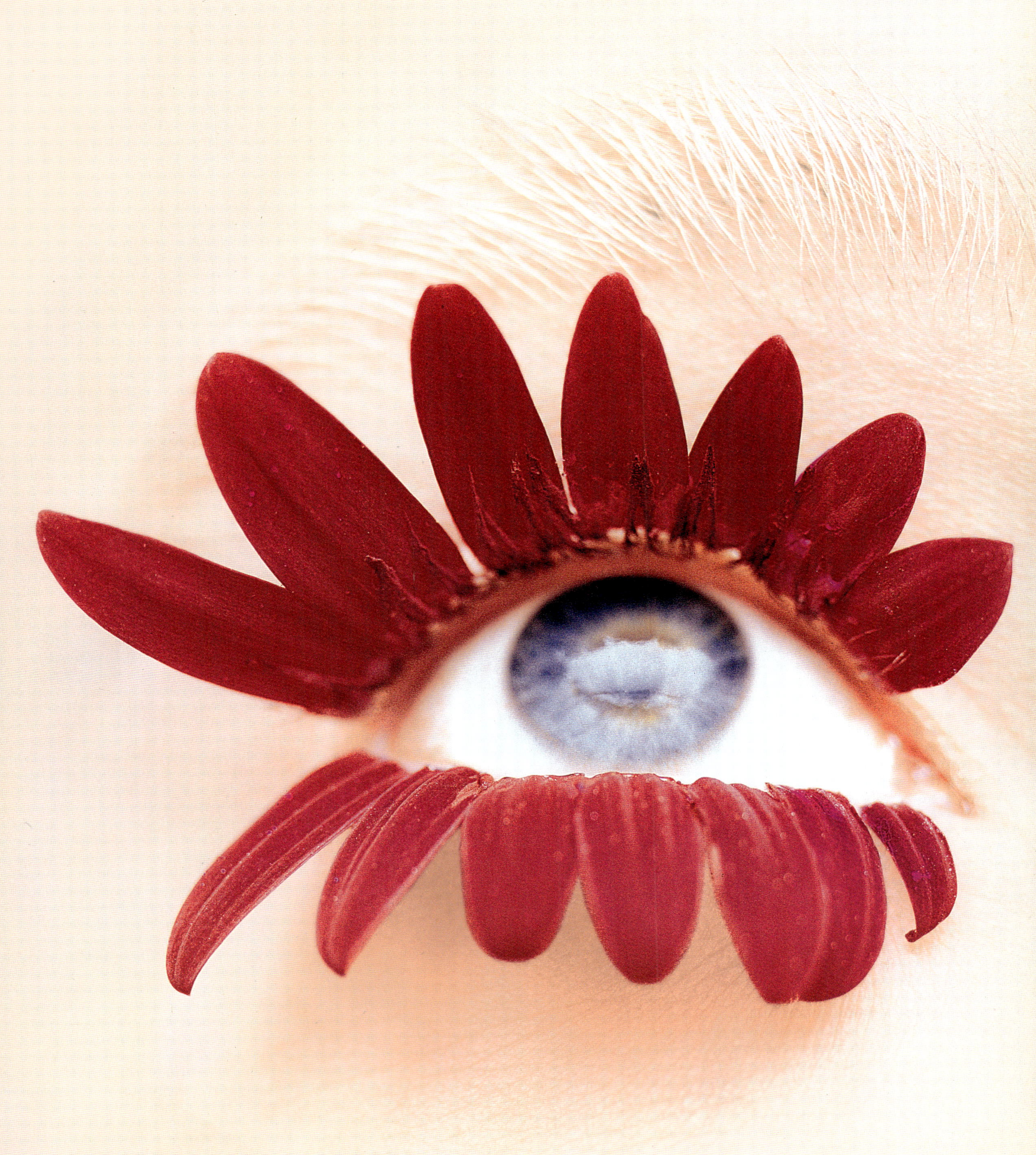

[134] *At my window,* photograph by André Kertesz.

[135] *Flower-eye,* 1987. Make-up by Topolino, photograph by Satoshi Sakusa.

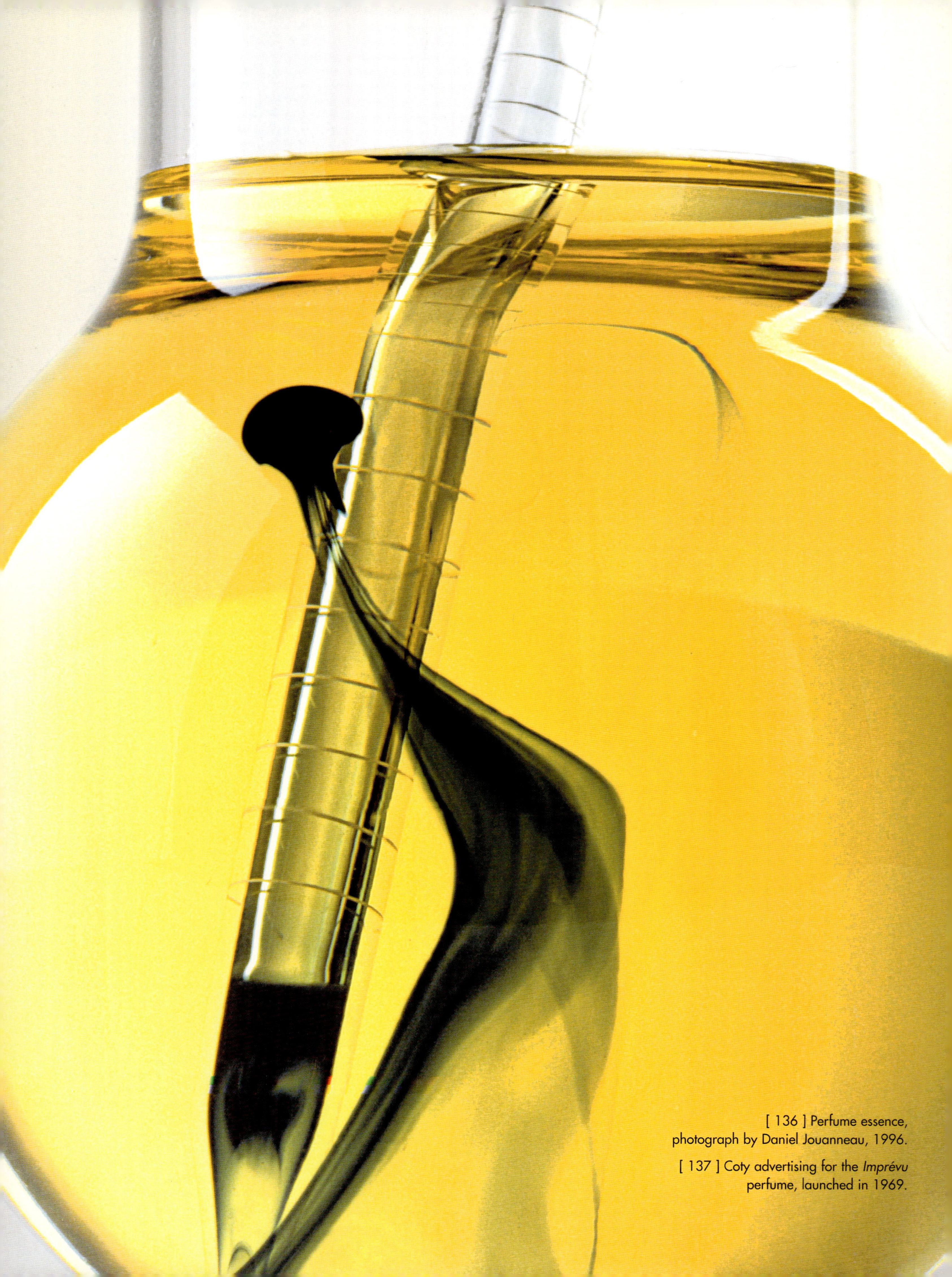

[136] Perfume essence,
photograph by Daniel Jouanneau, 1996.

[137] Coty advertising for the *Imprévu*
perfume, launched in 1969.

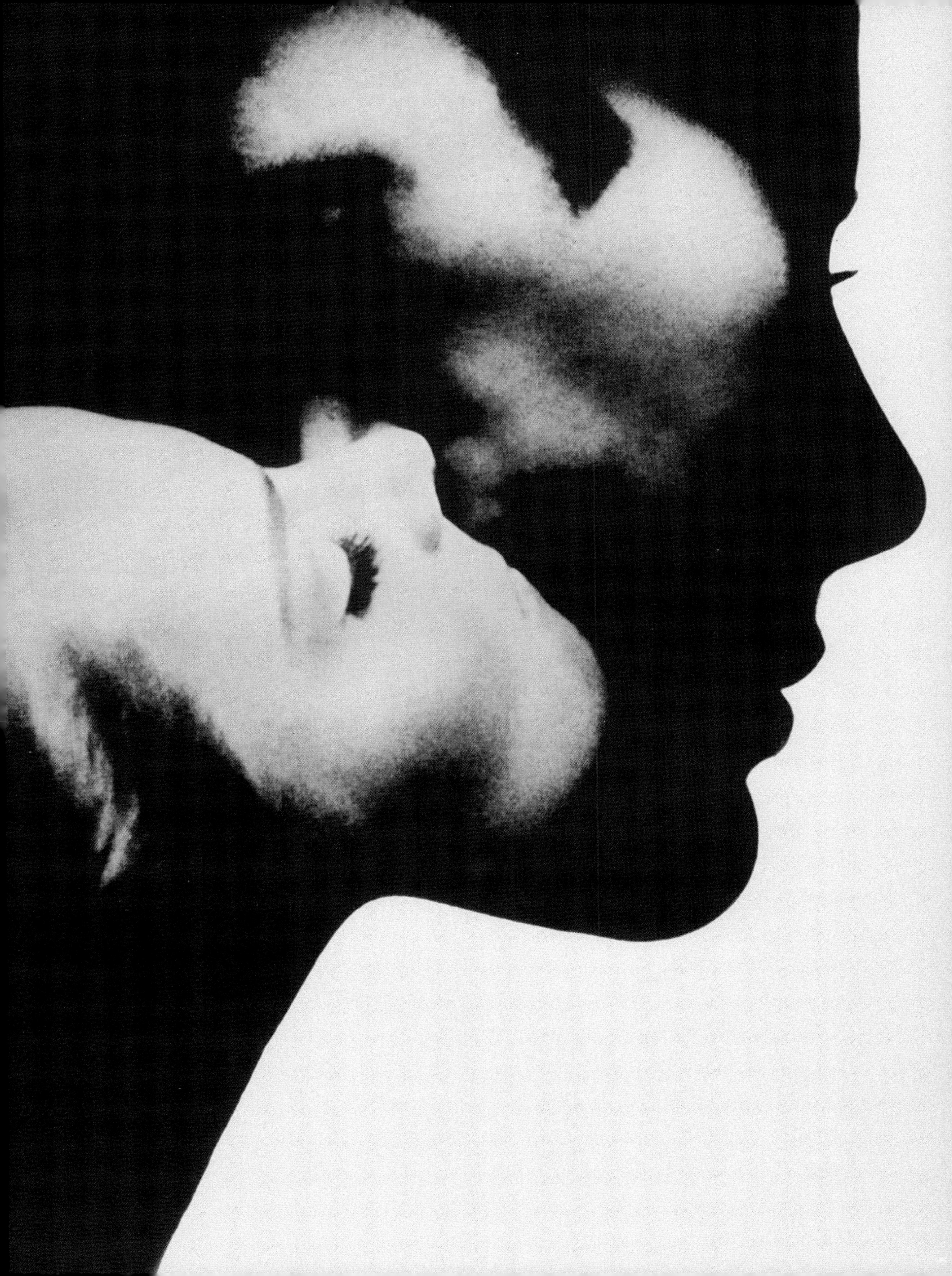

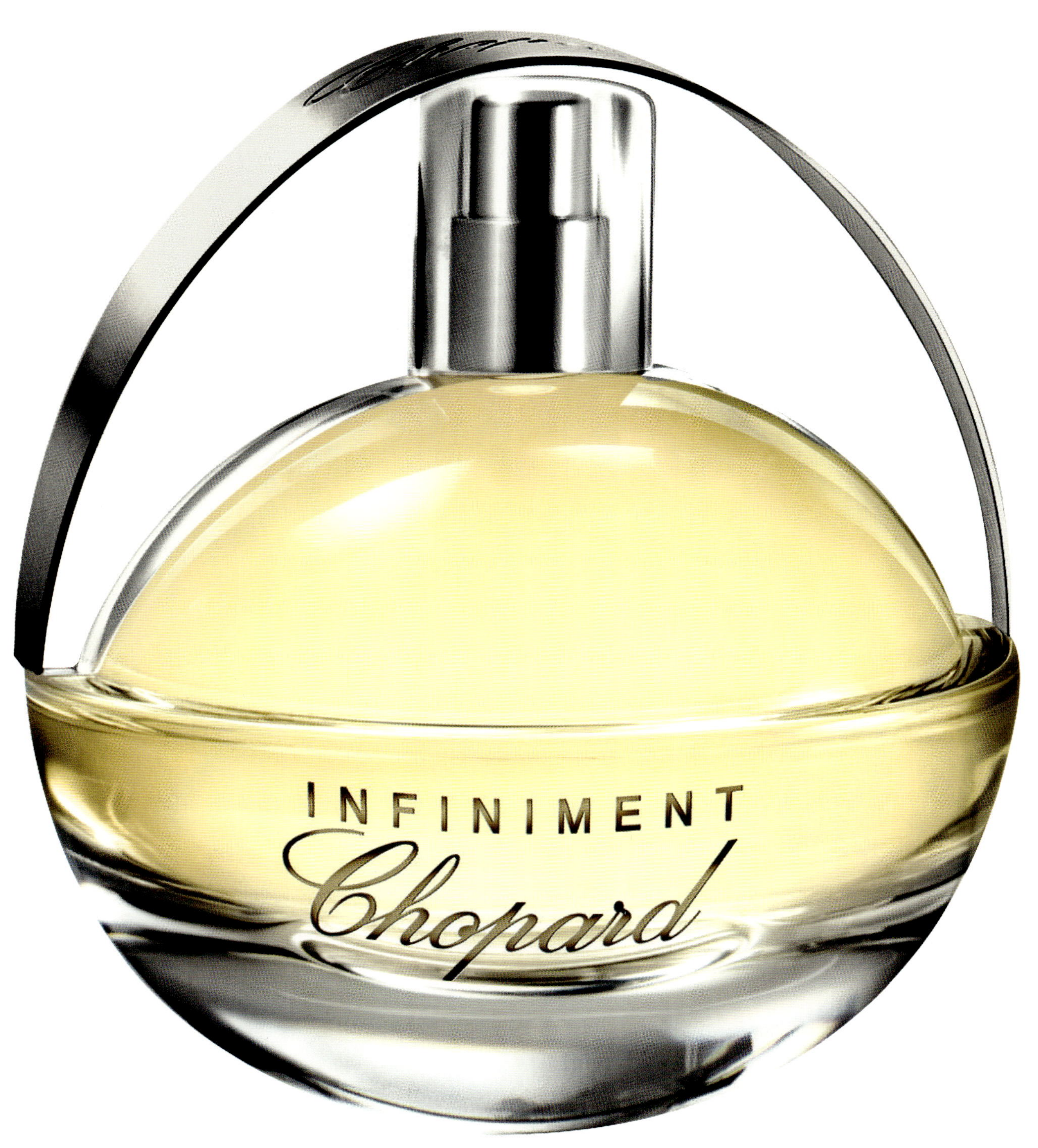

[138] [139] Campaign for the *Infiniment Chopard* perfume by Chopard, launched in 2004.

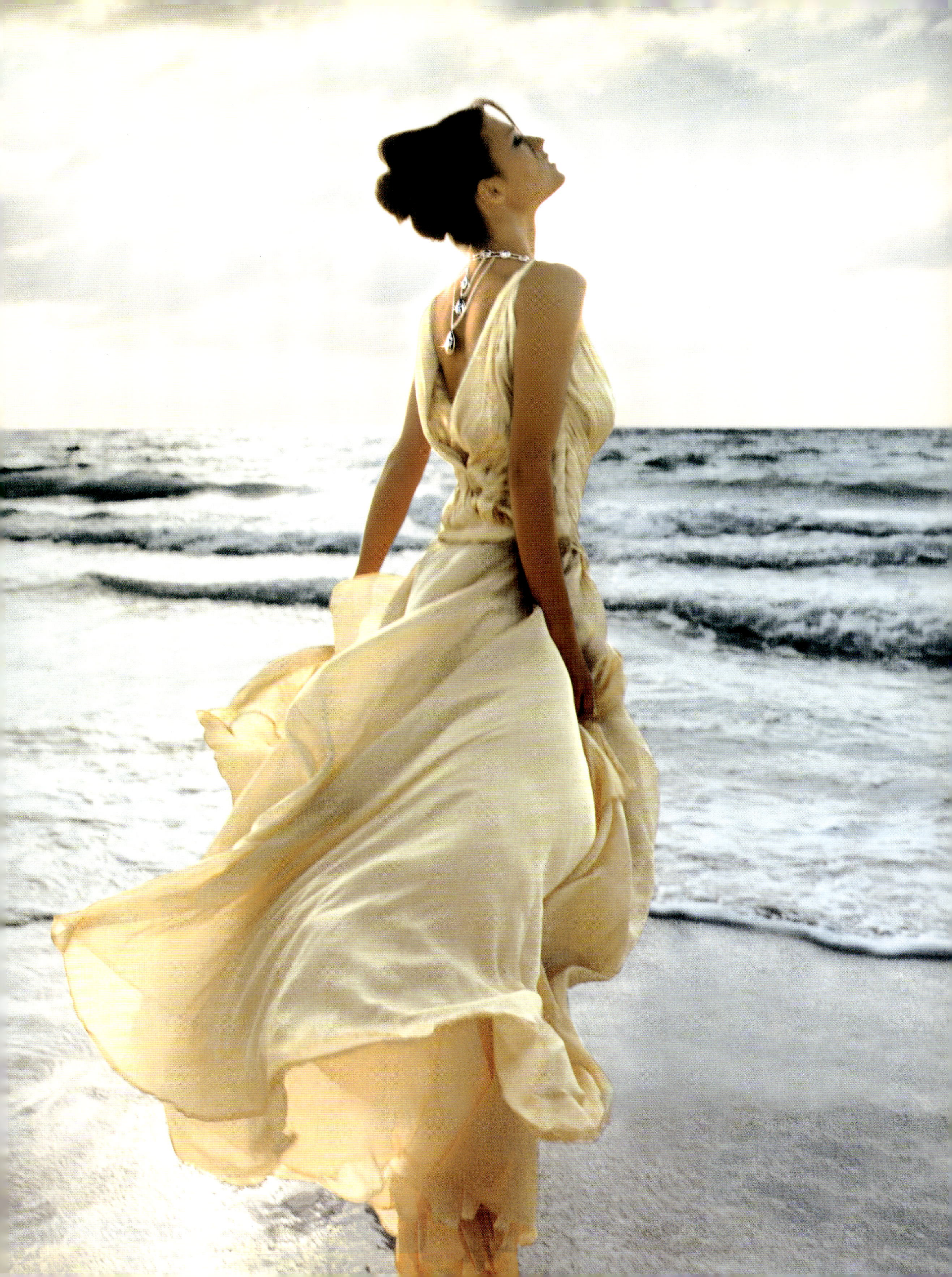

[140] Building on the success of her first fragrance, Coty Beauty launched in 2004 *Celine Dion Parfums Notes*.

[141] Gold record.

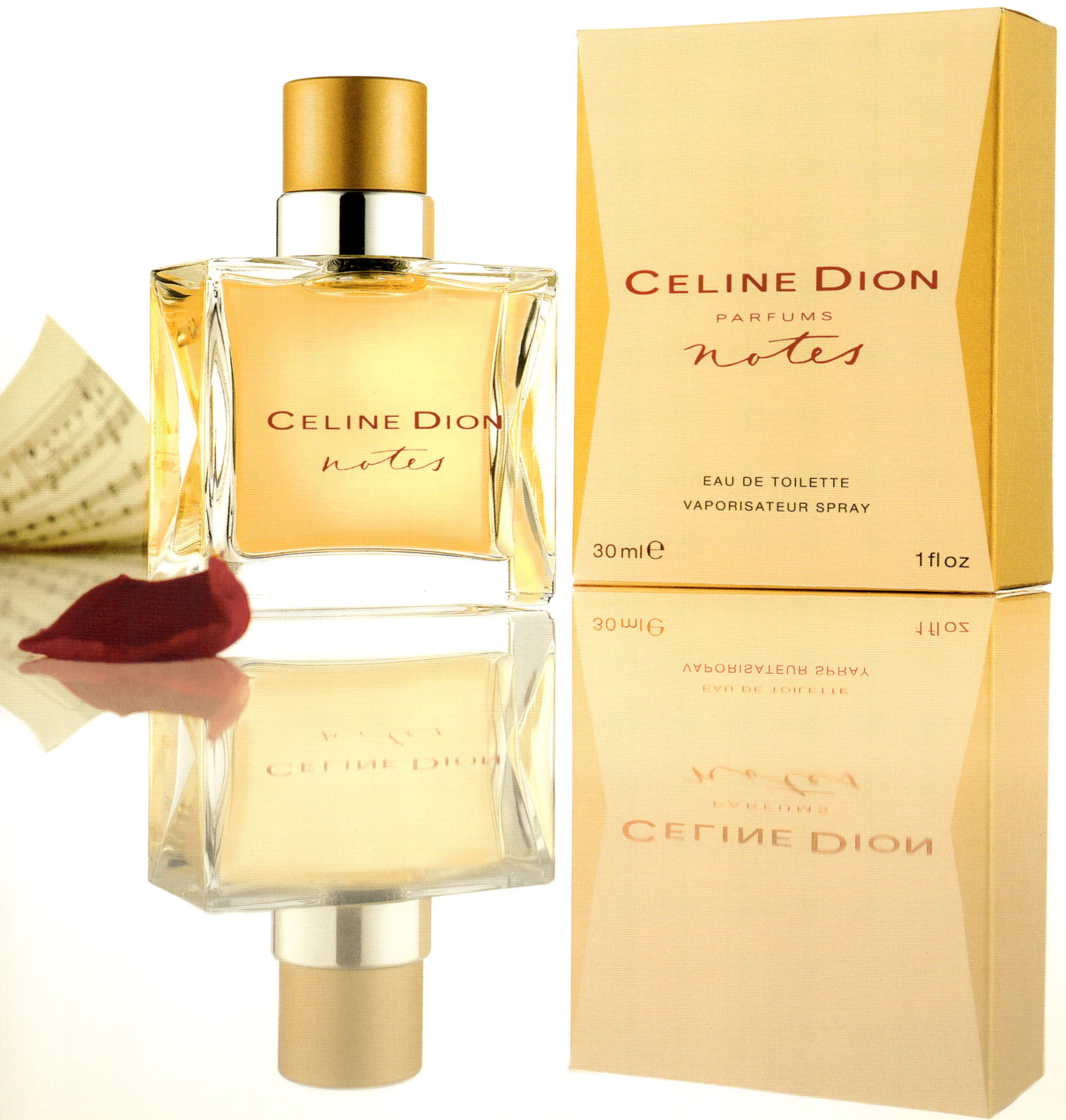

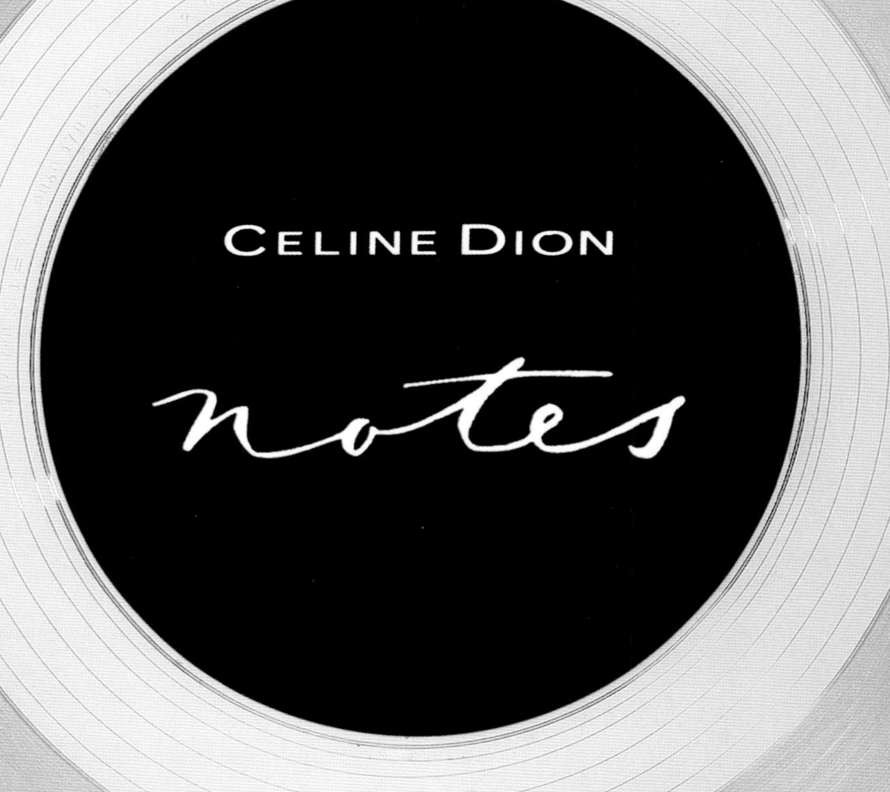
Celine Dion
notes

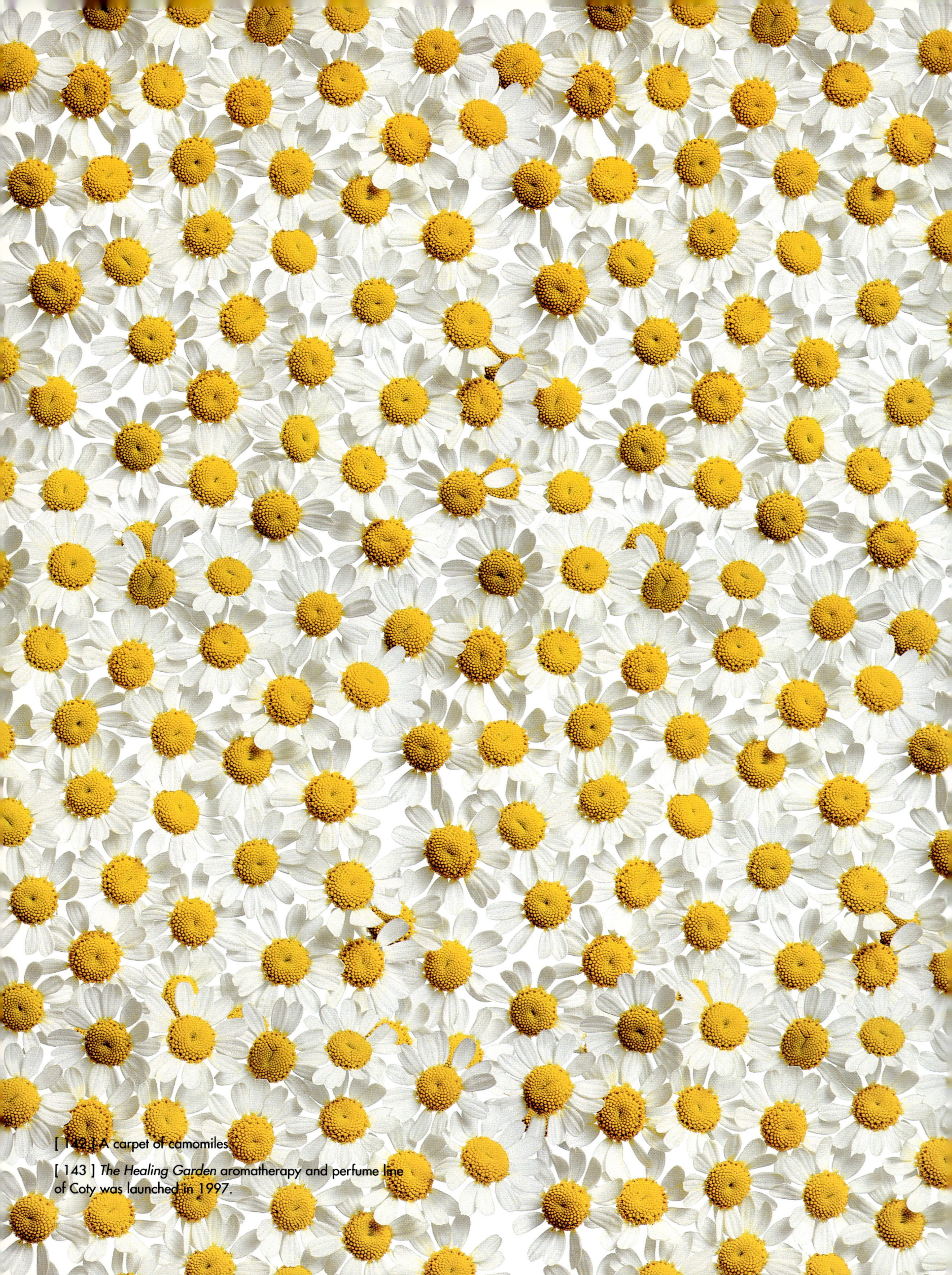

[142] A carpet of camomiles.

[143] *The Healing Garden* aromatherapy and perfume line of Coty was launched in 1997.

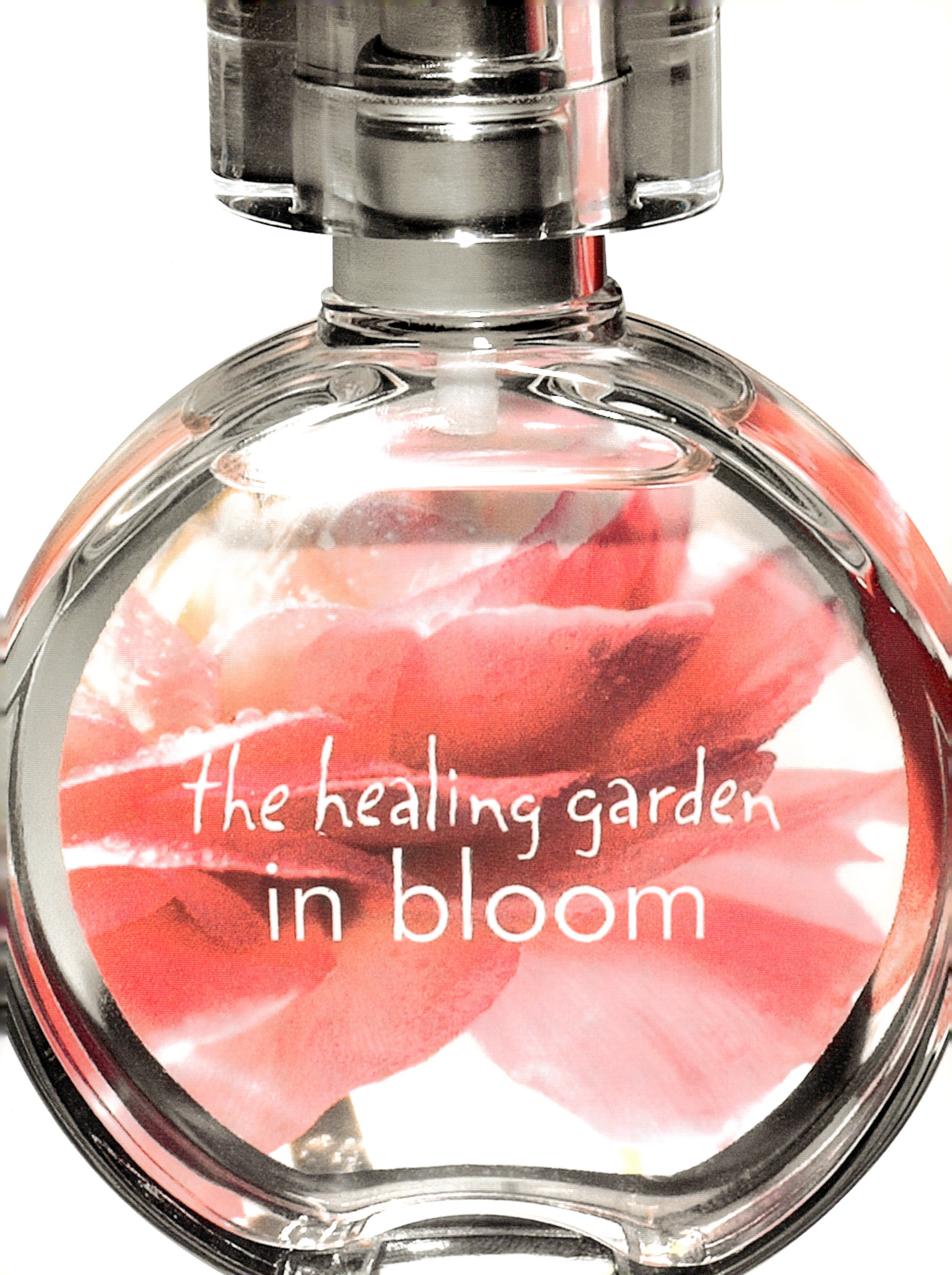
the healing garden
in bloom

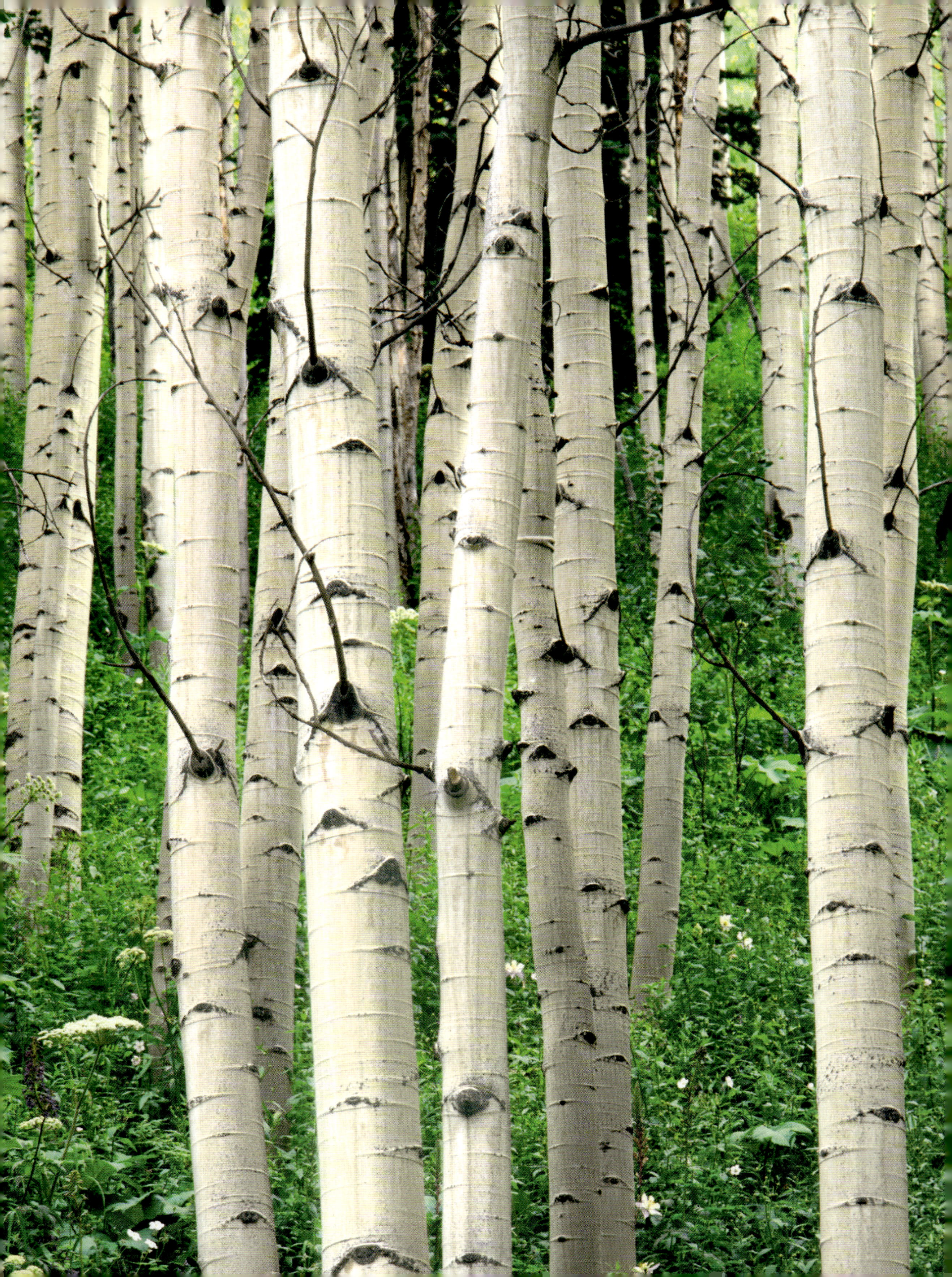

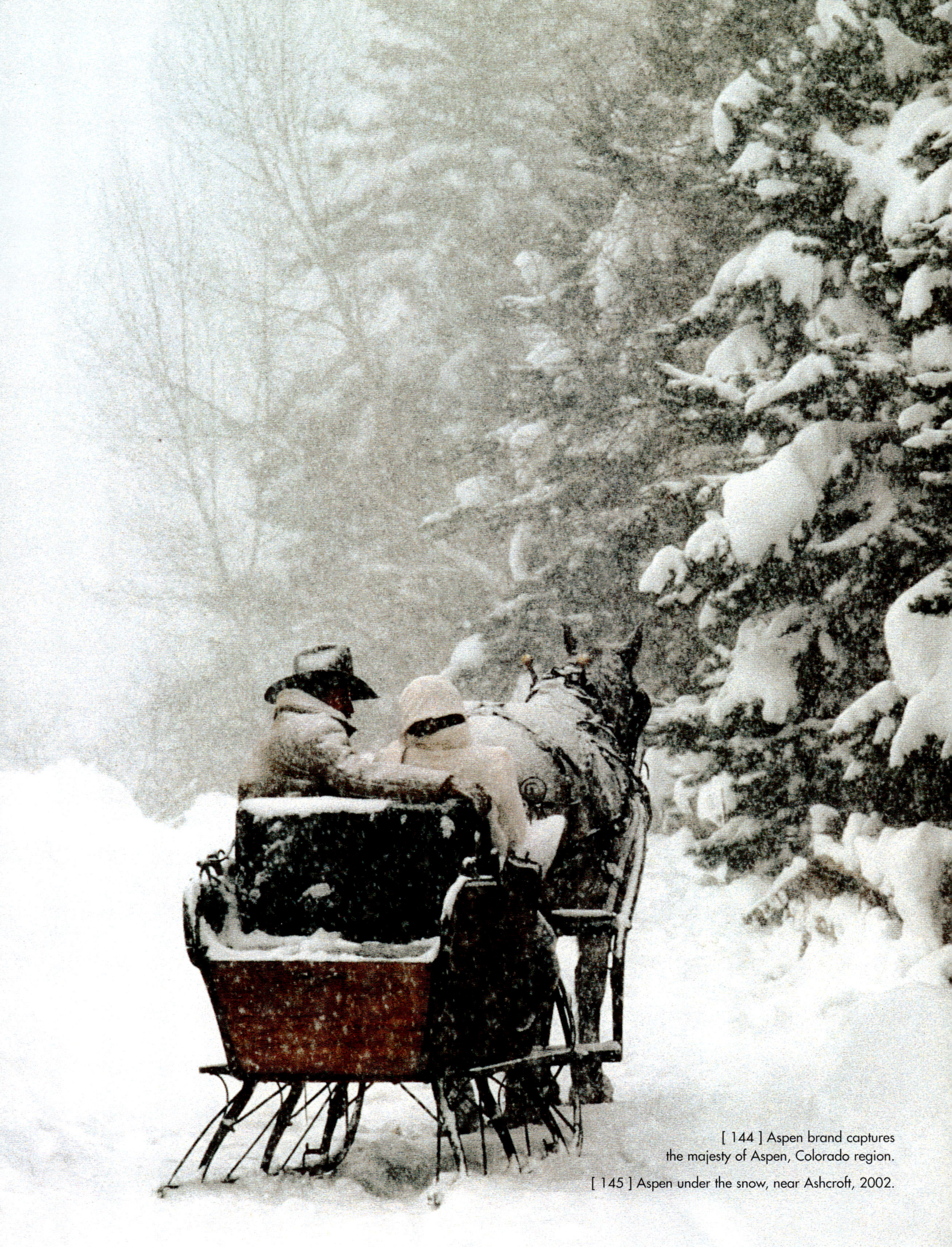

[144] Aspen brand captures
the majesty of Aspen, Colorado region.

[145] Aspen under the snow, near Ashcroft, 2002.

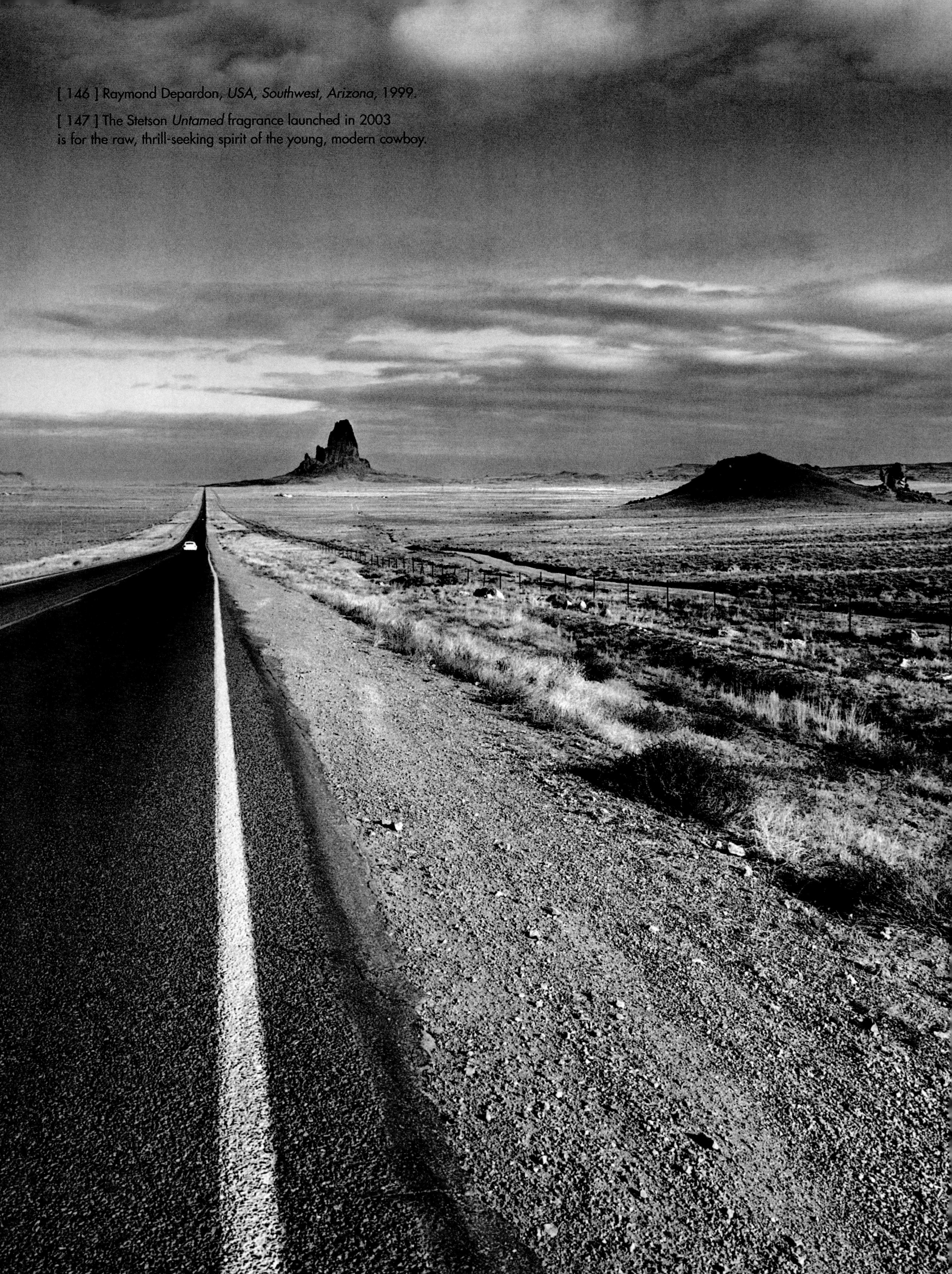

[146] Raymond Depardon, *USA, Southwest, Arizona*, 1999.

[147] The Stetson *Untamed* fragrance launched in 2003 is for the raw, thrill-seeking spirit of the young, modern cowboy.

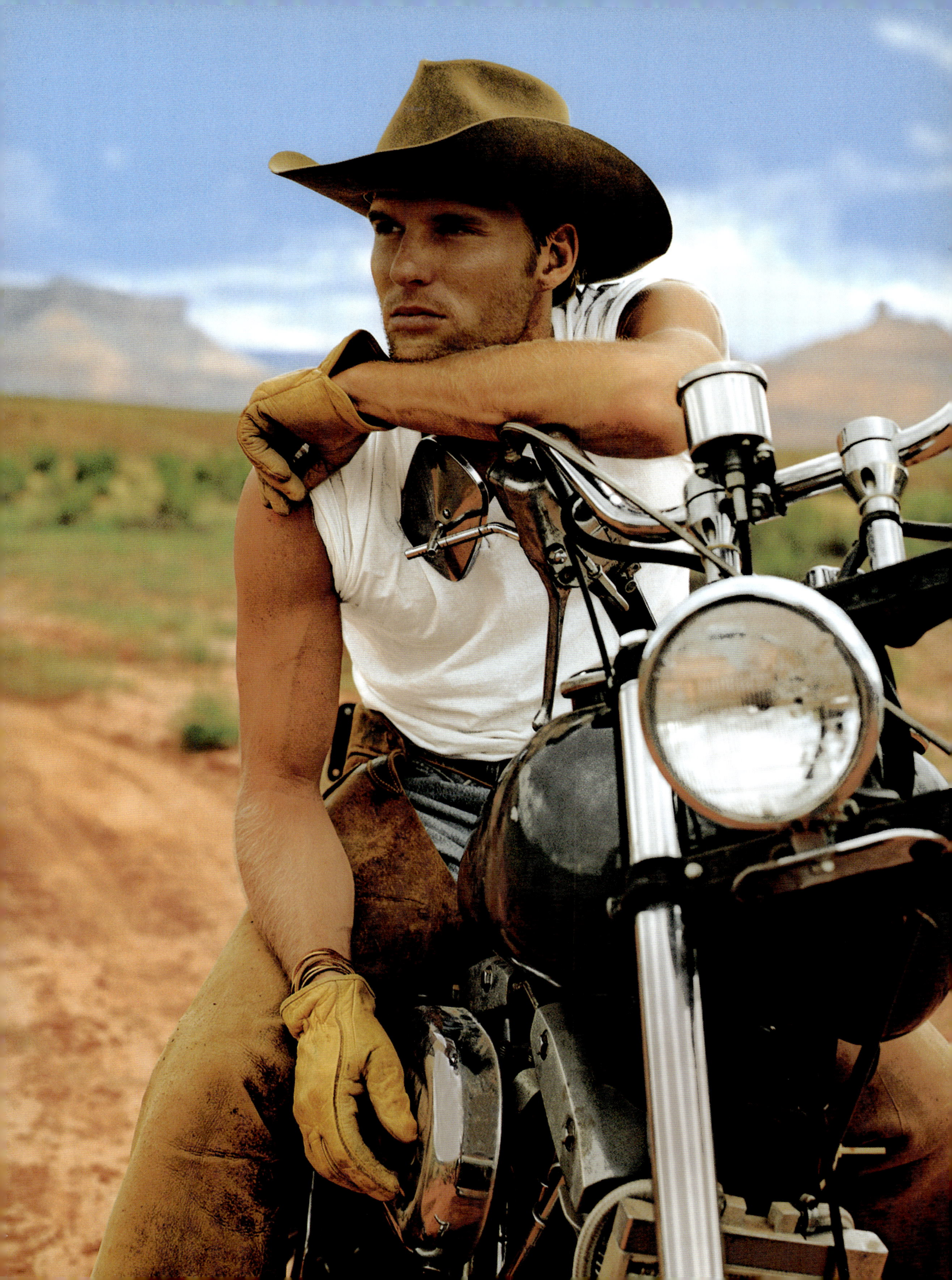

Photo credits

[1] © Private collection/All rights reserved; [2] © Keiichi Tahara; [3] © Arsenic; [4] © Keiichi Tahara; [5] © 2002 Esther van der Bie, courtesy gallery Synopsism Lausanne; [6] © Jean-Philippe Dume; [7] © Guido Mocafico; [8] © Lindsay Hebberd/Corbis; [9] © Guido Mocafico; [10] © Peter Lindbergh; [11] © Private collection/All rights reserved; [12] © Daniel Schweizer; [13] © Rick Goldberg; [14] © Elisabeth Peyton; [15] George P. Ide Company advertising, 1922, Paul Outerbridge © The Target Collection of American Photography, Museum of Fine Arts, Houston, Texas/Bridgeman Giraudon; [16] © Greg Delves; [17] © Franck Dieleman; [18] © Warren Bolster/Getty images; [19] © Private collection/All rights reserved; [20] Martial Raysse © Adagp, Paris 2004; [21] © Ora-ïto; [22] © Keiichi Tahara; [23] © Dove Allouche and Evariste Richer, 2000/Photo Philippe Chancel; [24] © Frédéric Godet; [25] © Collection Roger-Viollet; [26] © Solve Sundsbo; [27] © Derek Lomas; [28] © International Center of Photography, David Seidner Archive; [29] © Keiichi Tahara; [30] Andy Warhol © Adagp, Paris 2004; [31] © Plamen Petkov; [32] © Derek Lomas; [33] © George Silk/Time Life Pictures/Getty Images; [34] © Denis Scott/Corbis; [35] © James Turrell, 1991/Confort Moderne, Poitiers/Photo Jean-Luc Terradillos; [36] © Robin Broadbent; [37] © Nick Knight; [38] © Quentin Bertoux; [39] Live © S.I.N./ Corbis; [40] Erwin Blumenfeld © Adagp, Paris 2004; [41] © David Sims; [42] © Brigitte Niedermair; [43] © Quentin Bertoux; [44] © Thomas Nutzl; [45] © Craig McDean; [46] Man Ray © Man Ray Trust/Adagp, Paris 2004; [47] © Michael Thompson; [48] © Keiichi Tahara; [49] © Coty Archives/All rights reserved; [50] © Nick Knight; [51] © Craig van der Lende/The Image Bank/ Getty; [52] © Keiichi Tahara; [53] © Jorgen Ahlstrom/Klosslondon; [54] © All rights reserved; [55] © International Center of Photography, David Seidner Archive; [56] © Frédéric Maurel; [57] © Frans Lanting/Minden Pictures/J. H. Editorial; [58] © Guido Mocafico; [59] © Marie-Jo Lafontaine; [60] © Valérie Knight; [61] © Harry Meerson/All rights reserved; [62] © Nils Udo, courtesy Galerie Alain Gutharc; [63] © Peter Knaup; [64] © Keiichi Tahara; [65] © Alistair Taylor Young; [66] © International Center of Photography, David Seidner Archive; [67] © Eric Zeziola; [68] © Photo B.D.V./Corbis; [69] © Juergen Teller; [70] © Petre Buzoianu/Corbis; [71] © Laziz Hamani; [72] © Jean-Baptiste Mondino; [73] © David Sims; [74] © Nic Hudson; [75] Clifford Coffin © Condé Nast Archive/Corbis; [76] © Nathaniel Goldberg; [77] © Lancaster Archives, courtesy H.S.H. Prince of Monaco; [78] © Tyen; [79] © Gilles Bensimon; [80] © Kutlu Ertan; [81] © The Estate of Guy Bourdin/Art+Commerce Anthology; [82] Man Ray © Man Ray Trust/Adagp, Paris 2004; [83] © Nathaniel Goldberg; [84] Alexej von Jawlensky © Adagp, Paris 2004; [85] Gérard Martinet © Vogue Paris; [86] © Tyen; [87] © Liz Collins/Art+Commerce Anthology; [88] Robert Delaunay © L & M Services B.V. Amsterdam 20040509; [89] © Liz Collins; [90] © Roger-Viollet; [91] © S. Held/Stock Image; [92] © Société des Bains de Mer Archives; [93] © Société des Bains de Mer Archives; [94]: © Jean-Philippe Dume; [95] © Assouline; [96] © Mikael Jansson; [97] © Roger-Viollet; [98] © Musée de la Vie suresnoise; [99] © Musée de la Vie suresnoise; [100] © Musée de la Vie suresnoise; [101] © Keiichi Tahara; [102] © Keiichi Tahara; [103] © Daniel Schweizer; [104] © Nathaniel Goldberg; [105] © Pierre Boucher/ All rights reserved; [106] © Jean-Charles Recht; [107] © Bill Ling/Getty Images; [108] © Jean-Pierre Buscat Collection; [109] © Raymond Depardon/Magnum photos; [110] © Greg Delves; [111] © Frédéric Maurel; [112] © The Estate of Guy Bourdin/ Art+Commerce Anthology; [113] Man Ray © Man Ray Trust/Adagp, Paris 2004; [114] Raymond Meier © Vogue Paris; [115] © Private collection/All rights reserved; [116] © Corbis; [117] Erwin Blumenfeld © Adagp, Paris 2004; [118] © Hans Gissinger; [119] © Henri Dunoyer de Segonzac/Youpi la Création; [120] © Henri Dunoyer de Segonzac/Youpi la Création; [121] © Coty Archives/All rights reserved; [122] © Coty Archives/All rights reserved; [123] © Private collection/All rights reserved; [124] © Coty Archives/All rights reserved; [125] Man Ray © Man Ray Trust/Adagp, Paris 2004; [126] © Matthias Vriens; [127] © Private collection/All rights reserved; [128] © Raymond Meier/Vogue Paris; [129] © Private collection/All rights reserved; [130] Photo Guegan © L'Officiel/June 1964; [131] © Amy Neunsinger/Getty Images; [132] © Craig McDean; [133]: © Mario Sorrenti; [134] A. Kertész © Ministère de la Culture France; [135] Topolino make-up © Satoshi Sakusa; [136] © Daniel Jouanneau/SIC; [137] © Private collection/ All rights reserved; [138] © Enrique Badulescu; [139] © Enrique Badulescu; [140] © Frédéric Maurel; [141] All rights reserved; [142] © Robin Broadbent; [143] © Bryan Warakomski; [144] © David Muench/Corbis; [145] © Jeffrey Aaronson/Network Aspen/All rights reserved; [146] © Raymond Depardon/Magnum photos; [147] © Richard Phibbs.

Acknowledgments

The publisher would like to thank photographers Jorgen Ahlstrom, Gilles Bensimon, Laziz Hamani, Sam Klosslondon, Keiichi Tahara, as well as all those who contributed to this book, Adagp, Art+Commerce Anthology (New York), Samuel Bourdin, Galerie du Confort moderne (Poitiers), Corbis, Getty Images, Galerie Alain Gutharc (Paris), International Center of Photography (New York), Magnum Photos, Marie-Claire, Officiel de la Mode, Roger-Viollet, Jordan Shipenberg (Art Department, New York), Galerie Synopsism (Lausanne), Topolino and Satoshi Saikusa, Vogue Paris.
He extends his thanks to Coty for their relentless and outstanding collaboration, especially Marie-Sabine Leclercq, Caroline Fons, Maria La Gamba and Ève Leporq.

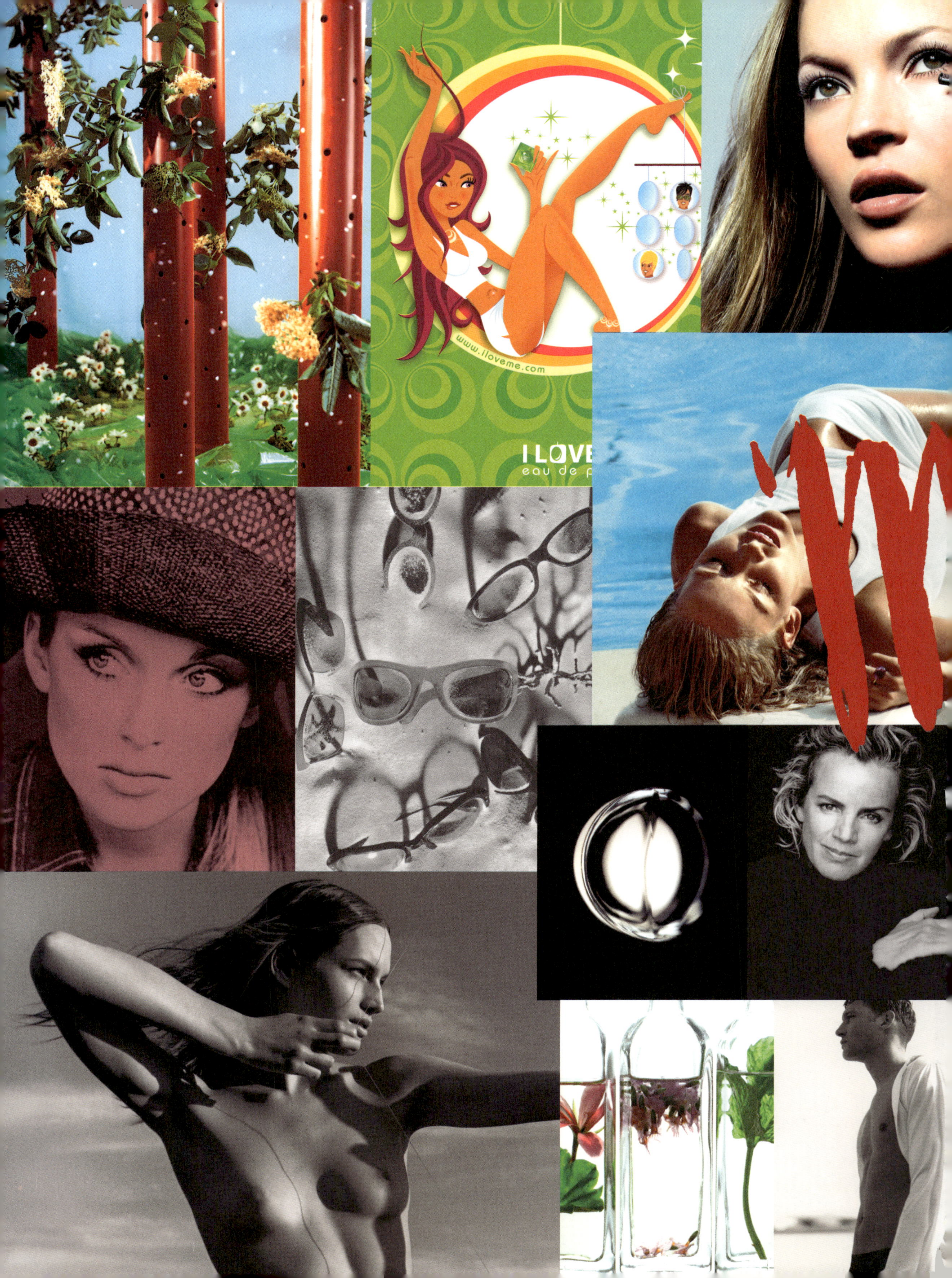
www.iloveme.com
I LOVE
eau de p